STATUS SYNDROME

STATUS SYNDROME

*How Your Social Standing Directly
Affects Your Health*

Michael Marmot

BLOOMSBURY

First published in Great Britain 2004
This paperback edition published 2005

Copyright © 2004 by Michael Marmot

The moral right of the author has been asserted

Bloomsbury Publishing Plc, 38 Soho Square, London W1D 3HB

A CIP catalogue record for this book
is available from the British Library

ISBN 0 7475 7408 1
9780747574088

10 9 8 7 6 5 4 3 2 1

All papers used by Bloomsbury Publishing are natural,
recyclable products made from wood grown in well-managed
forests. The manufacturing processes conform to the
regulations of the country of origin

Typeset by Hewer Text Ltd, Edinburgh
Printed in Great Britain by Clays Ltd, St Ives plc

www.bloomsbury.com/michaelmarmot

To Alexi, André, Daniel and Deborah

The success of an economy and of a society cannot be separated from the lives that members of the society are able to lead . . . we not only value living well and satisfactorily, but also appreciate having control over our own lives.

Amartya Sen, *Development as Freedom* (1999)

CONTENTS

INTRODUCTION

We have remarkably good health in the rich countries of the world. Malaria is long gone from Europe and the US. Parasitic diseases do not wreak havoc with our lives. When we give birth, we can reasonably expect that fewer than one child in a hundred will die in the first year of life. What a good time to be alive. Except that it is better for some than others – considerably so. Where you stand in the social hierarchy – on the social ladder – is intimately related to your chances of getting ill, and your length of life. And the differences between top and bottom are getting bigger, and have been for a generation.

Let me translate 'where you stand in the social hierarchy'. You are not poor. You are employed. Your children are well fed. You live in a decent house or apartment. You turn on the tap and drink the water in the secure knowledge that it is clean. The food you buy is not contaminated. Most people you come across in your daily round also meet this description. But, among these people, none of whom is destitute or even poor, you acknowledge that some are higher than you in the social hierarchy: they may have more money, bigger houses, a more prestigious job, more status in the eyes of others, or simply a higher-class way of speaking. You also note that there are other people lower than you on these criteria, not just the very poor or the homeless, but people whose standing is merely lower than yours, to a varying extent. The remarkable finding is that among *all* of these people, the higher the status in the pecking order the healthier they are likely to be. In other words health follows a social gradient. I call this the status syndrome.

This is really rather surprising. More, this is really astonishing. Why should educated people with good stable jobs have a higher risk of dropping dead than people with a bit more education or slightly higher-status jobs? Is living in a five-bedroom house with three bathrooms better for your health than 'crowding' the spouse and two children into a four-bedroom house with only two? Why, since I asked, should living in a four-bedroom house be better for your health than living in a clean, dry, warm, three-bedroom apartment? Why should someone with a master's degree have a longer life expectancy than someone with a bachelor's?

The answer that I shall lay out in this book, is that for people above a threshold of material well-being, another kind of well-being is central. Autonomy – how much control you have over your life – and the opportunities you have for full social engagement and participation are crucial for health, well-being and longevity. It is inequality in these that plays a big part in producing the social gradient in health. Degrees of control and participation underlie the status syndrome.

Sounds simple, I hope. But those two sentences about control and participation took more than twenty-five years of research to formulate. In the age of the genome and high-tech medical care, thinking about health typically turns to biology and technology. The discovery of how important control and participation are for health leads in a different direction: to the circumstances in which we live and work. In other words, this is health research that leads us to focus, not on access to the latest medical technology, but on the way we think about the sort of lives we want for ourselves, and the sort of society in which we want to lead them. What started out as a research programme into the causes of inequalities in health between social groups ended up as an inquiry into what is best and worst about the way we live.

These social inequalities in health – the social gradient – are not a footnote to the 'real' causes of ill-health in countries that are no longer poor; they are the heart of the matter. Status syndrome can be illustrated by a short ride on the Washington DC subway. Travel from the south-east of downtown Washington to Montgomery County Maryland. For each mile travelled life expectancy rises about a year and a half. There is a twenty-year gap between poor blacks at one end of the journey and rich whites at the other.[1] Men in Japan have the longest life expectancy in the world at 77; men in Kazakhstan in the former Soviet Union are way down at 57. Within Washington and its environs, we see differences as big. These are the ends of the spectrum – the rest of the developed world's population is ranged in between.

If I am going to argue that the way we organise society leads to inequality in the lives people are able to lead, then we must look at the health impact of how different societies organise themselves. It is not just that health researchers like to travel. We do, but I am such a nerd that when I travel I come back not with holiday snaps but with the heart-disease statistics. Have you seen the beaches in Cuba? Yes, and life expectancy there is 73.7 for men and 77.5 for women. What did you think of the Hermitage Museum in St Petersburg? Wonderful, but life expectancy in Russia has sunk to 57 for men and 72 for women. We shall have to travel to look at what we can learn from observation of how health in different societies may be related to features of those societies, and especially, how the social gradient in health varies from society to society.

The contrasts in Washington DC demand attention, because healthy and unhealthy live cheek by jowl. The findings of a health gradient are, however, remarkably general. The wide corridors of power of the British civil service are about as far as one can get conceptually from the down-at-heel streets of Washington DC as the developed world allows. But there, dramatically, is evidence of the status syndrome. I began my research on civil servants in 1976 with the Whitehall studies and found a social gradient in health.[2] Britain was and is a stratified society and no part of it is more exquisitely stratified than the British civil service. When I published the finding of higher rates of disease increasing progressively down the social ladder, the first reaction was: civil servants, who cares! But what was true in Whitehall was true in Britain as a whole. The barely concealed reaction from other countries was: Ah! The British! What else can you expect from class-ridden Britain? Americans and Australians believed their countries were egalitarian so there would be no social-class difference there. They were wrong. In North America and Australia the differences are as big as, if not bigger, than they are in Britain. Scandinavians said they had no class differences in health, until they looked and found that this phenomenon went deeper and wider than class-ridden Britain. Many continental European countries were slower at picking up on this story, because they did not have the data systems in place. When they looked, they too found a clear social gradient in health. When the doors opened on the former communist countries of Europe, we found big and growing social differences in health within those countries as well as a growing gap in health between them and the flourishing countries of Western Europe. Even in Japan, whose health record is the envy of the world, we find evidence of the status syndrome.

One of the lessons that I have learnt from examining health in different countries is that the factors responsible for the social gradient in health may be responsible for variations in health of whole countries. As we travel, we shall look at populations whose health has suffered badly, particularly those of the former communist countries of Central and Eastern Europe, where health has been at crisis level. We shall also look at whole populations whose health record is remarkably good, Japan most notably, but also relatively poor populations whose good health defies their lack of money, such as Costa Rica and Kerala.

Not rich and poor

I illustrated the massive size of the health inequality problem by contrasting the tragically foreshortened lives of poor blacks in the inner cities of the USA with the long lives of well-off whites in the comfortable suburbs. This should not lead us into thinking that the health gap is confined to poor health for the disadvantaged, 'them', and good health for everybody else, 'us'. We have many terms to describe the disadvantaged that betray 'them and us' thinking: poverty, social exclusion, the underclass, the disadvantaged, haves and have-nots. These all imply a clear division into poor and non-poor. Such a division does not describe our problem. I am addressing the gradient: it affects not 'them', but all of 'us'. Wherever we are in the hierarchy, our health is likely to be better than those below us and worse than those above us. The socially excluded are at the end of a health spectrum, but it is the social gradient in health, the status syndrome, that is the challenge.

I have just told you what the book is about. Let me emphasise what the book is not about. Michelangelo, apparently, looked at a block of marble and saw his task as liberating the masterpiece within. At a less exalted level, let me remove the extraneous pieces so that we can concentrate on the main story. First, this book is not about absolute deprivation and illness – important as that is. Few people who have experienced poverty would recommend it. Among its many disadvantages, it shortens life. As the cruel joke goes, the bad news is that it makes you miserable; the good news is that you won't have to survive it for too long. Vast swathes of the world's population live in absolute deprivation and their health suffers as a result. Living on $2 a day will mean malnutrition to add to inadequate shelter and unsanitary conditions. Viewed from this perspective, the 'poor' in Europe and North America are rich. They do not suffer the diseases of absolute deprivation. Even the most deprived indigenous groups in Australia and North America suffer from obesity, diabetes and heart disease rather than starvation, dysentery and malaria – the diseases we usually think of as related to absolute deprivation.

I am dealing with a different problem: why there should be a social gradient in health among people who are not poor in the sense of absolute deprivation that afflicts the poorest countries of the world. Karl Marx argued that there were two great classes in society and that the bourgeoisie benefited at the expense of the proletariat; the haves at the expense of the have-nots. Perhaps. But that won't do as a description of a stratified society where there are degrees of having and not-having. If it were the case that in rich countries those below a supposed poverty line had poor health and everyone else had good health, a division into two great classes might be appropriate, but it is not like that. The status syndrome is not about disease for the poor and good health for everyone else. It is a gradient. Marx's concept of alienation may well be relevant to our discussion of control, but it is a graded phenomenon: you can have degrees of it.

We are dealing, then, with the diseases that people get when the society is rich enough to have dealt with malnutrition and poor sanitation: heart disease, diabetes, mental illness. They used, wrongly, to be labelled rich people's diseases. This brings me to the second thing this book is not about: the problems of being rich. I won't bore you with all the misfortunes that wealth can bring.

In the novels of Henry James, it always seems to be the rich American heiress who gets tuberculosis. In the film versions, when a man gets TB, he looks like he has been on a bender, but the women

get more ethereally beautiful and elegant, and when they die, everyone wears black lace. Very moving and very misleading. Think of
Keats and the Brontë sisters and Thomas Mann and the picture of TB
ravaging the privileged and well-to-do. Again tragic, and again
misleading. Tuberculosis was devastating in all classes of society,
but it always hit the poor with greater force. In the 1830s, English
mortuary registers revealed that 'the proportion of consumptive cases
in gentlemen, tradesmen, and labourers was 16, 28 and 30% respectively'.[3]

But that was TB. We know now that TB is a disease of the poor.
The millions who die of TB today are in the poor countries of the
world. In the rich countries, we believe, we have solved the diseases of
poverty. Today our picture of the quintessential diseases of modern
life is of heart disease and mental illness affecting the rich and famous:
the politician and the chief executive, the football manager and the
ageing rock musician. We think we know why that might be so –
overindulgence in the good life and all the stress involved in the jobs
that carry responsibility.

This is not right, either. We may think of these diseases as those of
the rich in the sense that in Sierra Leone, where a quarter of children
die by the age of five and life expectancy is 37 for men and 39 for
women, there are not many who survive to get coronary heart disease
– the forces of the diseases linked to poverty are too strong. But in
wealthier countries, heart disease and diabetes, mental illness and
chronic respiratory disease, accidents and violence all follow the social
gradient – the lower the ranking in society the higher the risk. These
are not rich men's diseases.

The book is about how we in the 'rich' countries of the world play
out our lives. It sets out the evidence that the causes of the social
gradient in health are to be found in the circumstances in which we
live and work; in other words, in our set of social arrangements. That
is important. It is not the calamities that most determine well-being,
but the way we go about our daily lives, in offices, banks, factories,
houses and neighbourhoods. It is about the fact that control over life
circumstances and full social engagement and participation in what
society has to offer are distributed unequally and as a result health is
distributed unequally. The status syndrome is important as a public-

health problem, but it is also important because, as I will show, it gives insight into how social experiences affect health.

How do these experiences translate into illness? Quite simply, the key lies in that most important organ, the brain. The psychological experience of inequality has profound effects on body systems. The evidence we shall examine suggests that this may be a major factor in generating the social gradient in health.

Most people have no difficulty understanding that problems in their lives can make them ill. It sounds eminently reasonable: if your need to be a flourishing person with freedom to live a fulfilled life is frustrated, health will suffer. It sounds reasonable, but one remarkable aspect of the set of findings and insights that I shall lay out is that they are accepted by the small group of scientists who have studied the issue and almost totally ignored by everyone else: biomedical scientists who delve into the mysteries of the cell, policy makers who are concerned with the funding and organisation of health services, health educators who are concerned with why people continue to smoke and be slothful despite advice to the contrary. In my experience, the readiest audience for these findings is to be found among non-experts among whom the conclusions resonate with their experience of everyday life. My immodest aim is to help change understanding of the wider effects of having control over one's life and opportunities for full participation in society. A changed consciousness is an important step in leading to profound change for individuals and societies.

I shall, of course, have to deal with the more conventional ways of thinking of the causes of ill-health. In seeking explanations for the social gradient we shall round up the usual suspects: bad habits, lack of access to medical care, unlucky genes. We shall look at the possibility that health of the poor is worse because they smoke more and eat unhealthily, or have worse medical care, or were somehow unfortunate in choosing parents with a genetic predisposition for short rather than long lives. I shall also consider, only to discard, the proposition that the causal direction runs the other way: that it might be the glow of good health that leads to some becoming princes, and that those racked by illness end up paupers. In other words, it is your health that determines where you will end up, not where you end up that determines your health. Plausible as this proposition is, it does not account for the relation between social position and health. In our search for explanations of the status syndrome we shall need to look at the evidence for what is not explaining the health gradient as well as what is.

I have said that we shall need to travel. The comparative perspective is vital for our investigation. Take one obvious example. In the US when people think of health disparities, the intrusive fact that 40 million people or more do not have health insurance, despite a sixth of national income being spent on health care, leads to obvious attention on medical care; so, many believe that disparities in medical care are responsible for disparities in health. In Britain we have a National Health Service. While not exactly the envy of the world, it does provide health care for the whole population. And yet, both countries have a social gradient in health, despite such dramatically different arrangements for delivering health care. It suggests that the explanation for the status syndrome lies elsewhere.

Examining health, discovering society

I ask myself how, as a physician, I find myself up to my ears with the problems of society. I trained as a doctor, initially because of fascination with the sciences of biochemistry and physiology – the biological science of medicine. Then I met patients and loved the frontline experience of treating real people. But real people, as I discovered, have problems with their lives as well as with their bodily organs. Dealing with real people the connection between the two was inescapable. Starting in the psychiatric wards, I used to worry that our patients were homeless, came from dysfunctional families, were subject to crime and abuse. What was the point of patching them up and sending them back to miserable lives? Should we not try and do something about the misery outside? In the medical wards, too, people would come into hospital in cardiac or respiratory failure, we would treat the acute episode and send them home. There were two problems with this. They went home to a whole slew of social problems; and we used to see the same patients back again three months later.

As the sage said: one thing leads to another. Asking about causes of disease from the perspective of a physician soon led to my asking about the nature of society that leads to disease and particularly to the social gradient in health. A perspective of wishing to improve the public health led, therefore, to wanting to improve society.

In arguing that health can be used as a marker of a successful society, I have distinguished companions. The Nobel prize-winning economist, Amartya Sen, argues that the close link between health and economic and social development means that we can examine health to tell us if a society is fostering well-being in its members.[4] Although much of my concern has been with the social gradient in health within societies, the causes that give rise to this gradient, in the circumstances in which people live and work, could apply to whole societies.

Alistair Cooke, the veteran radio broadcaster, praised the independence of mind of the late Senator Daniel Patrick Moynihan, and his habit of saying what he believed to be true whether fashionable or not. One time this habit brought him not scorn but ridicule. In the late 1970s he looked into the economy of all the Soviet republics and examined the interesting fact that the overall mortality figure was rising spectacularly. At the end of his study he announced in the Senate that the Soviet Union was a sickening society and communism would collapse in the next decade. Gales of laughter roared through the Senate at this wishful thinker. Nine years later it happened.

The health records of the former communist countries were disastrous during the last years of communist rule and, in the former Soviet Union, health deteriorated further as the society slipped into chaos with the collapse of the command economy. Here we have whole societies where people had little opportunity for control over their lives or full social participation. Apart from the gradients in health within those countries, they lend support to the general thesis that the circumstances in which we live and work are vital for health, and thus for the status syndrome.

The gross inequality between the rich countries of the world and the poor and the resulting health differences is a calamity of massive proportions, but has not been the focus of my research for the last thirty years and is not what this book is about. This is not to say that the same general message may not apply. Sen's book, *Development as Freedom*, has as its central theme that people not only value living well but having control over their lives. He argues that the point of development is to ensure basic freedoms.[5] Paul Farmer takes up this theme and argues that it is precisely because people in the poor countries of Latin America have so little control over their lives that there are such gross inequalities in infectious diseases.[6,7] Farmer argues that it is time now to apply our insights, our will, and our money, to solve these problems.

Two more words of introduction. I have described a social gradient in health, but you know some rich people who die young – look at the unhappy Princess Di – and some poor people who live a long life. We may call this the Winston Churchill effect. Churchill famously smoked and drank to excess but lived a long life. It does not refute the argument that smoking is bad for health. In general smokers die at a younger age than non-smokers. The fact that some smokers outlive more careful abstainers does not weaken the link between smoking and disease. (It may, of course, be that Winston Churchill lived a long life because of his high social status and because no one had more control over their life, or a more flourishing life, than he.) There is almost no condition in medicine that has a single cause. If a plane crashes from 30,000 feet, all passengers will die; individual hardiness does not come into play. But if the black death came back, some exposed people would survive and others not. It does not mean that plague is not a cause of death. I shall describe trends, averages, general causes. Not everyone exposed to the conditions that I shall describe will have premature illness, but those exposed will be more likely to than those not exposed.

My second point is that the social gradient is telling us that large parts of our population are not achieving their potential in health or in length of life – they are suffering the consequences of the status syndrome. Commonly, we refer back to the biblical notion that the years of a man's life are three score and ten. Did the Bible realise that the years of a woman's are a bit more? In the rich countries that form the subject of my inquiry we have now achieved that lifespan and then some. My concern is that within these countries there are marked differences: some are short of the three score and ten, and some way past it. Our achievement of the three score and ten is incredibly recent – the last thirty years or so – and most of the world is far below it. I cited Sierra Leone as having an average life expectancy of less than 40. It is, regrettably, true of Africa as a whole that life expectancy hovers around the 50 mark, and is much lower for some countries. Many developing countries elsewhere fall well below three score years and ten. (Given that, I wonder how the biblical author arrived at the three-score-and-ten figure. Perhaps he had trouble counting, seeing as he told us that Abraham lived to 175 and Sarah conceived a child at 97.) Large parts of the population of the wealthier countries have not enjoyed the health benefits of their more fortunate fellow citizens. We have not reached the limits of what we can achieve in health by any means.

The book

I shall start by laying out the evidence for the status syndrome in different countries, their similarities and differences. I will make the case that everyone's health could get better. We have not reached the limits. Studies of whole countries are useful, in that they show that the problem is important. But we also need detailed studies of individuals. Much of the thinking about what might and might not be responsible for the health gradients has come from the Whitehall studies in the UK. The thirty years of research we have done with these studies provides much of our insight into what might and might not be responsible for the social gradient in health.

I then move to the question of whether this whole story is simply about money. If it were, what's the argument against simple redistribution of income? I know the answer to that question, by the way, but it is not just a matter of money, important as money is if you have not got enough.

We then need to look at the crucial question of relative inequalities: the importance of where one stands relative to others in the hierarchy. This may be more important for health than absolute level of resources.

If relative position is important, how does it operate? The next chapters deal with that. Autonomy, how much control one has over one's life has clear effects on health. There is good evidence, too, of its effects on biological stress pathways. This provides an explanation for how society affects biology. We then move to social integration. As indicated, the factors that seem important may affect whole societies. We look at examples of a rich population, Japan, that has remarkably good health, and of relatively poor ones that do as well. We then move on to the countries that have done remarkably badly in health, despite having a developed-country pattern of disease – the countries of Central and Eastern Europe.

The social forces that affect health of adults have their impact, too, on the next generation. The seeds of the status syndrome may, to some extent, be sown in early childhood, and the 'rewards' reaped in adult life.

I finish with why we should care, and what we can do. It is a fascinating scientific question – to understand how subtle differences in social standing can translate into important differences in life chances and health. It is more than that. If I as an individual am interested in my own health or, as a concerned citizen, I am interested in the health of people in my community, I need to understand what is responsible for the health gradient and what can be done about it.

As the phenomenon of the social gradient in health has been discovered it has started to become a central issue in most developed countries. Even the policy makers are starting to notice the status syndrome. The chapters that follow give insight into what we have learnt. The central message from the study of health inequalities is that the magnitude of the difference can vary across societies and within a society at different points in time. This variation is determined by the balance between two features of all societies: hierarchies and co-operation. These translate into how much control individuals have over their lives and how widely spread are the opportunities for social participation. The book will not tell you what to eat for breakfast or how many times a week to go jogging – important as these things may be. Its aim is to help, by understanding the causes of the status syndrome, change the way we think about what we can do to lead more fulfilling lives and how we can shape the society in which we live to achieve that end.

1. SOME ARE MORE
EQUAL THAN OTHERS

Of all the hokum with which this country [America] is riddled the most odd is the common notion that it is free of class distinctions.

W. Somerset Maugham[1]

In *La Bohème*, Puccini's wonderful operatic tearjerker, after the most brilliant pick-up line in all opera, Rodolfo and Mimi fall in love. He is the bohemian poet, she the poor embroiderer; he in freely chosen happy poverty with his educated bohemian friends, a 'millionaire in spirit', she in lonely isolation and destitution. She has consumption (tuberculosis) and Rodolfo, recognising that she is dying, complains to his friend, that she is 'blighted by poverty. To bring her back to life, Love's not enough'. Mimi, in her turn, says that 'to be alone in winter is death!'. Mimi, of course, dies. Rodolfo weeps, and so do we, and go home uplifted.

Apart from creating surpassing beauty Puccini and his librettists, Giacosa and Illica, were kindly providing an introduction to the essential themes of this book. Mimi and Rodolfo are both poor, in that neither has any money and both live in a freezing garret, but it is no accident that it is she who dies not he. (Quite apart from the fact that, in the opera, her death guarantees more tears.) What is the difference between her poverty and his? Poverty is more than lack of money. He and his educated bohemian friends, poet, artist, musician, and philosopher, are in control. They live the way they do by choice, in a way that the unfortunate embroiderer does not. The opera goes further. Love could save lives; isolation could end them. Important as love and isolation are, their effects on health are moderated by other influences; isolation is worse in the harsh environment of winter; love may be life-enhancing but cannot overcome the blight of poverty.

The important things of life, control over your life, love and important social relationships, riches that are not measured by money, are related to when, and how we die. I cannot pretend to match Puccini's power to move, but the scientific findings that I shall review move me in their own way as much as Puccini does in his. These findings suggest that Puccini got it about right. The circumstances in which we live – that foster autonomy and control over life, love, happiness, social connectedness, riches that are not measured by money – affect illness. It is precisely because these benefits of life are doled out unequally in society that we have inequalities in health and in death. Life and death are not opposites, they are intimately related.

For most of us, life and health are in separate spheres. We think about health as to do with genetics, health care or lack thereof, or our own personal lifestyle and habits: whether we are following this week's advice on which vitamins to eat and which to avoid or which exercise regime is currently in vogue. Then there is life: education, family, career, friends, getting and spending, spiritual and cultural life, and the nature of the society in which all this takes place. Whenever health researchers raise their gaze from the microscope and look around, they find the evidence that health and life are not two separate spheres. It is not that genes, medical care or lifestyle are unimportant for health, but they miss out on the major influences on health of the way we live our lives in society. The circumstances in which people live and work are intimately related to risk of illness and length of life.

Nowhere do we see this connection more clearly than in the social hierarchy. Imagine that we are witness to a grand parade. Everyone in the population is classified by their formal education and ranked from least to most. Starting with those who have the fewest years of education, they file past us. The parade begins with the unable and the unwilling, continues with those who did not complete primary school, goes on to the high-school dropouts, those who completed high school, and up through various stages of college or university education. As the parade progresses we note the changes in style and demeanour, of comportment and confidence, and of increasing affluence. We notice something else: a healthy glow increasing in radiance with those going past.

If we could but measure this glow, it would show us that this sorting of people according to their education, has also, in a remarkably precise manner, sorted them according to their health and length of life. The higher the education, the longer are people likely to live, and the better their health is likely to be. It is not just that the people who come first, those without education, have poor health and those who come last, the Harvard and Oxbridge graduates, have good health, but our parade sorts everyone in between. This is the social gradient in health played out across the whole society. In general, a few more years of education translates into longer and healthier lives. The big question is why.

Before I jump to the conclusion that education for all would lead to good health for all, let's repeat the parade. Take everybody back to the starting point, forget their education and this time, sort them according to income. We have a new ranking system – lowest income first – but, remarkably, the finding is the same. The lower the income the worse is people's health status, and the shorter their lives. It is again a graded phenomenon, running from the poorest all the way up to the richest. Should I now jump to the conclusion that more money for all would improve their health? No more readily than I should conclude the same about education. I am nervous: which is it, money or education? Now let's repeat the parade with parents' social class: we find the same thing. It's a bit more difficult to give people higher-class parents in order to prevent premature death. They should have thought of that before they chose their parents. Try occupation as the ranking system. It should not be too hard to assign some sort of prestige score to occupations – doctors and judges come higher than shop assistants, who are higher than unskilled workers. There it is again: the higher the prestige of the job the better the health. As we cannot make everyone into judges and doctors, thank goodness, one might really like to know if there is something about the job that is important in causing this gradient in health.

I conducted this parade four times: each time using a new ranking system and ignoring the previous one. But there is overlap in the rankings: for example people with university degrees have higher incomes in general than those without; people with higher-class parents are more likely to have university education than those without; those in top jobs have more education and income. There is overlap, but the rankings are not identical. The professor of oriental literature is above the plumber in education but way below in income; the trader in the bond market has several times the income of the priest but lower occupational prestige.

At the heart of my inquiry is an investigation of which ranking system is most important in determining the health gradient. Not because I am interested in rankings for their own sakes, but because I want to understand what education, income, parental background, occupation can tell us about how life circumstances affect health. By understanding whether it is money or education, for example, that are most closely related to inequalities in health we shed light both on causes of the differences and what we could do about them. As I indicated, *La Bohème* got it about right: love, happiness, riches that are beyond money, lack of money and, indeed, the education of Rodolfo and his friends may all be important to the social gradient in health. Much as I am moved by Puccini,[2] I would like to put some scientific precision on this inquiry. The first step is to look for the health gradient in different times and places.

Where do we see the health gradient?

Pretty well everywhere. As one example, Figure 1.1 shows for the US that the higher the household income the lower the mortality rate.[3] Figure 1.1 makes clear that poverty is bad for health but it is at the end of a spectrum. Those in the poorest households have nearly four times the risk of death of those in the richest – which in any case are not fantastically rich. It also drives home the point that the relation between income and health is a gradient – people in the second highest income group have higher mortality than those in the highest; those in the third highest have worse health than those in the second highest.

Figure 1.1 illustrates the problem that our parades threw up. Income and education are correlated: the higher-income groups are more likely to include people with more education. Income predicts health as the figure shows, but so does education; is the relation between income and health because high-income people have more education? Figure 1.1 says yes, in part, but not completely. The 'adjustment' for education examines the relation of income to mortality after taking into account the fact of education's ability to predict mortality. When this was done it shows that the apparent effect of income on death is reduced. This means that this study confirms that there is a social gradient in mortality, but it is difficult to be sure whether it is more closely related to income or education, or to something else that was correlated with both of them. The question of whether it is income, education or something else that is responsible will run through the book.

Figure 1.1 Relative risk of death in the US Panel Study of Income Dynamics

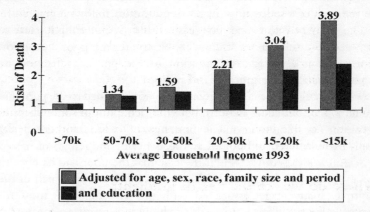

Note: A sample of 8,500 men and women were followed for a twenty-year period 1972–1991, or until they died. The study related the risk of dying to average household income in 1993 dollars. The figure shows the risk of death in each group relative to the best off group i.e. those with household incomes of $70,000 or more were arbitrarily assigned a risk of dying of 1, and all other groups were compared with them. The figure shows the gradient. Men and women second from the top had a relative risk of dying of 1.34, i.e. they were 34 per cent more likely to die in the twenty-year period. The next group were 59 per cent more likely to die, and so on until we get to the bottom income group whose risk of death was 3.9 times that of the top group. The figure shows men and women combined; the disadvantage of having an income below the top was similar for men and women. The differences between groups are 'adjusted' for differences in age, sex, race, family size and period. The second group of bars shows what happens to the relation between income and mortality, when the fact that income groups differ in their amount of education is taken into account. The effect of income on mortality is then reduced.

Source: Adapted from MCDonough, Duncan, Williams and House (1997).

I have been working with colleagues to study the health gradient in different segments of the populations in rich countries: UK, US, Canada, Finland, Japan, France, Sweden, Germany, Italy, Belgium, Australia and New Zealand. It is quite remarkable that wherever you look you find a gradient. Something equivalent to Figure 1.1 could be produced for each of these countries. For years, no one really paid much attention to what should have been obvious from the data. Perhaps they were too concerned with the effect on health of absolute material deprivation that results from lack of clean water or adequate nutrition. This understandable concern got in the way of seeing that rich and poor are the ends of a spectrum – in between, health follows a gradient.

The gradient is the issue. For reasons that are not entirely clear to me, people want to see things in binary terms: poor/non-poor, deprived/non-deprived. Recognition of the gradient changes the problem socially, scientifically and politically.

Socially, because health inequalities are not confined to the poor and the non-poor but affect all of us, whether rich, poor or somewhere in between. The status syndrome is about how you and I, neither rich nor poor, live our lives, and how that affects health and length of life.

Scientifically, because were it the case that the poor had bad health and everyone else had good health, we would focus on which of the multiple disadvantages associated with poverty might be most responsible for the damage to health. Absolute deprivation means the basics of food and sanitation are lacking along with adequate non-crowded housing, lack of medical care or other amenities. The social gradient in health is not only about absolute deprivation. It is about inequality, but not only that between top and bottom. The scientific question is as much to do with why people in the middle of the hierarchy have worse health than those at the top, as why those at the bottom have worse health than those in the middle.

Politically, it changes the way the problem is addressed. Politicians appear to be able to count up to two, actually zero and one: you are in or you are out, with us or against us. They can understand poverty as a discrete state and no politician is going to extol it. Many politicians, however, preach the virtues of inequality (set the wealth producers free). If bigger social and economic inequalities, i.e. a steeper social gradient, are related to bigger health differences, this might give the politician pause. A policy pursued for one reason – increasing inequalities as an economic policy – might have undesirable consequences for health. The gradient in health has the potential to change views of what constitutes the aim of social policy.

There is a strong tendency for scientific questions to get bound up with the political question of how the implications of the science might be implemented. As we go through the scientific evidence, the implications will be evident. We should, nevertheless, try and hold back the political question of what we would do with the findings until it is clearer what the science shows. The science is the place to start.

I said that we see the health gradient everywhere. When the environment is harsh and life-threatening, the socially advantaged fare better than the less advantaged; when the environment reeks of affluence and privilege, we still see a health gradient. I will illustrate with two dramatically contrasting situations: the South Pole for extremes of hardship and Hollywood for extremes of affluence.

As a schoolboy I was thrilled by the story of Captain Scott of the Antarctic. The tragedy of heroic English gentlemen failing to complete an expedition to the South Pole in 1911 trapped by a blizzard, and lying in their tents, running out of food, out of hope and out of luck, a mere eleven miles from their food depot. The weakest, Captain Oates, struggles to his feet and stumbles out of the tent into the blizzard, with the memorable words: 'I am just going outside and may be some time'. His self-sacrifice is to save rations for the others. Scott records in his diary: 'We knew that poor Oates was walking to his death, but though we tried to dissuade him, we knew it was the act of a brave man and an English gentleman.' Scott suggests in his diary that all four of them in this tent will be deemed to have died like English gentlemen.

How does this illustrate the gradient in health? It certainly shows that if conditions are severe enough, anyone will succumb whatever his social class – even an Edwardian English gentleman. There is a 'but'. On the final trek of Scott and his comrades, there was a fifth man, Seaman Evans. He was of a lower class than the 'gentlemen', a petty officer in the Royal Navy, chosen for his strength. Evans, the big man, was the first to weaken in the appalling conditions. He did not reach that final act of the drama in the tent. He began losing heart sooner. Why should the man who was, apparently, the strongest of the five be the first to succumb? Evans was, as Scott's diary records: 'nearly broken down in brain, we think'. His companions found him in the snow with a wild look in his eyes. The 'gentlemen' did what they could. They sledged him to the next camp, where he died. Scott and his remaining three men struggled on.

The story of Scott and his companions illustrates three pieces of the theory that I am laying out here. The first is that position in the hierarchy is important for life and death, whether toiling in the Antarctic, living in a bohemian garret in Paris, or coping with the crowds of Manhattan. It is not an accident that Evans, the lower-class man, would die first, just as it was no accident that Mimi, in Puccini's opera, died prematurely; it is consistent with what other data lead us to expect.

The second is that Scott was right in his diagnosis – he describes Evans as being broken down in brain. I shall argue that the brain is a crucial organ in generating the social gradient in health. To put the whole expedition in context, Scott was determined to be the first to reach the South Pole. He was second – beaten to the prize by Roald Amundsen, a Norwegian. Bitterly disappointed, Scott and his four companions had an 800-mile march back toward safety that destroyed body and soul. These explorers had made a massive effort without appropriate reward. Imbalance between effort expended and reward gained is psychologically damaging and hence damages physical health. As winners, they might all have had a greater chance of survival. My speculation is that what Evans, in particular, lacked was control over his own destiny. It was this lack of control that made him especially susceptible to the appalling conditions. The expedition was Scott's, not Evans's, in the sense that Scott was the one with control over who did what, when – to the extent that the environment allowed. I cannot say in Evans's case that it was his low control and not something more prosaic like the loss of a glove that did him in, but I will show you evidence that people of lower social position have less control over their lives and are more likely to be socially excluded, and that these two factors are important aspects of the status syndrome and play a big part in their worse health.

The third relevant feature of the Scott story is that exposure to an adverse environment is important. It is not simply that low-status people die earlier than high-status people regardless of the conditions to which each is exposed. Had Scott, Oates, Evans and the other two gone for a hike on a Southern California beach, rather than an 800-mile trek at the South Pole, it is highly likely that they would have been playing with their grandchildren years later. They would all have lived longer even if, predictably, Evans would have died first. Whatever differences in susceptibility to getting sick there may be between top and bottom social ranks, the environment to which people are exposed is crucial.

We see health gradients in harsh conditions; we also see them in agreeable ones. For a dramatic contrast, I want to move not to a Southern California beach but nearby to Hollywood to look for the health gradient among the most privileged and cosseted. The privileged are an interesting group to observe. We would like to know which is more important for generating the health gradient: differences in income, education or something else that we might call status, that is neither education nor income. Coming back to the parades with which I began this chapter, we saw that they are correlated: people with high education tend to gather more income and have higher status than people with less education. The problem is how to distinguish which is most important. One cannot do experiments; this is real life. You cannot simply assign people to different groups. Random assignment to high education or high income, interesting as it might be, is not an option. What we would like to have, for example, is a group of people where everyone has a high income, and where education matters little for success. If there were then differences in status we could observe whether it matters for health.

Successful Hollywood actors provide us with such a natural experiment. Two researchers from Toronto, Donald Redelmeier and Sheldon Singh, got the records of seventy-two years of motion-picture Academy Awards[4]. They reasoned that an actor who won an Oscar would get such a boost to her or his self-esteem and status in the world that, if these were important for health, Oscar winners should live longer than other film actors. The problem, of course, is finding an appropriate comparison group. Oscar winners will be richer than your jobbing film actor. Redelmeier and Singh needed a comparison group that was rich, even if not quite as gold-plated as the winners.

The researchers found two: actors of the same sex who had appeared in the very film which got the winner the Oscar; the second group comprised actors who had been nominated but never won.

The remarkable finding was that the Academy Award-winning actors and actresses lived an astonishing four years longer than their co-stars and the actors nominated who did not win. Four years might not sound like much. To give a flavour of how big an average of four years extension to life really is, we calculated how many years of life would be added to the population average if coronary heart disease, the major cause of death, was suddenly reduced to zero; i.e. no one died of coronary heart disease but their chances of dying of other diseases *at any given age* remained the same. The answer is that slightly less than four years would be added to the population's life expectancy. Four years, then, is enormous. Winning the Oscar is like reducing your chance of dying from a heart attack from about average to zero. Not bad. Winning the Oscar early in life changes the happy one forever. The average length of time between winning the Oscar and death was about four decades. If winning an Oscar did that it is a rather potent life enhancer.

I say 'like reducing your chance of dying from a heart attack to zero'. The winners had a lower risk of death from heart disease, but from other causes too. In fact, when the winners eventually died, the causes from which they succumbed were about the same as those affecting the other two groups. In other words, the reduction in death rate among the winners applied about equally to a number of different causes of death.

One argument that recurs is which way the causal process works: does social position affect health, or does health determine social position? We shall have occasion to examine this alternative argument at several points throughout the book. In this case, Redelmeier and Singh showed that it was not the case that the people who lived longer were more likely to win Oscars. Winning an Oscar prolonged life.

The potent life enhancer that added four years of life to the Oscar winners is unlikely simply to be money. The 'losers' in this study were hardly in penury. With an average 47.4 movies in their careers, they had little need to hock the Cadillac. The big questions are why and how Oscar-winning prolongs life. To answer those questions we need data that are only available from detailed studies of individuals that allow us to examine directly the effects on health of influences associated with status and prestige.

Before I go overboard about the effect of rewards on health, I should take note of the fact the effects do not stretch to scriptwriters. Scriptwriters who won Oscars do not live longer than scriptwriters who did not. I discussed with an acquaintance, a successful novelist who has had connection with films, why this should be. Was it a contradiction of the importance of status? His response was: not at all. People do not write for the movies for self-esteem, he argued, they write for money. For a creative person, writing for the big studios is an exercise in self-flagellation. Winning a prize will increase their money, but is more likely to increase their cynicism than their self-esteem.

Were I to argue that the actors' positive experience shows the effect of status on health, and the lack of benefit for scriptwriters is not counterevidence, it would not convince me, let alone you. It has a post hoc ring to it. The problem is that, neither in the case of the actors nor the writers was prestige or self-esteem measured. It is an inference, reasonable, but still a guess. To go further we need to measure the actual processes involved: autonomy and self-esteem, social participation. We need data that go beyond inference, that study more directly why and how status influences health. There is another rather obvious reason we want more data. For most of us, our lives no more resemble those of Hollywood actors than they do those of Antarctic explorers. We need evidence that more immediately relates to our own lives.

The status syndrome – which diseases follow the social gradient?

The easy answer is: most. In general, the lower the social position the higher the risk of heart disease, stroke, lung diseases, diseases of the digestive tract, kidney diseases, HIV-related disease, tuberculosis, suicide, other 'accidental' and violent deaths. The answer may be easy, but the questions it raises are difficult. Being low in the hierarchy means a greater susceptibility to just about every disease that's going.

We have to explain why there is a gradient, not only in how long one lives, but in risk of most of the major diseases.

I used to think that heart disease and cancer were diseases that people in rich countries got, when they no longer died of the things that people in poor countries now die of. Hence the thought that these were rich people's diseases. I was not alone in this thought.

More than twenty-five years ago, as I was beginning my research on heart disease in different social groups, my wife's mother – not the mother-in-law of low humour but an educated, insightful woman – asked about my research. When told that I was seeking to understand why, among office workers, clerks and messengers at the bottom of the office hierarchy had a higher risk of heart attack than senior managers at the top, she looked uncomfortable. She was thinking: 'My son-in-law – a doctor, no less – seemed like a sensible boy except for his interest in research. How do I point out to him that he has it upside down? It is well known that people in high-status jobs are more likely to get heart disease. How can he be telling me that *low*-status employees have *more* heart disease than those at the top?'

Her scepticism reflected the conventional wisdom of the 1970s and 1980s. 'Everyone' knew, many still do, that people in high-status jobs suffer stress and that stress causes heart attacks. This explained why the top people had their high risk of heart disease. It is still the case that whenever someone in the public eye has a heart attack, the newspapers are full of stories about how the stress of a high-status job brought him down. 'Everyone' was in good company, and had been for some time. In 1910, the great physician, Sir William Osler, described heart disease in his high-status patients and said that the typical heart-attack victim had the indicator of his engine 'set at full speed ahead'.[5] Research on the Type A behaviour pattern had suggested that business executives, striving for the top, were at particularly high risk.[6] My research flew directly in the face of that. Had it once been true that high-status people were at particular risk of heart attacks, it was no longer. Even heart disease then was more common the lower you were in the hierarchy.

My habit, born of years of medical training, of bowing to the wisdom of the great physician has long since lost out in the competition with habits of scientific scepticism. That said, such evidence as we have suggests that Sir William Osler, the greatest physician of his era, was right. When coronary heart disease emerged, in rich countries, as a major cause of death in the first quarter of the twentieth century, it probably did conform to Osler's description. Coronary heart disease caused death more commonly in richer than poorer people.[7]

The change in heart disease from rich man's to poor man's disease does not mean that the social gradient in disease is a relatively recent phenomenon. Not at all. If it was not heart disease it was something else. In the nineteenth century there was a social gradient in tuberculosis. In the US, for example, tuberculosis mortality was significantly higher in blacks, who were poor, than in whites, who were less so.[8]

The persistence of the social gradient in health from one century to the next raises two types of question that are rather fundamental. If there is always a social gradient, perhaps it is an inevitable part of living in society. The second issue is that if there was a social gradient in tuberculosis at the end of the nineteenth century and in heart disease at the end of the twentieth, how are we to think about causes of the status syndrome?

Reject: 'The poor are always with us'

Wherever we have had sufficient data to study the issue, we have found gradients in health. There appears to be certain inevitability to it. Indeed, my argument is that the health gradient is the result of social differences in society. All societies will have social rankings; ergo all societies will have health gradients. This leads to the statement, 'the poor are always with us', as a sort of counsel to go and study something else. I ask myself if I can envisage a society where all are equal. My answer is not in real life. Hence, health gradients are inevitable.

Yet I approach the challenge of the health gradient with optimism and invite you to join me in the same spirit. My optimism is not a personality defect; it is based on two arguments, both of which are illustrated in Figure 1.2. The first is that we should not accept as a given the current state of poor health of those lowest in the social hierarchy. Everybody's health can improve. In Great Britain, conscious of social class as we are, the government chief statistician known as the Registrar General has a system of classification of occupations into social classes. Class I is professional and includes accountants, engineers, doctors; II, managerial and technical includes marketing and sales managers, teachers, journalists, nurses; III (for simplicity's sake not shown in the figure) is divided into non-manual, clerks, shop assistants, and skilled manual, carpenters, plumbers; IV, partly skilled; V, unskilled. When originated it was thought of as a system of inferring social position from occupation and hence obtaining a measure of culture of different social classes.[9]

Figure 1.2 shows life expectancy by social class for the 1970s and 1990s. In both periods, there is a clear social gradient: the higher the social class the longer the life expectancy. But note something more. Between the 1970s and 1990s everyone's health improved. Life expectancy in all social classes went up. So much so, that if you were Social Class IV, partly skilled, in 1992–6, your expected length of life was *greater* than that for someone in Class I twenty years earlier. This can be seen by simply comparing the heights of the bars. The tallest bar in 1972–6, i.e. the healthiest, is not as tall as the second shortest, close to the unhealthiest, twenty years later.

Does this start to explain my optimism? Based on figures such as these, I take the view that there is no biological reason why today's bottom social groups should not, in the future, have the same good health as today's top social groups. That is what recent history teaches. And the means for this achievement? Read on.

Figure 1.2 contains a second reason for optimism, or pessimism: the gap between social classes is not fixed. Despite the improvement in life expectancy of Social Class V, Social Class I improved more. The gradient became steeper over the twenty years from the 1970s. The gap in life expectancy between top and bottom social classes increased from 5.5 years to 9.5 years.[10] A similar widening of the gap – steepening of the gradient – took place in the US.[11] The principle of 'to them that have shall be given' seems to be in operation. That is a reason for pessimism. Despite the evidence that inequalities are increasing, I remain optimistic. The gradient can change. It means that the health gradient is not a fixed property either of our biological natures or of the society in which we live, but it can change. It changed, presumably, as an unintended consequence of changes in society that happened for other reasons. If we can understand why the gradient became steeper, we should, in principle, be able to work out what to do to make it shallower.

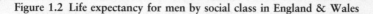

Figure 1.2 Life expectancy for men by social class in England & Wales

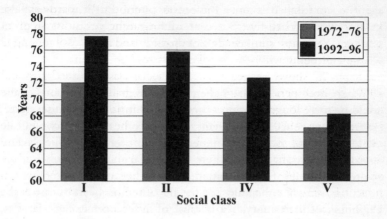

Note: The figures show life expectancy for two different time periods. I is the highest social class; V is the lowest – unskilled manual. Life expectancy for Social Class IV in 1992–6 was higher than for Social Class I twenty years earlier.

Source: Adapted from Drever and Whitehead (1997)

Explaining gradients then and now

A social gradient in heart disease in the year 2000, and in tuberculosis in 1900 – am I really going to look for a unifying explanation? Tuberculosis is such a different disease from coronary heart disease, which is different again from suicide and chronic lung disease, yet all show a social gradient. Despite their differences we can go about explaining the social gradient in a unified way, provided we take a full view of disease causation.

Epidemiologists, who developed their approaches studying infectious disease, think of host, agent, and environment.[12] The agent causing tuberculosis is the tubercle bacillus. Not everyone who becomes infected with the bug, the agent, becomes clinically ill, because people vary in their host resistance. The third part of the triad is the environment that can determine rates of exposure and, potentially, influence host resistance.

It is a little more problematic when applying this triad to non-communicable disease. For lung cancer, it is reasonable to think of the agent as smoking. It is not an infectious agent, but it is close to the main cause. Ninety-five per cent of lung-cancer deaths occur in smokers. Yet, most smokers do not die of lung cancer. We may label what determines why one smoker gets cancer and another not as variations in host resistance.

Where we see a social gradient in a variety of conditions, there could be three different approaches to searching out the causes: social gradients in agents, host resistance or environments. To complicate matters, environment can influence the other two. The 'agent' approach would suggest that there was a social gradient in tuberculosis at the beginning of the twentieth century because of differences in infection with the tuberculosis; a social gradient in heart disease at the beginning of the twenty-first because of differences in high-fat diet, smoking and slothfulness.

In my view this is not wrong; it is too limited. The links between a social gradient in tuberculosis a hundred years ago and in heart disease now is inequality of social conditions. This argument, agent versus social conditions, was played out with tuberculosis at an earlier period. It is so relevant to present concerns that I quote it in detail.

The tubercle bacillus was discovered by Robert Koch in 1882. Before that, tuberculosis was thought to be related to poor social conditions – hence its higher rates among the socially disadvantaged. Writing in 1921, two British doctor/epidemiologists, Collis and Greenwood, referring to the era before Koch's great discovery, put the social-conditions argument. They said:

> our grandfathers believed that in the case of consumption what was the matter with the poor was poverty, and that consumption (i.e. tuberculosis) would not be eliminated without the eradication of poverty; since they did not believe that poverty could be eradicated, they did not expect to 'stamp out' consumption.[13]

Koch wrote of his discovery of the agent, the tubercle bacillus:

> One has been accustomed until now to regard tuberculosis as the
> outcome of social misery and to hope by relief of distress to diminish
> the disease. But in the final struggle against this dreadful plague of the
> human race one will no longer have to contend with an indefinite
> something but with an actual parasite.[14]

We have, therefore, two quite different views about how to deal with
tuberculosis as a scourge of society: improve social conditions and
relieve distress; as opposed to taking specific action against the agent,
the tubercle bacillus. Collis and Greenwood, commenting on the
second, inspired by Koch, go on to say:

> The latter-day view is less pessimistic (or, if we look at it from another
> point of view, more pessimistic) and suggests that consumption might
> be eliminated without any obliteration of the distinction between class
> and class.

They conclude, however:

> that the general belief of our fathers and grandfathers is sound, and the
> policy which ought to have been, and to some extent was inspired by
> that belief is a sound policy. What is the matter with the poor is largely
> poverty. Not through any special intensive measures of campaigning
> against the tubercle bacillus, not even by the segregation of the actively
> tuberculous, does there seem any real hope of salvation. We have to
> improve the homes of the working classes in the first place . . .; in the
> second place, we have to ensure better factory conditions.

Thomas McKeown became famous and aroused the ire of many by
arguing that the fall in tuberculosis mortality in the twentieth century
had little to do with specific medical actions against the tubercle
bacillus.[15] In a simple graph he showed that tuberculosis mortality
dropped like a stone from the beginning of the twentieth century. By
the time streptomycin, the first effective anti-tuberculosis therapy, was
introduced around 1950, mortality from the disease had already fallen

to about 20 per cent of its 1900 level. McKeown thought the improvement was the result of improved nutrition. Others take issue with this part of his conclusion.[16] But the general proposition stands. It is hard to argue that knowledge of the agent was the key to reducing the disease. It is far more likely to have resulted from improvement of social conditions, and host resistance.

There need not, of course, be a stark choice between an approach that emphasises agent and one that points to social conditions. Effective treatment could make a big difference to tuberculosis among today's poor, provided it was made available. Paul Farmer, who has studied tuberculosis on the island of Haiti, argues that poor social conditions prevent those at the bottom of the social hierarchy, the disenfranchised and powerless, from receiving effective treatment.[17]

If we now turn to the situation in today's industrialised countries we are faced with the same dilemma. There is a social gradient in a wide range of different diseases. How can that be? One answer is to look for the different specific causes, the agents. Smoking and a rich diet cause heart disease; high blood pressure related to diet, alcohol and genes causes stroke; smoking causes lung cancer; infections, poor living conditions and smoking cause chronic lung disease; mental illness, caused by stressful life events and genes, causes suicide; aggression causes homicide; carelessness causes accidents; unsafe sex and dirty needles for drug use cause AIDS. All true. It may be that each of these specific causes follows the social gradient and, therefore, each contributes to the social gradient in a specific disease.

We should then ask why. What is it that leads each of these specific causes to affect people more the lower they are in the hierarchy? Why are lower-status people more exposed whatever is the agent that seems to be operating at the time? Twice is a coincidence, three times a trend. Even if we could explain the social gradient in diseases of the heart, lung and kidneys as due to social gradients in their specific causes (as I shall lay out I don't think we can), we still have to account for why there is a social gradient in these specific causes, and consequently in the deaths for which they are responsible.

There is another possibility. In addition to the operation of these specific causes, there is something more general associated with where you are in the hierarchy that is responsible for increased risk of a range of diseases. If we go back again to the nineteenth century, Booth wrote of poverty as follows:

> With regard to disadvantages under which the poor labour, and the evils of poverty, there is a great sense of helplessness: the wage earners are helpless to regulate their work and cannot obtain a fair equivalent for the labour they are willing to give; the manufacturer or dealer can only work within the limits of competition; the rich are helpless to relieve want without stimulating its sources. To relieve this helplessness a better stating of the problems involved is the first step.[18]

I am with Booth. What characterises being poor, and lower in the hierarchy, is a great sense of helplessness, or to use my language, lack of control over life circumstances. This will put people at risk of illness. The particular illness will depend on the noxious 'agents' to which they were exposed, be it the tubercle bacillus, or a crime-ridden neighbourhood. It will also put people under chronic stress, the effects of which, as we shall see, may be profound. In fact, we can resolve the dilemma of agent versus social conditions readily. The agent would determine which disease the individual got; social conditions would determine that it followed the health gradient.

The causes of cases and the causes of rates – the individual and the group

Following directly from this last discussion is an important distinction: that between individual cases of disease as against difference in rates between social groups. Booth could have asked why does one poor person get sick and not another. He didn't, or at least not primarily. He asked why poor people are more likely to get sick than the non-poor. Similarly, I am asking why a group of people with only primary-school education has a higher rate of illness than people who completed high school; and why they, in turn, have higher rates of illness than those who finished university. The causes of why one person with a high-school education dies sooner than another with the same education may be different from the causes of high-school graduates having higher rates of illness than those who went on to university. The causes of individual differences may not be the same as the causes of group differences.

We have no difficulty understanding this distinction between individual differences and group differences in other settings. Take a random day in December. If you were going to Boston, you would pack different clothes than if you were going to Miami Beach. Predictably, Boston will be colder than Miami. This average difference between the two cities tells you little about why one day is different from another within a city. A Miami winter's day can be balmy or unseasonably cold; a Boston winter ridiculously mild or impossibly freezing. We could study the causes of day-to-day variations in Miami's temperature and never quite figure out why Boston was so cold, unless we included it in our field of vision. We should not start by imagining that the causes of individual differences will be the same as the differences, in this case, between areas.

So it is with causes of disease. The reason why one San Franciscan gets heart disease and not another may be different from the explanation of why the heart-disease rate is higher in San Francisco than it is in Tokyo. Within medicine, the primary concern is with individual differences, the individual patient. Public health is more likely to be concerned with the health of groups. Geoffrey Rose, a physician interested in prevention, used to ask his students: why did this individual get this disease at this time? Risk factors, such as plasma cholesterol, were all about predicting individual risks of disease.

Geoffrey Rose had low levels of risk factors: he was lean and physically fit; a non-smoker who watched his diet, he used to joke that if one day he woke up to find that he had died of a heart attack, he would be very surprised. (He apparently worked on the practice attributed to the comedian George Burns: 'First thing I do in the morning is read the obituaries. If my name's not there, I get out of bed'.) Rose realised that by focusing on individual risks he had misled himself. It was true that if he compared himself to other Englishmen, his heart-disease risk was lower than most, because his risk-factor levels were low. But, and it is a big but, heart-disease rates in England are among the highest in the world. He may have been a low-risk Englishman, but compared to a Chinese or Japanese, Rose was high risk. The low-risk Englishman has a higher risk of heart-disease death than the average Chinese. The causes of why one individual gets sick and not another, may be different from the causes of why one group of people has a higher rate of disease than another.[19]

As physicians or as compassionate individuals, our field of vision is focused, understandably, on the individual person suffering. If we are only concerned with the individual case, however, we may miss the big picture. Take the case of traffic 'accidents'. You will see in a moment, why I put quotation marks around 'accidents'. Here is an item from my local newspaper: 'pensioner accidentally crushed her friend against a wall with her car after she mistook the accelerator for the brake . . . the friend died from multiple injuries later that day'. A human tragedy, an accident that killed the victim and devastated the driver to the degree that she never drove again and died a deeply traumatised woman, a few months after the accident. I have collected a whole series of these tales, each case more harrowing than the last.

To focus on individual cases misses the general picture. A predictable number of 'accidents' occur every year. This is tabulated in Table 1.1.

Table 1.1 Numbers of traffic fatalities in Great Britain in each of three years

	1994	1996	1998
Males	2535	2519	2535
Females	1098	975	1002

Source: Department of the Environment, Transport and Regions (2000).

These may be 'accidents' but they occur with near-constant frequency. Every year just over 2,500 men die in traffic crashes, and every year about 1,000 women die. Every year, there are two-and-a-half times as many male deaths as female. The individuals differ but the rate is the same. If we ask the early Geoffrey Rose question – why did this woman have this fatal crash, at this time – the answer may well be bad luck, accident, chance. If we ask a different question, why do two-and-a-half times as many men die in traffic crashes as women, you would not answer bad luck; not every year the same bad luck.

There are also regularities in the international variation. In the US, there is just under one fatality for 100 million car kilometres travelled. This is nearly twice the rate in Britain. The ratio between the two countries varies very little from year to year. I have once or twice caught a taxi in Brussels – I now avoid it if possible – the driver acts as if he is really annoyed that the whole world thinks Belgium is boring and he is going to prove it is not. Sure enough, year after year the Belgium traffic-fatality rate is 50 per cent higher than the US rate and nearly three times the UK rate.

There is then a social rate of traffic fatalities that shows regularities, whatever the circumstance of any individual tragedy. This is not to imply that nothing can be done to change it. When the US dropped the speed limits during the oil crisis, following the 1973 Yom Kippur War, the number of deaths in motor-vehicle crashes went down. When the state of Victoria in Australia toughened up on its drink-driving laws, the traffic mortality went down. When five years later, the state of New South Wales followed suit, its traffic mortality went down. There are actions that can be taken that change the rates, but the general point remains: the rate is predictable; which individual will succumb, much less so.

The social gradient in health, individual or group differences

I am arguing that an important cause of the social gradient in health is that people in different social groups are exposed to different social and economic conditions. It is these differences in the social environment that are responsible for the gradient. Pointing to the importance of the social environment does not in any way negate the importance of individual determinants of health. If you are exposed to dreadful conditions and your parents lived to 100, you will be more likely to be long-lived than someone else in those conditions whose parents died at forty-seven. On the other hand if your parents lived in dreadful conditions and died at forty-seven, and you live in more affluent circumstances, the chances are that you will live longer than they did.

Underlying my focus on the environment is the observation that individuals respond to the environment in predictable ways. If you reacted to high crime rates in your neighbourhood with a sense of foreboding and fear but your neighbour had a wonderful sense of well-being at all those muggings, burglaries and drive-by shootings, we could not avoid focusing on the reasons for individual differences in this response. To use a technical term, one of you might be a bit screwy. If, however, most people experience the high crime rates as a source of threat and have, therefore, predictable bodily reactions to that threat we can then study the effects of that environment on health.

Figure 1.3 Perpetrators of homicide in Chicago and England & Wales

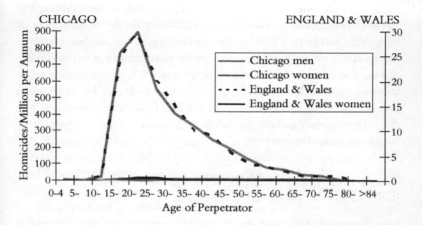

Note: The figure shows the age and sex of the perpetrators of homicide. The age and sex distribution of the victims is identical to that of the perpetrators. The figures on the left column are the rates per million for Chicago – the peak is 900 per million people of that age. The figures on the right column are the figures for England and Wales – the peak is 30 per million people of that age.

The interaction of individual propensities and environmental conditions can be illustrated by a study of homicide rates conducted by Margo Wilson and Martin Daly.[20] Their findings are shown in Figure 1.3. In Chicago young men kill each other. The figure shows homicide rates according to the age and sex of the perpetrator, but the victims are similar to the assailants. There is a remarkable peak in young men that we can barely discern in women. On the same graph we have the homicide rates for England and Wales. Same finding: young men kill each other. The peak of homicides is between the ages of twenty and twenty-four, in both countries. This suggests that there is something predictable about the state of young manhood that leads to violent behaviour. There is, however, an important question of the scale. In England and Wales the peak homicide rate is one-thirtieth of the Chicago rate: 30 per million in the population compared to 900.

The universality of the age sex pattern of homicide – young men killing each other – is a basic tenet of evolutionary psychology.[21] Where such universal patterns are seen, we are likely to be looking at an evolved characteristic of the species. In this case a tendency for young men to be aggressive. But what that evolved tendency leads to depends on the environment: the social conditions. It is likely that the environment of Chicago is either one that brings out this aggressive tendency and/or provides the means for this tendency to be translated into homicide.

I have a colleague in Chicago who asks why I am always carrying on about social conditions leading to differences in disease between social groups. Why, he wants to know, do I not ask why one individual flourishes in adverse circumstances where another goes under? Interesting question. I know people in Chicago who go for months on end without killing anyone at all. Instead of asking why the murder rate is so high in Chicago, I should ask why some refrain from killing. I should not trivialise his question. Murder is not randomly distributed in Chicago but occurs with greater frequency in deprived areas. It is important to ask why one person does and another does not commit murder but not at the expense of asking why the rate is so high in some groups compared to others. And then linking those differences in rates to the social conditions that are responsible for them.

Gradients in health abound. They run all the way down the social scale from the most to the least privileged, covering everyone in between. We see them in just about every society that has looked. Quite remarkably, we see them for diseases of poverty and for so-called diseases of affluence. The fact that the steepness of the gradient in disease varies gives grounds for optimism. If we can understand why health inequalities have got bigger, we potentially have the opportunity to make them smaller. I have reported that the lower the social position the worse the health, and left open the question of what it is about social position that may be responsible for the health differences. That is the task for the next several chapters.

2. MEN AND WOMEN BEHAVING BADLY?

Men at some time are masters of their fates: The fault, dear Brutus, is not in our stars but in ourselves, that we are underlings.

Shakespeare, *Julius Caesar*[1]

Throughout history there have been many average people. Some are born average, some achieve averageness and some have averageness thrust upon them.[2] By the standards prevailing in our community, you and I are about average; somewhat above average in some respects, a bit below in others. Our degree of departure from average in a social ranking matters for health. Does it matter how we got to our social rank – born to it, achieved it, or had it thrust upon us – or is it where we end up that is important for health? And if it's where we end up, why? What is it about being a bit higher than average in the ranking, or a bit lower, that leads to better or worse health?

The logical framework of this question, applied to differences in health, is no different from its application to other fields of human differences. If you play a recording down the phone to my music teacher, a successful professional string player, she can tell you if it is in the key of A minor or C sharp minor, or something else. (I could just about recognise whether it was fast or slow.) At fifty paces, she can tell you played an A natural rather than an A flat. How did she achieve her ability? Inborn talent, hard work, and the opportunity to develop her talent – music lessons when she was young; i.e. she was born to it, *and* achieved it, *and* had it thrust upon her. For every successful musician, there are many whose inborn talent and aptitude for achievement had no opportunity to flourish. What is true for musicians applies to athletes, mathematicians, chefs, and probably chartered accountants.

As with the musician, all three are important for the health gradient – where you came from, what you do, or what you have thrust upon you – but the relative importance of each matters. For example, were the social gradient in health due, in the main, to smoking or diet, that would lead us one way, in our efforts to reduce it. If, on the other hand, it were largely the result of unhealthy people failing to rise to the top, that might lead us in a different direction entirely. As it turns out, the evidence suggests that neither of these gives an adequate account.

Rank ill-health

There are not many people who would confess to this in public, but the British civil service changed my life! I am no Kafka, I was not enmeshed in the bureaucracy, but I have spent a good part of the last three decades studying the health of civil servants in two large studies, known as the Whitehall studies. Whitehall being the wide London street that houses many of the key government departments and whose name is shorthand for the civil service. By gathering information on how these government employees work and live; what they eat, drink and smoke; what they think and do; where they came from and where they are going, we can test hypotheses on the reasons for the social gradient in health.

I am interested in the social gradient in health across the world from Finland to Tierra del Fuego, and parts in between. The corridors of power of the British civil service might, therefore, seem an odd place to go to find insight. Why study British civil servants if the interest is in how the status syndrome appears through all societies?[3]

The first answer is because the social gradient in health in Whitehall is huge. Figure 2.1 shows quite how big it is.[4] The data come from the first Whitehall study, begun in 1967, of 18,000 civil servants, all men, classified according to their employment grade, i.e. their ranking in the occupational hierarchy. (At the time that the first Whitehall study was set up, these studies, mostly, studied men only because it was thought that was where the main problem of heart disease lay. Later it was recognised that heart disease is a major killer in women. Whitehall II, our second study of civil servants included men and women. It showed that the status syndrome applies to women as well as to men.) These are all non-industrial, office-based jobs.[5] The men at the bottom of the office hierarchy have, at ages forty to sixty-four, four times the risk of death of the administrators at the top of the hierarchy. More dramatic than the difference between top and bottom is the gradient. The group second from the top has higher mortality than those above them in the ranking. Everyone dies in the end; and you might have imagined the differences between social groups to become less at older ages. The social gradient does become shallower, but even at the oldest age, the bottom group has twice the mortality rate of the top group.

Figure 2.1 Mortality over twenty-five years according to level in the occupational hierarchy

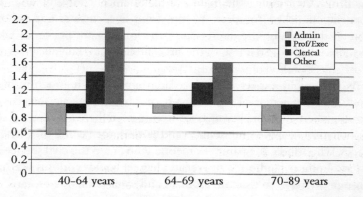

Note: The figure shows mortality in each grade relative to the average for the whole civil service population. The Administrators have about half the average mortality at age 40–64; the other grade about twice the average. Hence a four-fold difference between bottom and top grade.

Administrators are the top grade who set policy; executives carry it out, and professionals and technical staff are of equivalent rank; clerical grades are of lower status; then come the office support grades.

Source: Calculated from data in Marmot and Shipley (1996).

Both the gradient and the four-fold difference between top and bottom are dramatic. National figures at the time showed a 1.8-fold difference between top and bottom social classes, formed by grouping occupations together.[6,7] What is this civil-service organisation that there should be a steeper gradient in Whitehall than in the country as a whole? One might have imagined the civil service to be rather homogeneous. It excludes the richest and poorest in society; there are no private jets, and no unemployed or unemployable. Everyone has high job security.

This superficial homogeneity belies the exquisitely stratified nature of such an organisation. The civil service is like a big white-collar corporation, only more so. It is your stately bank or insurance company, not your high-tech start-up. No metal-bashing; all office jobs. It is, in my experience, like public bureaucracies in the US, Australia, Canada and the European Union. The similarities among the civil services in these countries are greater than the differences. All are highly stratified, as are big corporations. How many times have you called the telephone company, the airline, the bank, the insurance company and, in exasperation, asked to speak to the front-line person's supervisor? You do this because the discretion of the lower-status person to take decisions is limited. So it is with the large public-sector bureaucracies, of which the British civil service is typical.

As you might expect of such a large employer, it is a mix of a meritocracy, where ranking depends on ability; and age-based seniority, where there are rewards for having been there a long time. At the bottom end are the messengers and porters; then come the clerical grades, who handle the paper. Someone who enters the civil service as a clerical officer, without a university degree, could work his way up through the ranks to executive officer and even to the lowest rank of administrative grade before he/she retires. The executive grades implement policy; the professionals include scientists, statisticians and economists.

At the very top of the civil service are the high flyers who become the mandarins – the permanent secretaries. The people who come from glittering student careers at Oxford and Cambridge, sail through the entrance exam, and go into the civil service on a fast track, destined for great things. The top mandarin was once described to me as: 'That's R. Reached the top without touching the sides.' They both run the great departments of state and are responsible for working with elected politicians, the ministers, to develop and implement policy.

The very characteristics that I have just described both explain why the social gradient in health in Whitehall is steeper than in the country as a whole, and why Whitehall has been an ideal study in which to take further investigations of the status syndrome. White-collar organisations, and the civil service is best at this without question, are brilliant at stratification, better than the national social-class system. The national social-class system in Britain groups together occupations with similar social standing.[8] It is less adept than the civil service at classifying people precisely into ranks. In Whitehall, there are sharp differences between grades in income, education and the nature of the job. An executive officer is quite like another executive officer and quite different from an administrator. This does not apply nearly as neatly to national social classes. For example, in the national system, managers are grouped together into Social Class II: it means that the captain of industry and the proprietor of the bed-and-breakfast, who cooks your bacon and eggs in the morning, will be in the same social classification, despite their differences in income, power and perhaps education. Whichever measure of status we take (and it is my task as the book progresses to decide between income, occupational prestige and education), there will be a great deal of variability within national social classes; much less within civil-service grades. Hence Whitehall provides a clearer demonstration than national data that social ranking is strongly linked to health.

It is not difficult to see why the more precise a classification system, the stronger will be the relation between social position and ill-health, where such a relation actually exists. Misclassification leads to under-statement of associations. Think of the parades we conducted in the last chapter that demonstrated that social rank is related to health in a step-wise way. If some people with low status (and hence poor health) were wrongly put in with the high-status people, they would bring down the average health of the high-status group – by 'diluting' the good-health group with some who have worse health. Conversely, if some of the high-status people (and hence good health) were wrongly put in with the low-status people, they would bring up the average health of the low-status group. Result: less difference between top and bottom than is really the case, and an apparent shallower gradient in health.

Given the precision of the Whitehall ranking system, the health gradient in Whitehall is probably closer to the 'real' size than would be given by a less accurate classification system. Despite missing out on the richest and poorest in society, despite being confined to a white-collar organisation, Whitehall is an ideal 'laboratory' in which to discover how subtle differences in social ranking can lead to dramatic differences in health, in people who are neither very poor, nor very rich.

Separate books need to be written about the contribution of differences in medical care to inequalities in health. Another advantage of the Whitehall studies is that they show this cannot be the main explanation of the social gradient in health for two rather crucial reasons. First, we see a social gradient in incidence of disease.[9] Incidence of disease is a first occurrence. While it is plausible that differences in medical care could lead to differences in survival and recovery once someone became ill, it is a good deal less likely that differences in medical care could lead to differences in the rate of new occurrence of disease. Technically, control of blood pressure and cholesterol could be more adequate in the higher group, but as we shall see in a moment, these do not explain the social gradient in disease.

Second, we studied the medical-care issue directly in relation to heart disease. We showed that people in the lower ranks of the civil service were *more* likely to be investigated and treated for coronary heart disease than people in the higher ranks.[10] They had more treatment because they had more disease; the excess of the one matched the excess of the other. When we looked at people who had evidence of heart disease, the lower grades were just as likely to have investigation and treatment as the high grades.

High-quality medical care should be available to all in a rich society. Differences in access are unjust. But the evidence from Whitehall shows differences in access are not major contributors to the health gradient.

I noted in passing that the first Whitehall study was confined to men. At the time Whitehall was set up, most studies of heart disease were in men. The data from elsewhere are quite clear, however: the status syndrome applies to women as well as to men: the lower the social position of a woman the worse her health. There is the possibility for confusion because, in Britain, where the first studies of health inequalities took place, social position was defined on the basis of formal occupation, i.e. excluding domestic roles. The question then was how to classify married women who were 'not working' in the formal sense. Classified by husband's occupation, they showed the same gradient in health as did men[11]. More recently, Amanda Sacker and Mel Bartley have shown similar inequalities in health for men and women, but interesting differences in the way these are best demonstrated.[12] A socioeconomic measure that reflects the nature of the job best predicts the social gradient in mortality in men. A measure that reflects general social standing best predicts the social gradient in women.

Lifestyle and the social gradient

At the time, 1978, that I started to report from the Whitehall study, the gradient in health was a minority interest; it still is. No one was marching on Washington, protesting the unfairness of middle managers having worse health than their bosses. No committees were being convened to tell policy makers how to bring the health of college graduates up to the level of those with a master's degree. There was a general view that, in the words of one commentator: 'the burden of ill-health and premature mortality has shifted from the diseases of poverty to those related to individual behaviour'.[13] The general view was that when the killing diseases were due to poverty, social conditions could be held responsible, but now the major diseases such as heart disease could be attributed to freely chosen lifestyle.

A summary of this view would run as follows. Differences in health status between groups at different levels of the social hierarchy are the result of individuals making autonomous choices to smoke, to refuse to take exercise, or to persist with an unhealthy diet. To put it plainly, the lower the social status, the more likely are people to behave badly – in ways that damage their health. If they chose to do that, it is no business of anyone else. To argue otherwise is to 'slide imperceptibly into a form of determinism which appears to leave little scope for what used to be known as free will and is now fashionably known as "agency"'.[14]

I am in complete agreement with the importance of autonomy, but disagree with the concept expressed in the previous paragraph and find it to be inconsistent with the evidence. It is certainly true, as any reader of this book knows, that high-fat diet and high-plasma cholesterol are bad for heart disease. Smoking is a killer, in a variety of ways. Little exercise and too much food lead to obesity, diabetes and heart disease. High blood pressure, in part due to diet and obesity, increases risk of heart disease and stroke. Whitehall confirmed all of these findings and, further, showed that the lower the employment-grade position in the hierarchy, the more adverse were these health behaviours.

Why is this not the whole story? Stop people smoking, substitute some lettuce and tomatoes for the fries and hamburgers and everybody would be healthy. The job would be done. Indeed some think that is all there is to it. Rid the world of smoking and concerns about people's place in the social hierarchy would have little to do with health.

The problem with this approach is that the evidence is against it, whatever one's view of determinism and free will. These differences in lifestyle provide only a modest explanation of the social gradient in health. This is shown in Figure 2.2. The mathematics behind this figure is not very complicated; the logic even simpler. If low-grade men died earlier from heart disease because they had higher levels of risk factors – smoking, blood pressure, plasma cholesterol, short height and blood sugar – then 'adjusting' for these would make the risk in the 'other' grade not 1.8 times that of the top grade, but the same; the relative mortality would be 1. But it is not 1. It is just under 1.5. 'Adjusting' for these risk factors explains less than a third of the social gradient in mortality from heart disease.

It is not, in any way, to imply that these risk factors are unimportant. To repeat, Whitehall confirms the importance of these factors in predicting mortality. What is behind Figure 2.2 is that whatever the level of risk factor, being of low grade is worse for your health than being of high grade. A smoker who is low employment grade has a higher risk of heart disease than a smoker who is higher grade. A non-smoker who is lower grade has a higher risk of heart disease than a non-smoker who is higher grade. In the case of lung cancer, 95 per cent of the deaths occur in smokers. The question of a social gradient in lung cancer in non-smokers is not highly relevant. For mortality as a whole, taking all causes together, the social gradient in mortality was nearly as steep in non–smokers as it was in smokers. A similar conclusion applied to other risk factors.[15]

Figure 2.2 Mortality from coronary heart disease over twenty-five years in the first Whitehall study showing the contribution of risk factors to the social gradient

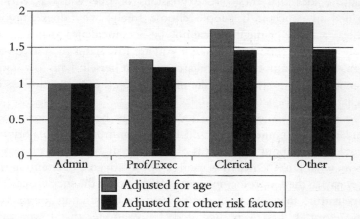

Note: Administrators are taken as having relative mortality of 1 and the other employment grades compared with them. The first group of bars allows for age differences. The second group, in addition, allows for differences in smoking, systolic blood pressure, plasma cholesterol concentration, height and blood sugar.

Whitehall shows clearly that there are two questions. The first is why should smoking and other features of lifestyle be more and more common as the social hierarchy is descended. This finding is not unique to Whitehall but is clearly evident in national data from the UK and the US, although not in some other countries such as France. The second is, if these aspects of lifestyle account for less than a third of the social gradient in mortality, what accounts for the other two-thirds? The second question occupies the rest of this book. Before we turn to it, the question of social differentials in lifestyle claims attention briefly.

Not if, but why behave badly?

As Figure 2.2 shows, health behaviour is not the main reason for the social gradient in health. I described its contribution as modest.

Nevertheless, if the social gradient in health could be reduced by a third by changes in lifestyle, that would be a wonderful achievement. It is therefore a highly important question: why should behaviours such as smoking, exercise and diet appear to be more unhealthy in lower-status groups than higher? I suggested, above, that the idea that these are expressions of free will was wrong-headed in concept. If people choose freely, why does smoking follow a social gradient? It cannot be a coincidence that you are more likely to choose to smoke if you are low status than if you are high. Is a single mother on welfare saying to herself: I am low status, therefore I choose to smoke like most of the other single mothers on welfare?

Smoking does not follow a social gradient because of ignorance. Studies in the United States and Britain confirm that a majority of people know about the hazards of smoking. It is almost as if people know what is in the health warnings, but the degree of attention that they pay to these warnings increases as they go up the social scale. The explanations that have been put forward for this finding are not very satisfactory. It has been suggested, for example, that lower-status people have less orientation to the future. Quite possibly, but why is that?

A rational-choice model of human behaviour suggests that people make choices that maximise their utility. This does not strike me as very helpful either. It is saying: people smoke because they like it. Well, of course. But it does a lot of harm as well, not just lung cancer and heart disease in years to come, but real problems in the short term, financial, for example. In Britain, households in the lowest tenth of income spend, as a proportion, six times as much of their income on tobacco as households in the highest tenth.[16] Alarmingly, over 55 per cent of single mothers on welfare benefits smoke, smoking an average of about five packs a week.

Hilary Graham has done careful observational studies of the lives of these women on low income.[17] Almost every penny that these women spend is for someone else, for the household, the children, the boyfriend. The only personal expenditure they allow themselves is cigarettes. Without that indulgence, the whole of life would be about keeping it together for others. Simple exhortations not to smoke are unlikely to have much impact on these low-status women, and men. Improving their social conditions might.

Where they came from?

If it's not what people do, in the realm of health behaviours, that causes the health gradient, then what? In fact, I have made no mystery of the search for the culprits responsible for the social gradient in health. On the first page of the Introduction, I told you the butler did it: social conditions affect the degree of autonomy and control individuals have and their opportunities for full social engagement. These needs, for control and participation, are more adequately met the higher your social position. As a result health is better. The next several chapters will show the evidence supporting that explanation, and what it means in practice.

I cannot reach that conclusion without first dealing with an obvious concern: People are not allocated randomly into positions in the hierarchy. A coin is not tossed at entry into employment and the luckless applicant assigned to porter or senior manager in the civil service. Where you come from must influence where you end up in the hierarchy. Al, from an affluent background with a good college degree, is more likely to end up in a high-status job, than Del who did not complete high school. And if Del's brother, Bert, from an unpromising background, does make it up to a top job, there must have been something really special about him, to triumph despite his lack of social advantage. In arguing, as I do, that it is the social conditions acting on people that determine their health, I have to take into account the alternate explanation: Al and Bert are healthier than Del because of who they are, not because of the positions they achieved.

This could work in two ways. First, a mix of social, psychological and biological attributes could determine your social voyage: Al's intelligence, vitality, social and psychological skills, and general robustness are all higher than Del's and determine that Al will land in a higher position in the social hierarchy than Del. These same characteristics may determine that Al has better health than Del. In other words, it is who you are that determines your place in the

hierarchy and your health. The social conditions attached to position
in the hierarchy are bystanders, not causal agents. The first part of this
has to have some truth to it: who you are has a big effect on where you
end up socially. We shall look at the evidence for this. (As shorthand, I
shall label this the 'who you are leads to where you end up'
explanation.) There are several pieces of evidence, however, that
suggest that this does not imply the second part of the argument: social
conditions attached to where you end up are far from innocent
bystanders; they are important causes. The explanation of the social
gradient in health does not come down to resilient, highly able people
having good health *and* ending up in high social positions.

The second way it could work is slightly different from the first and
it, too, is not right. It argues that ill-health leads to low social position,
good health to higher, and this is the reason for the health gradient.
While this also has plausibility, and must be true to some extent, the
evidence suggests that in practice it is not the explanation of the health
gradient either.

Some are born . . .

Rather than step gingerly around the edge of the issue, I propose to
jump in with both feet. The 'who you are leads to where you end up'
explanation leads without too much difficulty to an argument that
people in different social positions are genetically different, and the
social gradient in health reduces to genetic differences among social
groups. Certainly, it is not politically correct to argue that social classes
differ genetically and that is why they have different health.[18] But the
reason to eschew a genetic explanation of the health gradient is not
because it is unfashionable, but because it is untrue. To be more
accurate, genes are fundamental to everything that all living creatures
do and become, and how they live and die; but so is environment.
Variability in genetic endowments is not the explanation of inequalities in health and simply cannot do justice to the evidence before us.
This may sound as though I am going to enter the nature/nurture fray
– the tussle about is it genes or is it environment that is the principal
determinant of human characteristics. I shall enter it only far enough
to remind us that an explanation of the reasons for individual

differences in a human characteristic that affects health may be quite different from explanations for differences between groups or variation over time. The mix of genes and environment may be different in these different types of variation.

We can deal with the 'who you are leads to where you end up' explanation by looking at two markers of who you are, one physical/biological, and one psychological, i.e. cognitive function or intelligence. To start with the physical/biological, I have a tall story to tell. It is about height. In Britain, there was a famous TV sketch about social class. Three actors lined up in descending order of height. The tallest, dressed smartly, says: 'I am upper class; I look down on him, and on him.' The one in the middle, less smartly dressed, says: 'I am middle class; I look up to him and down on him.' The little chap, dressed in workman's overalls and a cloth cap, says: 'I know my place.' It confirms what everyone knows about class-ridden Britain. Not only do the social classes have different accents, different clothes, they even have different heights. The height differences are confirmed by national figures. But the differences are similar in the US. There is a clear relation between height and social position. It is as if the higher people stand, the higher their standing. We confirm this in Whitehall: the taller go further. To be more precise, men in the top grade are, on average, 5 cm (2 inches) taller than men in the bottom grade. The differences are a bit smaller for women but, as with men, the high grades are taller than the lower.

Before we turn to the most obvious reason for how social position and height could be linked, for completeness, let us consider two others. Height could determine social position. As the TV sketch suggests, people look up to someone taller than themselves. This is not altogether fanciful. Height could lead to promotion and greater success. Height is likely to correlate with physical attractiveness, athletic performance, and general bearing, which, in turn, influence success in life, at school, university, and in interview panels. When Michael Dukakis was a presidential candidate against George Bush senior, such was his height disadvantage that one only had to see the two of them on TV to realise that Dukakis did not have a chance.

More fanciful, is that it is the other way round: people in high-status jobs are taller because they grow into the job. This is unlikely to be more than metaphorical. In adult life, there may be an effect of posture on apparent height, 'walking tall', but this would not account for the link between occupational prestige and height.

No, the likely reason for a link between height and social position is a common factor underlying both: the same set of factors that determine height, determine social position in adult life. Height is highly relevant to our concern with 'who you are leads to where you end up'. It can be thought of as a marker of biological fitness, in that in the Whitehall and Whitehall II studies, shortness was associated with increased risk of coronary heart disease. Men over 6 feet tall have about 40 per cent lower risk of heart disease than men less than 5 feet 9 inches.[19] Here, then, is the issue: height is a marker of biological fitness and height shows a clear correlation with adult social position: height and high status are correlated; is this not a clear demonstration that it is biological fitness that determines why some people end up low status and in poor health, and others high status and in good health? The answer is no, for the reasons that I set out below.

At first glance, height might seem to lead rather naturally to the argument that the differences between social groups are genetic. Studies of twins reared apart and of children who were adopted show that 90 per cent of the variability in height, *among individuals*, can be attributed to inheritance – known as heritability.[20] This fits with everyday observation: tall parents have tall children. It would appear that I have a steep mountain to climb if I am going to reach the point of arguing that the social gradient in health cannot be attributed to genetic differences.

Actually my climb up the mountain is not at all difficult. Two related facts make it a shallow climb. Height is also influenced by environment. And the above conclusion about heritability applies to individuals in a particular environment, not to differences among groups in different environments. I can illustrate the first with my own family. My father was the second oldest of nine children. His was a typical story of Jewish immigrants who left the pale of settlement in Eastern Europe and arrived in London penniless to make a life in a new country. At my grandmother's funeral, I had the opportunity to see nearly all her sons and daughters – my aunts and uncles – together. For the seven men, there was a remarkable gradient: with the exception of the youngest, the younger the man, the taller he was.

How do I account for this? The two oldest sons were born in the old country into conditions of great poverty: their nutrition was likely to have been restricted both during their mother's pregnancy and in infancy. Son number two might have had a slightly more adequate nutritional environment because he came to London at six months. The family was still in poverty after they arrived in the slums of the East End of London. As their circumstances improved, the nutrition available both to the pregnant mother and to the children would have become progressively better. What of the youngest child? Why should he not have been the tallest? His father died six weeks before he was born, leaving my grandmother a widow with eight children, and a ninth imminent. Setting aside the effect of stress of bereavement on the growth of the foetus she was carrying, the family's dramatically reduced financial circumstances would have had an effect on child number nine. The nutrition and care available to the new baby were likely to have been less adequate than for number eight.

My uncles, dear as they are to me, hardly constitute a sufficient case for the importance of the environment, but there are more systematic observations. Robert Fogel, has shown how average heights have increased over the last 150 years or so.[21] More recently, John Komlos, working in Munich, has compared heights of males in Germany and the US. In the mid nineteenth century the average height of adult men was 174.1cm (5ft 8½in.) among American whites and 167.3cm (5ft 6in.) among men in Bavaria, in what is now Germany.[22] At the end of the twentieth century adult men in their twenties averaged 178cm (5ft 10in.) in the US and a shade under 180cm (5ft 11in.) in Western Germany. Tall fathers may indeed have tall children. When conditions are changing, however, there may be big changes in average heights – 13cm (5 inches) increase in the case of the Germans. They went from being shorter than Americans, on average, to being taller.

There seems to be a paradox here: a statement that up to 90 per cent of the variability in adult height is heritable would appear to be at odds with such a huge growth in average height in 150 years. There will be no wholesale change in the genetic makeup of the population in such a short time – apart from what may be accounted for by migration. The resolution of the paradox comes from recognising that there are two different questions. If you go into a typical American college classroom, and measure the heights of all the young men and women, much of the variation in height that you will find will be the result of differences in genes. The taller ones are likely to have taller parents than the shorter ones. This is a question of individual differences – why one person differs from another. A different question is why Americans with a college education are taller than Americans with only elementary education. This is a question of group differences. The fact that individual differences are largely the result of genetic variation tells us little about the causes of group differences. They could be genetic, environmental, or a mix of the two.[23]

This is not simply playing with statistics. In a contemporary college classroom, few of the young men and women have been exposed to any significant degree of malnutrition, in utero, or in childhood. In the extreme, if there are *no* differences in nurture among them, all the differences have to be due to nature, i.e. genes, or measurement error.

Where the differences in nurture are likely to be substantial, it would be incorrect to attribute the differences between groups to genes. As an example, I reported above the nineteenth-century heights of US white men as 174.1cm (5ft 8½ in.). For 'slaves' in 1860, average height among adult men was 168.7cm (5ft 6½ in.) – more than 5cm shorter than US whites. Does that mean that the average difference in heights of blacks and whites in the nineteenth century was due to genetic differences between blacks and whites? That is one possibility. Far more likely is that blacks were nutritionally deprived compared to whites. An individual black man may have been short or tall because of his genes, but blacks on average were shorter than whites because of nutrition. In support of the nutrition argument are more contemporary figures for height. The figure of 178cm (5ft 10in.) for average height of American men in their twenties, now, is the same for blacks as for whites. In other words, the average height of white American men increased by about 1½ inches from the mid nineteenth century to the present, and of African-Americans it increased by about 3½ inches. The environment can have a big impact on average heights.

In sum, this distinction between group differences and individual differences is vitally important. Height may be 90 per cent heritable but a conclusion, in the nineteenth century, that the shorter average height of blacks was due to genes would have been quite wrong. In contemporary America or Britain the differences in height among social groups may have as much or more to do with nutrition in early life as they do to any supposed genetic differences between groups.

Showing that variability in height relates to variability in both genes and environment does not, by itself, knock on the head the 'who you are leads to where you end up' explanation. It changes it. Instead of arguing that who you are is determined by your genes, it could take the form that 'who you are' is a mix of genes and nutrition in early life. We still need to ask the question if who you are is more important for the social gradient in health than the social conditions that are related to where you end up. This is especially true because I reported above that short height was related to risk of heart disease in the Whitehall studies. However, we did deal with this 'who you are' question. Squirrelled away in Figure 2.2 (p. 45) is the word 'height'. The figure shows clearly the higher mortality as the social hierarchy is descended. It also shows that this social gradient in mortality was not greatly changed by adjusting for the effects of a number of different influences on health. Among these was height. Social position in adulthood is strongly related to health in adulthood, even after taking account of the differences in height that occur along the social hierarchy.

To be clear, I am not arguing that endowment from early life is unimportant, neither genes nor environment. Height as a marker of such endowment predicts heart-disease mortality. I am arguing, however, that they are not the major reasons for the social gradient in health in adulthood.

Another way of looking at the 'who you are leads to where you end up' explanation of the health gradient, involves health of parents. If your parents were blessed with long life you are likely to be. You and your parents share genes, and tend to share habits and environments. If these are harmful to the health of your parents, they may well be harmful to your health. Achieving high social status in adulthood, with the favourable circumstances that go with it, can change the destiny predicted by your parents' fate.

To illustrate, one senior manager that I interviewed told me his own story. His grandfather and father, both in blue-collar occupations, had died of heart attacks at age fifty-four. He was the first member of his family to go to university, and had ended up in a top job. As he moved into his fifties he felt the sword of Damocles hanging over his head – death at fifty-four. Within days of his fifty-fourth birthday he suffered crushing chest pain, sweatiness and faintness and was admitted to hospital with a heart attack. All this was in accord with his genetic destiny, but what happened next was not. In his words, he took control over his life. He stopped smoking, changed his diet, became a fitness fanatic, lost weight, and used his high-status position to take control of his work life to suit his needs, rather than simply the needs of others. I interviewed him a decade after his heart attack and he was hale and hearty. Parents' medical history is a potent predictor of illness, but so is the complex of factors related to current circumstances.

The message of this anecdote is confirmed by a more systematic study of Whitehall II civil servants. Whitehall II included women as well as men. The question was whether low-grade men and women are at higher risk of heart disease because they were more likely to have unhealthy parents. As with height, the logic was to take a measure of heredity and family background that is known to predict disease and ask if it was this that accounted for the social gradient in disease. A simple way to do it was to chose participants in whom neither parent had died before the age of sixty-five (we repeated it for seventy, with the same results). Among these people, none of whose parents died 'prematurely', the social gradient in incidence of heart disease was undiminished.[24] The assumption here is that your parents bequeath you both genes and an environment of poverty, affluence or something in between. If your parents did not die prematurely it suggests that neither genes nor your early environment were particularly toxic. Social circumstances in adult life predict health independent of whether your parents were long-lived or short-lived. Adult social position is crucial.

Justice will not have been done to the 'who you are leads to where you end up' explanation, unless I consider another measure of who you are that is likely to be a potent determinant of where you end up socially. I refer to intelligence or cognitive function. In the British civil service, there is a social gradient in scores on standard tests of cognitive function: the higher the grade the better the performance.[25] It is hardly earth-shattering news that those whose jobs are more demanding of intellectual function are better at it. It would be rather upsetting were it not the case. If the people who got first-class degrees from top universities and are now charting economic and social policy for the nation had no more intelligence than a porter, we would worry for the country.

Intelligence then is related to social position; it has to be. Yet, it would be wrong simply to take this as evidence for the 'who you are leads to where you end up' explanation. The line of reasoning could be: a favourable genetic profile leads to better cognitive function, higher status and to better health. Plausible, but there are drawbacks. For a genetic explanation of inequalities in health to work, people in different social classes would have to be genetically different *and*, it is a vitally important 'and', these genetic differences would have to account for the health differences seen among social groups. In the case of height, we saw that it failed the second test, quite apart from the fact that the height differences between social groups are likely to be environmental as well as genetic.

A plausible way that intelligence could lead to inequalities in health is indirect; i.e. higher intelligence leading to higher social position, and the circumstances associated with higher social position affecting health. In other words who you are leads to where you end up, but it is where you end up in the social hierarchy that is responsible for your level of health. I know of no evidence that intelligence itself, independent of its link with adult social position, is related to health. It is conceivable that such evidence could be forthcoming, it is therefore worth having a brief look at the first test: do differences in intelligence between social groups mean that they are genetically different?

The argument is similar to the one we have just looked at with height. Twin and adoption studies show that intelligence is highly heritable. Some estimates suggest about 50 per cent heritable,[26] others say it could be as high as 75 per cent.[27] That conclusion applies to *individual differences*. But environment plays a big role in determining average intelligence levels. For example, as William Dickens of the

Brookings Institution in Washington DC and James Flynn of the University of Otago in New Zealand report: in every one of twenty countries analysed, there have been sizeable gains in IQ since about 1950. It is a real effect, not simply a result of making the tests easier. We are all getting smarter; or, to be more accurate, our children are smarter than we are. In Holland, for example, eighteen-year-old men tested in 1982 scored twenty points higher on a standard IQ test, than did eighteen-year-olds in 1952. Twenty points is huge. Variation can be measured by the standard deviation. One standard deviation either side of the mean includes about two-thirds of the population. The standard deviation of this test was 15. This gain over time in IQ cannot be attributed to genetic change; genes in the population do not change so quickly.

As with height, we have the phenomenon that individual differences appear to have a big genetic component, but group differences, in particular improvements over time, are surely the result of environmental changes. Dickens and Flynn point out that twin studies that attempt to separate the effects of genes and environment may have difficulty doing so, because genes and environment are correlated. A child who, because of genetic predisposition, is good at maths ends up in an environment that fosters his maths ability. A child who is predisposed to be athletic is likely to end up in an environment that fosters his athletic ability. Thus twin studies may over-estimate the genetic contribution to intelligence.

Sandy Jencks from Harvard had reached similar conclusions to Dickens and Flynn. He suggested that if red-haired children were discriminated against in school and, as a result of that discrimination, performed worse on cognitive tests, one might conclude in a study that genes, associated with red hair, caused low performance. It would in a sense be correct, but not because the genes were a direct cause of IQ.[28] The genes caused the hair colour, the hair colour 'caused' the discrimination, and the discrimination, not the genes, was the culprit.

The finding of a social gradient in intelligence does not therefore mean that the social classes are genetically different in ways that could lead to health differences. As Sandy Jencks argued, everyone who has studied the issue concludes that some of the 'test score' (i.e. intelligence) difference between rich and poor is due to genes and some to environment.[29] He thought the social differences more environmental than genetic but the insights of Dickens and Flynn into the matching of genes to environment make it difficult to come up with a precise figure.

Genes and environment, mutually reinforcing, will both be responsible for a social gradient in intelligence. As I argued above, this will be of importance to the social gradient in health in an indirect way. Intelligence is correlated with education and that, in turn, leads to different sorts of jobs. Different jobs with different pay mean different social conditions. Intelligence, then, plausibly leads to different social conditions. It is for this reason that there is a likely link between intelligence and social differences in health. There will be some societies where low intelligence leads to destitution because that is the fate of the ill-educated low-paid worker, and others where it does not, because the link between lower intelligence and worse social conditions is not as strong.

Whatever role 'who you are' plays in determining who ends up where, it does not cancel out the effect of social conditions for the reasons that we reviewed in Chapter 1: health for everyone can improve and the magnitude of the health gradient change on a time scale that is much faster than any genetic change.

In other words, where people come from is important for health, and the social gradient, but not to the exclusion of where they end up. To make it concrete, picture two people, Bob and Ted, both successful managers in a bank, insurance company, or in the public sector. Bob's father worked on a building site, the family were poor, and Bob went to the local school, did well, went to college, and had a good career in the bank. Ted's father was a university-educated accountant; Ted went to a private school, and a small private liberal arts college. With his good college degree he went to the bank and did well. He ended up alongside Bob. They are then of equivalent employment status and income, but the background of one was more favoured than that of the other. Does this difference in background matter for their health?

The simple answer from the second Whitehall study, Whitehall II, is: yes, but. Where you come from does matter for your health, but it is not the reason for the health gradient.[30] Family background, measured as parents' education and father's social class, are related to risk of heart disease. In the above example, Bob, from humble origins, is at higher risk of heart disease than Ted, from a more privileged background, despite the fact that they have the same occupational prestige. Background matters. There is then a different question: given that people in lower-status jobs are likely to come from more humble origins than those in high-status jobs, is this the main reason why low-status people have higher risk of heart disease? Whitehall II shows that it is not. Even taking into account differences in family background, your position in the job hierarchy is closely linked with your risk of heart disease.

Some achieve . . .

We have just been looking at how social and psychological characteristics affect social position. An argument that people float up and down the social scale because of their health, psychological or social characteristics is perilously close to social Darwinism. This comes from Herbert Spencer in the nineteenth century and has been described thus:

> The theory that persons, groups and races are subject to the same laws of natural selection as Charles Darwin had perceived in plants and animals in nature . . . The theory was used to support laissez-faire capitalism and political conservatism. Class stratification was justified on the basis of 'natural' inequalities among individuals, for the control of property was said to be a correlate of superior and inherent moral attributes such as industriousness, temperance, and frugality. Attempts to reform society through state intervention or other means would, therefore, interfere with natural processes; unrestricted competition and defence of the status quo were in accord with biological selection. The poor were the 'unfit' and should not be aided; in the struggle for existence, wealth was a sign of success.[31]

Stirring stuff, if you have a strong stomach. Leave the poor to rot, otherwise their survival would weaken the gene pool. Surely I am exaggerating. I fear not. Spencer opposed state-supported education, postal services, regulation of housing conditions, and even public construction of sanitary systems. This thinking penetrated many of the great industrialists of the swashbuckling era of growth of American industrialism in the nineteenth century.[32] In a less harsh form, the people who today say that social classes are segregated on the basis of natural inequalities are subscribing to the first part of social Darwinism. Those that say that social action is therefore unjustified are subscribing to the second.

Echoes of social Darwinism are, thankfully, faint today. Some hear those echoes when they hear the argument that the 'cream rises to the top'. The assertion is that the biologically fit are upwardly mobile; those less fit sink down the social hierarchy. It could be intelligence that makes you rise up, or it could be health itself. Earlier I introduced Bob and Ted who both had achieved successful high-status jobs, but Bob was from humble origins, compared to the comfortable conditions that Ted enjoyed. The relevant comparison now would be with a third person, Jim, who had the same humble origins as Bob, but had recurrent bouts of illness. Could it be that Jim's illness meant that he was slower to climb the social ladder than Bob? More generally, could it be health that determined one's social position rather than social position determining health?

You can hold to this position without being a social Darwinist and wish to leave the poor to rot. If ill-health leads to poverty, we might wish to have in place social programmes that tried to break that link — better medical-care provision, support for disabled people and so on.

There are some well-documented examples of ill-health causing downward social mobility. It has been shown, for example, that patients admitted to hospital with schizophrenia are likely to have achieved a lower social class than their fathers.[33] They were, in other words, downwardly mobile because of their health. This is known, technically, as health-related social mobility. There will be other examples such as ill-health interfering with earning possibilities.[34] The evidence shows, however, that this is not a general explanation for the social gradient in health: it cannot be, in the main, attributed to health determining where you end up socially.

This is the conclusion of two medical sociologists, Mel Bartley and David Blane, who have separately looked at this issue.[35,36] They show that health-related social mobility exists but it is not the reason for the social gradient in health. They do find that people who are downwardly mobile are less healthy than people in the social class they left. Going the other way, people who are upwardly mobile are more healthy than those in the class they left behind. It may look like an open-and-shut case. Health determines where you end up: the healthy rise up, the unhealthy sink down. Bartley and Blane conclude precisely the opposite: far from health-related social mobility being the cause of the social gradient, it serves to narrow it. How can this be?

It is true that people who rise up the social scale are healthier than those in the social class they left behind. But these upwardly-mobile people are *less* healthy than others in their class of destination. Conversely, those who are downwardly mobile are, indeed, more unhealthy than those who stayed in a high social class, but not as unhealthy as those who were always in a lower class. It works the same way as misclassification. The healthier top-rank people are having the average health of their group reduced by recruitment to their ranks of some people who were less healthy. The less healthy low-rank people are having the average health of their group improved by recruitment to their ranks of some who are healthier than they were. This health-related social mobility is blurring the social gradient in health, not increasing it. This effect works precisely because social position is related to health.

Blane and Bartley looked at social mobility during adulthood, i.e. at adults who changed social class. Michael Wadsworth has been studying a group of people who were all born in one week in 1946, and has traced the social-mobility effect all the way back to childhood. He shows that sick children are less likely to be upwardly mobile than children who are well, but the effect is small. After taking account of this health-related social mobility, there is still a clear social gradient in health in adulthood.[37]

What these studies show clearly is that health-related social mobility does exist: healthier people are more likely to be upwardly mobile; unhealthy people more likely to be downwardly mobile. The effects of this are to reduce the social gradient in health not to increase it. Were it not for this effect, the health gradient would be steeper, not shallower. This is not to argue that other forms of social mobility are irrelevant. Far from it. The evidence shows clearly that the social position in which you end up is crucial for health. If your father had little education and you have a PhD from Harvard, the chances are that your health will be better than someone from a similar background who had the same low level of education as his father. Not because your good health determined your success, but because your success led to social conditions that in turn led to your good health.

. . . others have it thrust upon them

The rest of this book looks at what those social conditions might be. As the discussion in the earlier part of this chapter showed, it is not only that people in higher socioeconomic groups are less likely to smoke or are more likely to eat well. There are aspects of conditions in which people live and work that are important. One way of enquiring into the relevant aspects of these social conditions is to ask more precisely what we mean by high rank. The next three chapters will look at three aspects of socioeconomic position and examine their relevance for health: money, status and power. As we shall see, enquiring after the causes of the status syndrome, the social gradient in health, is not only of interest itself, but is a way of asking what in the way we live in society is important for health and well-being.

3. POVERTY ENRICHED

By necessaries I understand not only the commodities which are indispensably necessary for the support of life, but what ever the customs of the country renders it indecent for creditable people in the lowest order to be without. A linen shirt, for example, is, strictly speaking, not a necessary of life. The Greeks and Romans lived, I suppose, very comfortably though they had no linen. But in the present times, through the greater part of Europe, a creditable day-labourer would be ashamed to appear in public without a linen shirt, the want of which would be supposed to denote that disgraceful degree of poverty which, it is presumed, nobody can well fall into without extreme bad conduct. Custom, in the same manner, has rendered leather shoes a necessary of life in England. The poorest creditable person of either sex would be ashamed to appear in public without them.

Adam Smith[1]

If a poor man eats chicken, one of them is sick.

Yiddish saying

Society can favour its privileged in different ways: more money, more status, more power. Each could be related to the social gradient in health. Money, at first blush, seems the easiest to think about and measure. It is an obvious way to characterise social position, and its distribution is finely graded from richest to poorest. If the social hierarchy in health were entirely attributable to how much money one had, the explanation and solution would appear simple – until one thought about two problems. First, what is it about having a thick wallet, or more electronic impulses in a bank account, that leads to better health; what does money buy? A nonchalant assumption that it buys more medical care will provide little in the way of explanation in those countries where personal income bears little relation to the medical care received. Second, if money were most important in creating the social gradient in health, what would you propose be done? Organise society so that everyone had the same income? I do not see you getting elected on that programme. Nor would it work, at least not completely. The data that we shall look at in this chapter suggest that even if everyone were to have the same income, there would still be a social gradient in health. The status syndrome would remain.

The problem is this: for those who are poor, nothing is so important as their poverty.[2] In a poor society, problems of ill-health, among others, can be laid fairly directly at the door of poverty. It would be reasonable to suspect that an increase in income, for people who have little, should have a direct effect on improving health. If it were simply that income solves material problems that lead to poor health, then in rich countries, there would be no relation between income and health. But there is. Why should that be?

The importance of money for health depends on how much money you had to begin with. If you have little of it, more money will improve health by meeting basic needs of food, shelter and sanitation. Above that level, when the problems of privation have been solved, how much money you have is not as important as how much you have relative to others in society. It is this relative income that determines what you can do with what you have. We need a richer understanding that poverty and wealth are not only about money. At a higher level of income, if you are really swimming in it, money may still appear to be important for health because it is a way of keeping score – a marker of success. But it is not the money that is important, it is the score.

We tend to think of income as something we have individually or, equally important, that the person next door has. But it matters crucially where we have that income: whether the surrounding society is rich or poor in a way that will affect health.

Money matters if you have little –
the importance of material conditions

At the beginning of the twentieth century, in Europe and North
America – in countries that we now think of as rich – dying was
almost as easy an option as living, particularly for the poor. This was
especially the case for infants and young children. It is at this young age
that the grim effects of poverty on health are seen most starkly. A study
in the English town of York in 1900, for example, found that in the
poorest part of town one child in four died before the age of one.[3]
Compare that with the poorest people in England at the end of the
twentieth century: fewer than one child in a hundred dies before the
age of one.[4]

The explanations for this dramatic loss of life among the poor at the
beginning of the twentieth century are readily apparent. For a vivid
description of poverty in the North of England, I turned to George
Orwell's descriptions of mining communities in *The Road to Wigan
Pier*. He found squalor that we can scarcely imagine.[5] Toilets were a
fifty-yard walk from the house. Houses with three rooms contained
four beds for eight people. For lack of privacy, a miner would not
wash the lower half of his body for six days of the week. In one house,
three teenaged girls staggered their shifts at work, so that they could
each have shifts in the one bed they all shared. A typical family would
eat meat once a week, fruit never, and aside from potatoes, little in the
way of vegetables. Damp, cold, crowded houses, with poor sanitation,
unclean water and lack of nutrition give ample explanation for the
high death rate of children and high susceptibility of adults to chronic
respiratory disease and tuberculosis.

Today, with an infant mortality rate of 8/1,000 among the poorest
members of society, we can say that it is over: poverty of material
conditions – in the Orwell/York 1900 sense – has been solved in
England. The same is true throughout Europe and Australasia, with
the exception of a few pockets of material deprivation. In the US, too,
in 1999, infant mortality among babies born to black mothers was 14/
1,000. Although this compares unfavourably with infant mortality
among babies born to white mothers, which was 5.8/1,000[6], the gap
is tiny compared to the figures of a century ago.

Though there was not much good to be said for being poor 100 years ago, the rich did not fare so well either. The richest people of York in 1900 were the servant-keeping class. Mortality among their babies was just under one in ten.[7] This figure is considerably better than that of the poorest of York in 1900 – one in ten versus one in four. But the richest people, then, had infant mortality an order of magnitude higher than that of the poorest people now: 94 versus 8 per 1,000 live births.

Would you rather have been rich and had servants in York in 1900 or been poor and had a vacuum cleaner in 2000? If your criterion was not having your babies die, it would be a good deal better to be poor now than rich a century ago. Material conditions for good health improved for everybody. We should not think about income and health only as it relates to individuals. We have to ask what the community provides. If having a great deal of money does not guarantee clean water for your children, your money will not buy better health. Conversely, if the standards of the community have risen, even children of the poorest families will have better survival chances.

In examining the relation of income to health, we therefore have to take into account not only the income of individuals but also the wealth of the community. The first conclusion applies to whole communities: if a country is poor, a little extra income can make a big difference to health. For example, several African countries, Sierra Leone, Malawi and Zambia, have gross national product (GNP) less than $1,000 per capita and have life expectancy of 45 years or less. The biggest contributor to this loss of life is the death of children. To take the worst case, in Sierra Leone around 30 per cents of children die before the age of five. By contrast, in Sweden the rate of child death is less than 0.5 per cent. Children die because of poor sanitation, malnutrition and a range of infectious diseases – a direct effect on health of poor material conditions. In Sierra Leone, the World Bank reported that 57 per cent of the population subsisted on less than $1 a day, 75 per cent on less than $2.[8] A small increase in income for the country, if spent wisely, could lead to dramatic improvements in health.

I added the caution 'if spent wisely'. Sudhir Anand and Martin Ravallion showed that the relation between GNP and life expectancy depends on how the national income is spent. If spent on reduction of poverty and on improving health specifically, then life expectancy is improved, not otherwise.[9] Even in Haiti, one of the poorest countries in the Americas, infant mortality is 68/1,000. The servant-keepers of York had infant mortality (94/1,000) comparable to Uganda or Equatorial Guinea today. A small amount of money, spent on public health and education, could make infant mortality lower in one of today's poor countries than it was among the rich people of York in 1900.

After material conditions have been improved

If water is safe to drink, it is safe. If sanitation is adequate, it is adequate. In other words, it is important for a country to get rich enough to provide these basic resources for life, and adequate calories to eat. Once it provides those things, a larger national income is unlikely to provide better health for the country as a whole. Table 3.1 shows this to be the case for the rich countries of the world.[10] All these countries have low infant-mortality rates, precisely because all have good nutrition and material conditions for children. The table shows that although there is substantial variation in life expectancy and in income, there is little relation between the two. Higher national income does not result in higher life expectancy.[11]

For example, the US, which has the highest GDP (gross domestic product) in purchasing power (except for Luxembourg), ranks twenty-sixth in life expectancy. The four-year difference in life expectancy between first-place Japan and the US would be as if the Japanese all won Oscars and the Americans were all also-rans. Israel, Greece, Malta and New Zealand – all countries with GDP under $20,000 per person – have higher life expectancy than the US. Among these developed countries, there is simply little relation between average income and health. Greece with a GDP of a little over $17,000 per household has longer life expectancy than the US with twice the national income. Once a country has solved its basic material conditions for good health, more money does not buy better health. When comparing whole countries, there is no gradient in the relation between income and health.

On the face of it, there is huge contradiction here. Within the US, people whose household income is $17,000 have worse health than those whose income is $34,000; and those whose income is $68,000 have better health still. There is a health gradient. And the gradient stretches way above the level of income that makes any difference to a whole country. Yet for a country, having a national income of $34,000 per person does not seem to buy better health than having one of $17,000. How are we to reconcile these?

Quite easily; with the first two parts of my proposition. If you have little of it, more money will improve health by meeting basic needs of food, shelter and sanitation. Above that level, when the problems of privation have been solved, how much money you have is not as important as how much you have relative to others in society. How much money Greeks have compared with Americans is of far less interest and importance to Greeks than what having a low income means for a Greek compared with a Greek having a high one. This relative income determines what she is able to do in life, more than whether the Swedes or Japanese are richer or poorer than the Greeks.

Table 3.1 Life expectancy at birth and GDP (gross domestic product) in $US in 2001 adjusted for purchasing power

	Life expectancy at birth	GDP per person
Japan	81.3	25,130
Sweden	79.9	24,180
Canada	79.2	27,130
Spain	79.1	20,150
Switzerland	79.0	28,100
Australia	79.0	25,370
Israel	78.9	19,790
Norway	78.7	29,620
France	78.7	23,990
Italy	78.6	24,670
Netherlands	78.2	27,190
New Zealand	78.1	19,160
Malta	78.1	13,160
Greece	78.1	17,440
Cyprus	78.1	21,190

Germany	78.0	25,350
UK	77.9	24,160
Costa Rica	77.9	9,460
Singapore	77.8	22,680
US	76.9	34,320
Ireland	76.7	32,410
Cuba	76.5	5,259
Portugal	75.9	18,150

Source: United Nations Development Programme (2003).

For further dramatic evidence that income itself is not the issue, look beyond the figures in Table 3.1 for the US, at those for African-Americans. One estimate puts the average, US black income at $26,000 per person.[12] They are, by world standards, rich. Yet, life expectancy for US blacks is 71.4, way below that of poor countries such as Costa Rica (77.9) or Cuba (76.5). The UN Human Development Report classifies fifty-five countries as 'high human development'. Many of the countries in the next category, 'medium', also have better life expectancy than US blacks: Tunisia, Jamaica, Panama, Libya, Lebanon. In dollar terms, and in terms of what they can purchase with those dollars, Costa Ricans and Cubans and residents of these other countries are far poorer than US blacks, but their life expectancy is considerably longer. This is not to argue that US blacks are not disadvantaged compared to US whites. It is to argue that their disadvantage is not well captured by absolute income.

That health disadvantage is considerable. Consider two typical American teenagers of fifteen: a young white man in an urban area of Michigan, and a young black man living in Harlem in New York City. Michigan is about as close as you can get to the statistical average for life expectancy in the US.[13] The white teenager has a 77 per cent chance of still being alive at age sixty-five. The black teenager has a 37 per cent chance.[14] Two out of three black fifteen-year-olds on the streets of New York will not see their sixty-fifth birthday. Three out of four white fifteen-year-olds in Michigan will.

Poverty of income leading to poor material conditions is an inadequate summary of the life conditions that lead to the early death of these young black men. To see this, look at the causes of death. The three major causes of death contributing to this tragic waste of life were HIV–related causes, homicide and cardiovascular disease. We do not think that heart disease is related to poor sanitation, malnutrition and overcrowded conditions in houses without gardens. Heart disease is not, in other words, related to material deprivation in the sense that I have been using it. Nor do we think that poor sanitation causes HIV or that bacteria in the water supply predispose men to commit, or become victims of, violence. Circumstances of impoverished lives might lead to these causes of death, but we have to enlarge our notion of poverty.

There is more to poverty than low income and poor material conditions

Here is a more contemporary picture of poverty. In an American city a young woman, let's call her Patty, sits and contemplates her life. She recalls that a researcher, doing a health survey, came to the local grocery store, where Patty works as a cashier, and asked her how much exercise she did. She laughed. Most of the day is spent sitting or standing behind the till. What about exercise at home? She lives in a crowded, inner-city tenement building. She won't let the children play on the strip of asphalt surrounding the buildings. Apart from broken glass, she is worried about the violence in this part of town.

Patty's reverie continues. The children come home from school and ask if they can go swimming. It would certainly relieve the long oppressive hours from Friday night to Monday morning that is the lot of a single mother with two children. But joining a fitness club had been out of the question. They might as easily have a vacation on the moon. There is the Y. But it is an hour on the bus. With the bus, entry, snacks and sodas for the kids, the trip would cost $30. A king's ransom, but it would fill a couple of hours at least. Then what? She and the children sit cooped up in their two-bedroom apartment going quietly stir crazy. Not so quietly. The children yell at each other and start to fight again. Patty lights another cigarette.

As she contemplates the week ahead, she thinks that the boy needs new sneakers. Why they have to be the ones with special laces, when he never does them up, is beyond her. Something about all the other kids having them. The girl has been to three different friends for dinner and a sleepover in the last month. She wants friends home to her place. Four children, pizzas all round . . . Where is that money going to come from? Patty lights another cigarette. She remembers when she splashed out and bought herself a pair of designer jeans. It was Mother's Day before last. Gallows humour of the single mother to buy herself clothes that she could not afford on Mother's Day.

As she thinks about it, she realises that the only money she spends on herself is the cigarettes. When she took the children to the clinic the other day, the nurse told her, for the umpteenth time, that she shouldn't be smoking: bad for her health and a bad example for the children. The hell with that, thought Patty, take the cigarettes away and what am I left with? That clinic nurse should try leading my life, and see if she still worried about lung cancer in thirty years' time. I have enough trouble getting through next week.

Is Patty poor? Her world is an order of magnitude different from a miner's wife in George Orwell's account of Northern England. Patty's apartment is small, but she sleeps in a separate room from the children. They have a bathroom in the apartment. The idea of not having toilet facilities on the premises is unthinkable. The apartment is warm and dry. Undernutrition is not their problem. It is malnutrition of another kind. Patty is overweight and the children are already showing signs of going the same way. For Patty, lack of money is a problem. Material deprivation, in the sense of lack of sewage facilities or undrinkable water, is not. For Patty, the issue is being able to participate fully in society, which includes giving her children what the other kids have. She smokes, takes no exercise and is overweight – all bad for her health. But to focus on these, and blame her for her poor lifestyle, is to focus on symptoms rather than the cause. If smoking, being over-weight and lack of exercise are causes of ill-health, then we have to look at the causes of the causes.[15]

This view of poverty starts to give us a way in to the gradient. Once we are no longer discussing material deprivation, it is less appealing to think in terms of a threshold, i.e. below it you are deprived, above it you are not. In the Whitehall studies, we asked why people second from the top had worse health than those at the top. Material deprivation of those second from the top is not the first thing that comes to mind. I think it unlikely that having a small three-year-old

car is worse for your health than a new large one because of worse
material conditions. Lack of participation fully in society, or relative
deprivation might start to get closer.

The many faces of inequality

On rare occasions, one comes across an idea that changes the way one
sees the world. If the idea is truly important, you cannot imagine that
there was ever a time when you did not know it. The idea seems so
self-evidently true. This particular one made such a strong impression
that I remember exactly where and when it became part of me. The
brilliant light of a cold early autumn day lit up the sleek, clean Nordic
design of the hotel in Helsinki. Sitting at breakfast, I was too engrossed
in the book in front of me to bother with the morning session of the
meeting.

The book was Amartya Sen's *Inequality Reexamined*.[16] He wrote:

> The major ethical theories of social arrangement all share an endorse-
> ment of equality in terms of *some* focal variable, even though the
> variables that are selected are frequently very different between one
> theory and another. It can be shown that even those theories that are
> widely taken to be 'against equality' turn out to be egalitarian in terms
> of some other focus. The *rejection* of equality in such a theory in terms
> of some focal variable goes hand in hand with the *endorsement* of
> equality in terms of another focus.

This makes sense of everything! If that sounds a trifle overenthusiastic
as a reaction to a piece of densely written prose, an illustration may
help. Take politics, for example. We tend to see it, at best, as serving
class interests, and at worst, as a corrupt pandering to the greed of
those who put the politician in office. The political right argue for low
taxes and the freedom to pursue their own profit-making; the political
left, for care for the downtrodden and disadvantaged, protection from
the ravages of economic inequality. That is when each side is arguing
'ideologically', rather than from tribal loyalties or greed.

How does the insight from Sen clarify this? Rising above naked self-
interest, or wickedness, both sides may be arguing for equality of

something. They clash because they are arguing for equality of different things. A libertarian agenda that rejects equality of incomes or happiness as a goal of public policy as it entails too much state interference is, in fact, arguing for equality of individual liberties. As equality of rights is central, equality of other things, such as income or happiness, is peripheral. By contrast, a political philosophy that argued that equality of condition is paramount may pay less attention to the rights of individuals. The right to amass a fortune unbridled may bow to the demand for equality of quality of life or health, or, at least, of opportunity. The battle between politicians may be about tribal loyalties or class interests, but the battle between political philosophies may have to do with which measure of equality should have precedence.

These arguments have been played out in public health. The right of individuals not to have to drink fluoridated water, against the desire of the community to prevent dental caries; the right of individuals not to wear seat belts, against the aim to prevent traffic fatalities. (The language of rights is sometimes misused. I heard a lawyer interviewed who complained that her client had been denied the most funda-mental right of all: to talk to a lawyer. More fundamental than breathing? A TV advertisement for an analgesic told me that it was my right to be free from pain. Really?)

Sen coins the idea of the 'space' in which you measure equality. The primary concern may be with justice, or social welfare, or living standards, or quality of life. Each of these will require a different space in which to measure inequality and to evaluate policies and pro-grammes. In which space, then, are we to measure poverty and inequality? Income is one such space; it is this that we have been exploring. A different 'space' is that of capabilities. Sen argues that more crucial than what we have, in terms of income, is what we are capable of doing, physically, psychologically and socially. Income should not be thought of as an end in itself. It is a means to some other end. Most would accept that that end has something to do with quality of life. Sen would argue that the end is capabilities, or freedom. Income is only one means to that end.

Income and capabilities are conceptually distinct, but related in practice.[17] An excellent way of depriving people of capabilities to lead the life they would wish to lead is to make them low income. Patty is deprived of the necessaries, in Adam Smith's sense that the 'customs of the country renders it indecent for creditable people' to be without.

What are these necessaries? How shall we define them? An approach that has been taken in Europe is to think of absolute and so-called 'overall' poverty where overall poverty is defined as 'not having those things that society thinks are basic necessities and, in addition, not being able to do the things that most people take for granted either because they cannot afford to participate in usual activities or because they are discriminated against in other ways'.[18]

If you ask people what it means to be poor, they will tell you. There has been a series of surveys, under the title *Breadline Europe*, in which people were asked just that. Researchers then looked at those items without which at least 50 per cent of people said they would consider themselves to be in poverty. Let us look first at the items related to adults. If people have insufficient money for the following they would define themselves as poor:

- Replace or repair broken electrical goods
- Home in a decent state of decoration
- Contents insurance
- Telephone
- Appropriate clothes for job interviews
- Carpets in living rooms and bedrooms
- A small amount of money to spend on yourself
- Television
- Roast joint of meat once a week
- Replace worn-out furniture
- Clothes to wear for social or family occasions

There were also a series of adult activities, without which people would define themselves as poor:

- Celebrations on special occasion
- A hobby or leisure activity
- Friends or family round for a snack
- Presents for family or friends once a year
- A holiday away from home

There were then two series that related to children. Here, first are the items:

- Toys and dolls
- At least seven pairs of pants (underwear)
- Bike
- Leisure equipment

Here are the children's activities which, if you could not afford them, would define poverty:

- A hobby or leisure activity
- Going on a school trip
- Swimming
- Holidays away from home
- Friends round for tea

If not being able to buy children new trainers or have a holiday away from home defines poverty, it sounds awfully relative. A *New Yorker* cartoon showed a man saying 'I thought I was poor because I had no fax in my car, and then I saw a man with no mobile phone'. Under this type of relative definition of poverty, there will always be poverty. If everyone but me has a Mercedes or its equivalent then I with my bicycle am poor. This can take us down the road of cultural relativism. The prevalence of poverty could be the same in Boston as in Bogota, despite the fact that in terms of material possessions and purchasing power, the people of Boston were far richer than the people of Bogota.

To repeat; if you have little of it, more money would benefit health, but if you have more of it, then it is how much you have compared to other people in your society that is more important for health.

Absolute poverty is of great relevance to the 2.5 billion people in the world who live on less than $2 a day.[19] This is for all the reasons we discussed in relation to the low life expectancy in poor countries. In richer countries, it is more usual to define poverty as income relative to the median. If the median income for the society rises, the dollar amount that defines poverty will rise. Poverty is defined relative to others in society. For example, the United Nations *Human Development Report* produces a set of figures for higher 'development' countries, showing the proportion of people whose income is below 50 per cent of the national median income. The proportion of poor ranges from 3.9 per cent in Luxembourg to 17 per cent in the US.[20] These figures tell us not so much about absolute standards of living but about how income is distributed. In Luxembourg, the spread of incomes must be narrower than in the US. Implicitly, if someone has less than half median income, they will have less of the necessaries that custom dictates, even if their absolute needs are met.

Once people are above the threshold of absolute deprivation, are we always to think of poverty as a relative concept? Amartya Sen's answer to this question is with regard to his notion of the spaces in which we measure poverty. The primary 'space' of interest should be capabilities – not so much how much a person has but what he or she is able to do.

> Relative *deprivation in the space of* incomes *can yield* absolute *deprivation in the space of* capabilities.[21]

We have to think of income in two ways: how much the individual has and what the society has. Individual income may relate to people's capabilities to participate fully in society and to take control over their lives. The degree to which this is so will be influenced by what the society provides. If transport, medical care, education, recreation, quality housing, a safe neighbourhood in which to raise children all depend on individual income, then individual income will be an important measure and, indeed, a determinant of control and capability to participate in society. If, on the other hand, these were all provided by the community, individual income would matter less. Individual income will be an uncertain guide to the conditions under which people live and their opportunities to participate fully in society.

I have left one issue hanging uncomfortably: the relevance of material conditions for the gradient in health. In discussing the decline in infant and child mortality, I offered the conclusion that the material problems that lead to ill-health have been solved in the rich countries of the world. This is not a proposition that has met with universal acclaim. Some argue that material conditions play the dominant role in generating inequalities in health, even in rich countries.[22] This contention appears to contradict the case that I am developing here of the importance of participating in society without shame and of having the capabilities to lead the life you most want to lead.[23] Telephones, carpets, clothes for a job interview sound rather 'material'. Can I really argue that they are irrelevant? They are, indeed, relevant. But how does lack of home decoration act to cause an increase in heart disease? We need to distinguish conceptually between material problems that lead to infection, malnutrition and exposure to toxins in the environment, and material conditions that prevent participation or add to the difficulty of getting through the day. If your child does not have the trainers he needs to hold his head up high, or you cannot entertain your daughter's friends for a meal, these are, in a sense, material problems. But they cause disease in a different way from an infection. Trainer deficiency is going to have a different biological effect from vitamin deficiency.

There are credible pathways by which lacking the necessaries, in the Adam Smith sense, can lead to ill-health. Lack of social participation and inadequate control over your life, in the sense of not being able to lead the life you want to lead, will lead to chronic stress, which in turn increases risk of a number of diseases, heart disease among them. The evidence for this will be laid out in Chapters 5 and 6. Lack of social participation is also likely to change behaviour. Patty's argument to the clinic nurse was: 'Why should I worry about smoking or obesity that might increase my disease risk in thirty years, when I cannot see how to get through next week?' A young black man on the streets of Harlem has, as quoted above, a two-in-three chance of dying before his sixty-fifth birthday. What do you imagine your reception would be if you turned up with the message that smoking was bad for his health? Informing him that if he did not moderate his smoking behaviour he would not live to a ripe old age will not be a forceful argument.

To the extent that possession of material goods defines or allows participation in society, they are important. It is not difficult to see, however, a situation in which such goods lose their importance.

Income as keeping score

When I was a graduate student in the US, I was a little shocked when faculty would refer to how much another professor was being paid. Why, I wondered, would a full professor at a prestigious university, with two cars, an attractive house with a view of the Bay, and two perfect children, care if another professor earned more than them? To return to Adam Smith, by no stretch of the imagination did they lack the Berkeley, California equivalent of a linen shirt or whatever the custom of the day rendered it indecent to be without. They had prestige and, surely, full participation in society. Why should income matter? These university professors, at Berkeley in the 1970s, were not, for the most part, addicted to conspicuous consumption. Income was a way of keeping score. If you were paid more, it was not so much that you could do more with the money, but you were more highly valued.

Does money still predict health at this rarefied level? I know of no data, like the life expectancy of Oscar winners, correlating the life expectancy of tenured professors with their income. But Robert Erikson, a leading Swedish social scientist, has done the next best thing. Intrigued by the Whitehall studies of British civil servants that showed a gradient in health in people who were not poor, he looked for a way of testing out the importance for health of social position in people who were not materially deprived.[24] He has used Sweden's remarkable record systems to match the whole population of Sweden aged 25–65 at the national census in 1990 to subsequent mortality.

Sweden may be egalitarian compared with other countries (6.6 per cent poverty in the Human Development Report figures, compared with 17 per cent in the US) but income is still related to mortality: the higher the income, the lower mortality. Erikson was concerned to rule out the possibility that poor health leads to low income. He used education for precisely this reason. The argument is that ill-health in later life may reduce earnings and hence induce a relation between health and income that has little to do with low status causing illness. Such an effect cannot lead to a reduction in education. (We have already, in Chapter 2, looked at the possibility that ill-health could lead to downward social mobility, and ruled this out as a main cause of the social gradient in health, see pp. 59–61.)

Figure 3.1 Mortality according to level of education in men in the Swedish
population 1991–6

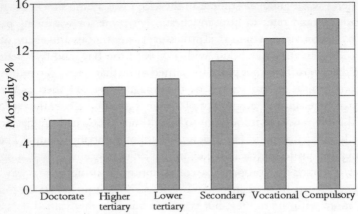

Note: The graphs shows the percentage of men aged sixty-four in 1990 who died in
the period up to 1996 according to level of education. Education is listed in graded
order – compulsory is the lowest. Similar results were observed at each age.

Source: Adapted from Erikson (2001).

Erikson's findings for male mortality according to level of education
are shown in Figure 3.1. It is not surprising that men with the
minimum (compulsory) education had higher mortality than men
with a doctorate – more than double. What captured Erikson's
attention was that men with a PhD had 50 per cent lower mortality
than men who had higher tertiary education. (Higher tertiary was
more than three years of university education and included physicians,
higher-level engineers and lawyers). The gradient in mortality continues up to the highest level. In women, similarly, low education was
associated with higher mortality. Erikson did not, however, find
women with PhDs to have lower mortality than women with higher
tertiary education. The reasons for this difference from the results in
men is not clear. It points up the necessity to go beyond simple
classifications, such as 'education', to look at the reality of people's
lives. In this case we would want to enquire whether women with
PhDs were in a different situation from their male counterparts.

Erikson considered the possibility that influences from early life could account for these findings. Interestingly, taking into account father's social class made little difference to the results. This is consistent with the results from Whitehall II (reported in Chapter 2: see p. 57) that adult social position is related to health, even after taking into account the social background from which people came.

One interpretation of these findings is that the categories of education actually represent income groups and the figure is showing a relation between income and mortality. Indeed, it was true that, for men, even within the groups of PhDs and professional education, income was still related to mortality. But the findings in Figure 3.1 could not all be attributed to income. The difference in mortality between the PhDs and the higher tertiary was still in evidence even after taking into account income, marital status and the type of job people did.

Erikson interpreted his results in a similar way to my interpretation of the Whitehall findings. He thought it most unlikely that the relation between income and mortality among these university graduates had anything to do with material conditions. His view was that higher educational status gives people more control over their lives. He had no data to test this hypothesis, but I do and as I shall report in Chapter 5, the data support Erikson's view.

We had similar results from the Whitehall II study of British civil servants. Higher-grade civil servants have higher incomes than lower-grade civil servants: the higher the grade the higher the income. Grade of employment is, however, a better predictor of health than is income.[25] When we have other measures of social ranking, the power of income to predict health diminishes.

Income inequality and health

There is one more question suggested by the first two parts of my proposition: income matters for health if you have little; above that it is how much you have relative to others in society that matters. Is the magnitude of income inequality in a society important for the health of that society?

Looking first at infant mortality: many international studies have shown that the greater the degree of income inequality of a country, the higher the infant mortality rate, even after taking the country's average income into account.[26]

One way this could work is fairly simple and related to the first part of the proposition. The absolute loss of health from reducing a rich person's income is likely to be less than the absolute gain from increasing a poor person's income.[27] Therefore, a more egalitarian distribution of income – meaning fewer rich people and fewer poor people – will raise up the average health of the society. This follows simply from the health of poorer people improving and the health of richer people staying much the same.

Therefore, a policy of redistributing income from rich to poor should have health benefits. It is not that simple, of course. Angus Deaton, a leading economist at Princeton, points out that economists worry about deadweight loss. It costs money to take $1,000 from a rich person and give it to a poor person. Apart from administrative costs, rich people go to some lengths to find ways to avoid or evade tax. Right-wingers tend to exaggerate the effect of this deadweight loss; left-wingers, to minimise it; but it does exist.

Richard Wilkinson, working in Britain, suggested that income inequality was related to poor health but not simply because more inequality implied more poor people. He looked at some of the countries included in Table 3.1 (p. 67), where average income appears not to matter for health, and reported that the degree of income inequality was related to life expectancy – more inequality, shorter life.[28,29]

Wilkinson's findings could be interpreted in three ways. First, more income inequality implies more poor people, and poor people have worse health. Wilkinson showed that income inequality appeared to be bad for health, despite the link between inequality and poverty.[30] Second, the distribution of income may itself be important. Unequal incomes, *per se*, may be the cause of societal problems such as crime and social unrest that affect the health of everybody in society. Third, the actual distribution of income may not be at the root of the ill-health that seems to follow larger income inequalities; there may be other features of society that are correlated with income inequality, and these features lead to ill-health, not the inequality of income. For example, a society that has bigger differences in income may be less socially cohesive and more hierarchical and these may be bad for health. In this way of reasoning, income inequality is not a cause of a society's health problems, it is a marker, i.e. a less cohesive society tolerates, or even encourages, larger income inequalities. This could happen by excluding some groups from full social participation and, through tax and other benefits to the rich, encouraging their incomes to rise.

Wilkinson's thesis is that an area characterised by greater inequality is bad for health because it is likely to be one with more severe hierarchies and less co-operation. Put bluntly, does income inequality cause the hierarchies and lack of co-operation or do these features cause the income inequality?

If income inequality itself were a cause of Wilkinson's findings, one would expect the relation of income inequality to health to be found widely. At this point the picture becomes clouded. Angus Deaton, at Princeton, reviewed a wide body of evidence and concluded that Wilkinson's original observations, comparing countries, could not be replicated.[31] An extension of the analysis, from comparison of countries to comparison of provinces within Canada, found little relation between income inequality and mortality.[32]

Within the US, however, there is a clear relation found between income inequality and mortality. Comparing states and metropolitan areas, the higher the degree of inequality, the higher are the mortality rates.[33] Which of the two explanations is most likely: that income inequality is the cause of the high mortality, or that an area that is bad for health, in some other way, is one that tolerates or encourages high income inequality? Angus Deaton comes down firmly on the second of these two explanations. In his comparison of income inequality across areas, he finds that the states with the highest income inequality are also the states with the highest proportion of black people. Both income inequality and the percentage of black people are correlated with mortality. In fact, when both are analysed at the same time, income inequality fades to insignificance and per cent black continues as a predictor.[34] Statistically, when two measures are highly correlated it can be difficult to judge which, if either of them, may be more important for health.

Nevertheless, if income inequality ceases to be a predictor of mortality when per cent black is examined at the same time, it casts doubt on whether income inequality is a cause of increased mortality. But the percentage of black people is unlikely to be a cause of mortality either – because the per cent black is correlated with mortality among whites. Black people are not killing white people. Something else must account for the link with white mortality. That something else is likely to be linked to the social environment. I suggest that both income inequality and per cent black indicate the degree to which people have the opportunity to participate fully in society, in the Adam Smith sense. Society does not allow their capabilities – psychological, physical and social – to be fully developed. A society that excludes high proportions of its population from full social participation is one that does not value all its people equally highly. Such a society is likely not to provide the conditions that favour good health.

The thrust of my argument in this chapter is not that money is unimportant either for individuals or societies. On the contrary, with low levels of income, increases will allow for the improvement of the material conditions for health. When these material conditions have been met, income plays a different role. It determines people's capabilities, in the sense that Amartya Sen uses the term. Capabilities will not only be affected by individual income, but by the general prosperity of the society and, crucially, by the set of social arrangements that determine how this prosperity is used to impact on the life of members of society.

We need now to put flesh on the concept of capabilities in relation to health. If capabilities are to provide the insight into how position in the hierarchy leads to the social gradient in health, the status syndrome, we need to understand more specifically what these relevant capabilities might be. We shall examine this question once we have explored the nature of status or relative position.

4. RELATIVELY SPEAKING

*Who can say for sure that the deprivation which afflicts him with hunger
is more painful than the deprivation which afflicts him with envy of his
neighbor's new car . . .*

John Kenneth Galbraith[1]

This chapter looks beyond the influence on health of absolute level of
resources to consider what we mean by status or position relative to
others, to ask why status distinctions are so widespread, and to
examine their implications for well-being and behaviour. It brings
an uncomfortable memory. A Canadian colleague, Bob Evans, presented a paper at a British Association of Science meeting, reviewing
the social gradient in health. He described his evidence as coming
from two long-term studies of free-living primates: Sapolsky's studies
of baboons in the Serengeti ecosystem and Marmot's studies of civil
servants in the Whitehall ecosystem – both showed that higher status
was linked to better health. The newspapers had fun, more fun than I
did. 'Making a monkey out of Whitehall', teased one headline. My
fears of the press coverage threatening the future of our Whitehall
studies were, happily, groundless. Civil servants did not take umbrage
at being compared to baboons.

There were two serious points to come out of this comparison.
First, it exposed as doubtful some of the theories as to why there
should be a gradient in health. Low-status baboons don't smoke, eat
hamburgers, or fail to keep appointments with their doctors; high-
status baboons don't read the health pages of the *New York Times* or
belong to fitness clubs. Yet there is a social gradient in health among
baboons. The health differences are more likely to be due to something else related to position in the hierarchy, rather than to health
behaviours or medical care.

The second point is also fundamental. If we find health to be related to position in the social hierarchy, everywhere from British civil servants to baboons, from Swedish university graduates to average Americans, then is the whole enterprise of understanding health inequalities with a view to doing something about it not doomed? The thrust of the previous chapter was to argue that above the minimum level of resources it is what you have, relative to others in society, that is crucial for health; and what you have relative to others is related to your position in the social hierarchy, it may even define it. If there will always be hierarchies, there will always be some who are relatively deprived compared to the top dogs (or baboons, or macaques, or Swedes with PhDs), and hence always a social gradient in health.

If you thought that anything that was part of our 'nature' was fixed it would, at first, seem a bit of a challenge to a view that the social environment is responsible for the social gradient in health; and that by changing social conditions we could change the gradient. It is hard to argue that social inequalities in health are due to capitalism, or globalisation, or totalitarianism, or income inequalities if the baboons have them. I have to confess: the baboons rocked me. The baboon studies solved one problem – the gradient could not be attributed to failure to follow health advice – while introducing another. If wherever animals live in groups, they form hierarchies, perhaps it is a consequence of the evolved nature of social animals and hence there is a biological inevitability about the social gradient in health. Out with society; in with biology.

I was wrong. Status syndrome is not due to biology or society; it is the result of both. Our evolved nature may indeed include characteristics that lead to the emergence of hierarchies, but the consequences of those hierarchies are not inevitable, or fixed. What it means to be high and low in a hierarchy varies. My mistake was to continue to see the biological world as divided into the two great camps of biology/nature and environment/nurture: if we are evolved to be a certain way nature must be operating, if the gradient varies in different times and places it must be nurture. Quite wrong. As we look, in this chapter, at why hierarchies should be so widely seen, and why their consequences for health vary, it will be apparent that evolution programmed animals, including us humans, with predispositions to respond to environments in particular ways. It is imperative to understand both: the features of the environment and the ways humans are predisposed to respond.

The previous chapter provided the lead-in to this one by making the distinction between absolute level of resources and the amount one has relative to others. Research on happiness is useful in showing the importance of this distinction. As we shall see, relative income is a more important determinant of happiness than absolute income. Level of happiness is one way of determining if social needs are being met.[2] I shall argue that health is another such measure that may work rather better. I endorsed Amartya Sen's view that we need to look, not only at what people have, but at what they can do – their capabilities. Much of my argument in this book is that the level of health of a group is a good measure of the degree to which those capabilities are being enhanced. If population health is high, then our set of social arrangements must be meeting important human needs. By examining health, we therefore learn something about the quality of our social arrangements. Others would make the same argument for happiness. There are interesting parallels, and some differences, between the findings of this happiness research and that on health. They relate to the different effects of absolute standard of living and relative position.

Relative position and well-being

Rumour has it that money does not make you happy. A convenient myth, if you are rich, is that the poor are happy down there in the slums. This folk wisdom is a half-truth. It has its origin in the observation that, over the last thirty or forty years, as countries became richer, people in them did not become happier.[3] In the US for example, during the period of 1965 to 1990, the economy grew by 1.7 per cent a year, but happiness did not change at all. Similar results have been reported from all the major industrialised countries that carry out these surveys. In Japan, during 1965 to 1990, economic growth was a staggering 4.1 per cent a year, and, again, happiness did not rise. (Happiness is commonly assessed as 'subjective well-being', using a question such as: 'All things considered, how satisfied are you with your life as a whole these days?' or, 'Thinking of your life as a whole, would you consider yourself a) very happy; b) fairly happy; c) not happy.')

Can it really be true that money does not buy happiness? What are people working for if the extra money does not bring satisfaction? Highly sceptical of this proposition, I looked at measures of happiness and meaning in life (as measured by response to a simple question), in the Whitehall II study of British civil servants (p. 39). Sure enough, the higher their position in the hierarchy, the more happiness they enjoy. This is not a quirk of the British civil service. Colleagues in Wisconsin looked at two American studies – a study in Wisconsin, and a US National Study of Families and Households – and found exactly the same thing: the higher the social position the greater the level of happiness.[4] Other studies have looked directly at income and have found a similar relation. When individuals within a country are surveyed, the higher the income, the higher is the level of subjective well-being.[5]

We have, then, an apparent contradiction: two very different results, depending on how we ask the question. As a country gets richer over time, the rise in average income does not go along with an increase in happiness. Comparing individuals at one point in time, within a country, the relation of income to happiness is quite clear. H. L. Mencken put it aptly: 'a rich man is one who earns $100 more than his wife's sister's husband.'[6] Absolute level of resources is not the crucial influence, relative position is. Happiness levels are determined by where we are in relation to others. If everyone in the society is richer, some will still have more than others. The financially favoured are happier. Average happiness levels do not rise with increasing average of the society, because whether societies are rich or richer, there will always be those who are better off, and those who are worse off; there will always be relative inequalities. This is one of the differences between the findings on happiness and those on health. In the USA and Japan, there were marked improvements in average health over the same period when happiness was not changing. Relative position appears to be important for both health and happiness, but if we take health as a measure of well-being, it was improving when happiness was not. Possibly because other things were offsetting the benefits to happiness, an increase in crime, for example.

The importance of relative position fits with everyday experience. We are all concerned with where we stand. We may choose the criterion by which we compare ourselves to others, but that does not mean we are unconcerned. Like most academics, my self-esteem or my status in the eyes of others has little to do with the size of my car, for example. (I see my fifteen-year-old, non-trendy bicycle as relative insurance against theft.) This does not mean academics are insensitive to where we stand in the hierarchy, however. Far from it. We are being judged all the time. Whether it is a paper for publication or a grant application being peer-reviewed, an invitation to a meeting, election to a professional body, simply having one's ideas taken seriously or a rise in professorial salary, we are highly sensitive to others' opinions of us. It all matters and it's all evidence. We simply choose the hierarchy that is important to us.

This concern with status underlies conspicuous consumption. The idea goes back to Thorstein Veblen's *The Theory of the Leisure Class*. (J. K. Galbraith says that the first time he went to an academic conference in a nice place, some wag dubbed it 'the leisure of the theory class'[7].) Veblen argued that in modern urban society – his book was published in 1899 – where people came and went and did not know each other well, wealth was advertised by conspicuous consumption. In a small English village, for example, everyone knew who had the wealth and who did not. When this local knowledge was not available, it was important for people not just to have the wealth but to flaunt it. Veblen argued that consumption for show, to achieve status and recognition, was important in addition to whatever comforts were afforded by the goods thus acquired.

Self-esteem

So important is this concern with relative position that we appear to have psychological mechanisms to boost self-esteem by appraising ourselves as having high standing relative to others: self-enhancement bias. To illustrate, ask yourself how you compare to other people. Chose a criterion – intelligence, sympathy, creativity, industriousness

– and then rate yourself in relation to others. If you are an average American, the answer is probably: I rate myself better than average. (Modesty was not one of the qualities assessed.) Your frame of reference was probably not the richest or most famous people, nor those down on their luck, but people more like you, in your profession or circle of acquaintances. I hasten to say that I am not being especially insulting about the hubris of Americans. We once asked British civil servants in the Whitehall study how fast they walked compared to other people of the same age. Most people claimed they walked faster than average. I had this wonderful image of civil servants whizzing round the corridors of power – each going faster than the last.

My evidence for self-enhancement bias comes from the type of study where college students are asked, for each of twenty different characteristics, what proportion of their peers are better than themselves. If students had an accurate perception of where they stood, some would, correctly, rate themselves as better than others; some would correctly rate themselves worse. Summing up all the rankings, you would expect the overall mean for a group of people to average out at 50 per cent. On average, people are average.

But the study turns out to be a bit like the civil servants' walking speed. American students, on average, judged only 32 per cent of their peers to be better than themselves.[8] In other words, most American college students think they are better than most other American students in the same college. Interestingly, when the same study is performed on Japanese students the result is strikingly different. Japanese students, on average, judge 50.2 per cent of their peers to be better than they are. The Americans enhanced their worth. The Japanese got it about right, perhaps because of a desire not to stand out from the group. Such group solidarity may be important for health. I shall have more to say on this in Chapter 7.

There is a Western tendency to rate yourself higher compared to others than could be supported by an objective assessment. It seems to cover a range of characteristics: sympathy, trustworthiness, sincerity, sensitivity, intelligence, attractiveness, creativity and many others. (With one delicious exception: decisiveness. It came out exactly at 50 per cent. You can imagine the question and answer. 'Are you more decisive than most people?' 'Gosh. That's a tough one. I'm really not sure.' Or even better: 'Not in the slightest. Absolutely not more decisive than average!')

This self-enhancement bias may be a way of psyching oneself up for competition: 'I'll show 'em'. Desire for status and competition are closely linked.

Status and hierarchies – a universal phenomenon?

Times are changing. I can hear Bob Dylan's nasal whine and mournful harmonica and am tempted to wallow in nostalgia for the idealism of being a university student in the 1960s. Being all grown-up and serious about that time, now, may be intellectually rigorous and reflect greater experience, but it misses the passion and excitement of then. It was a time when we thought that the old social structures would be broken down; we would do away with hierarchies and create an egalitarian world that would bring a new approach to everything. You would meet someone and ask the usual 'what do you do?' question. 'Preparing' would come the answer. Occupation was a guide to social status. People were not going to admit to being a trainee bank manager and be assigned a social rank and status. Since then, of course, the once-young people of the 1960s have sorted themselves into senators and local-government officials, professors and lab assistants, CEOs and temporary office workers, engineers and factory hands, venture capitalists and failed entrepreneurs. I am not the least bit cynical, or world-weary, about all this social differentiation. It is just that our idealism was all a bit naïve. Wherever we look, we have hierarchies, people varying in their social status.

Given the ubiquity of hierarchies in humans, and other social animals, it is likely that evolution played a part in their appearance. The question is how. If you are not signed up to evolutionary psychology, a word of explanation is in order. It applies evolutionary principles to the mind and human behaviour.[9] The general approach is that just as other bodily mechanisms – for example, for heat conservation or cooling – are an adaptation to environmental demands, so are functions of the mind. This is not to say that all psychological characteristics of humans are the product of evolutionary forces. In fact, those that show the most individual variation are least likely to have been programmed by evolution. It is unlikely that the fact that some people like train-spotting, and others like collecting jam-jar labels, or ballroom dancing, or going to art galleries, has much to do with evolution.

By contrast, it is highly likely that when confronted with a threat we choose to fight or flee has much to do with evolution. Fighting or fleeing is an adaptation that led to survival in the environmental conditions in which we evolved. It appears to be a universal adaptation of humans and other animals. The more a characteristic is universal of a whole species, the more likely is it that it is shaped by evolutionary forces.

There is an important message in the fighting or fleeing example. It may be a universal characteristic of humans, and some other animals, but we do not go around fighting or fleeing all day. We do it in response to threat, and that threat comes from the environment, and our appraisal of it. We are programmed to respond to environmental challenges in particular ways. It is true that each person who has ever lived is unique. If, however, every individual had a unique response to an environmental challenge, we could predict nothing about what would happen to you in the future. Confronted with a threat, instead of responding predictably with a flight or fight reaction, you might start collecting jam-jar labels. It is precisely because, although unique, we share characteristics in common, that we react in predictable ways to environmental challenges. As usual, Shakespeare finds the words. Shylock, as a Jew, in *The Merchant of Venice*, tries to make the point of the universality of man, and in particular that Jews and Christians share the same common humanity. He asks, is not a Jew

> fed with the same food, hurt with the same weapons, subject to the same diseases, healed by the same means, warmed and cooled by the same winter and summer as a Christian is? If you prick us, do we not bleed? if you tickle us, do we not laugh? If you poison us, do we not die? and if you wrong us, shall we not revenge? If we are like you in the rest, we will resemble you in that.[10]

He sums up the central point. There are predictable responses to environmental challenges, precisely because humans share characteristics in common. This will cover not only bleeding when pricked, or dying when poisoned, but taking revenge when wronged; i.e. not only physiological reactions but behaviours. You may well ask, as I did, if Christians, Jews, Hottentots and Eskimos, high social classes and low, share characteristics in common, why is there so much variation in disease rates? The answer is akin to British Prime Minister Harold Macmillan's answer when asked what determined success in politics: 'Events, dear boy, events.' One major reason for systematic variation in disease rates is that environments differ. The reaction of all human groups to an external threat may be similar, but if one group is more frequently exposed to threat, it will suffer the consequences more frequently than another.

Philosopher Helena Cronin has emphasised that 'environment' is not an invariant concept. If the Minister of Finance changes the tax rate it may be a threat to humans, but not much to their pets. The environment for humans is different from that of other species living in the same place. Even within a species, what constitutes a threat may be different for men and women.

Does the evolutionary psychology perspective help with the question of why there should be hierarchies? There may be a built-in motivation to seek status. The argument is that males seek status in order to have privileged access to resources, above all, females. As a result of this striving for status, hierarchies emerge. The hierarchy is a by-product of the motivation for status.

In species where successful males have multiple partners, there will be competition for females. Some males will miss out altogether, and their genes are consigned to oblivion. Other males will mate successfully with several females – their genes will be more numerous in the next generation. A genetic predisposition for characteristics that led to successful mating will flourish in the next generation. This is sexual selection.[11] Status will be a characteristic linked to mating success for two reasons: fighting off other males and appealing to female choosiness.

Fighting off other males seems straightforward. If we were bull seals, the characteristic that would get all the females would be bulk, sheer size. The biggest male would beat all the other males and protect his harem. We aren't bull seals, although our species is no stranger to fighting off the competition. But one characteristic of humans is that children need nurturing for a long time before they achieve independence. Having a man around to contribute resources and even to share in child-rearing is helpful. Males who are high in status will not only beat off other males, they are likely to have more resources to contribute to the union with a female and the children that are the products of that union. Females will, it is suggested, therefore favour males of status who appear willing to contribute resources to their offspring. This combination of female choosiness and male status and access to resources is a combination that is likely to increase reproductive success. Both characteristics, female choosiness and male drive for status will have been passed on to us the descendants of these hunter-gatherer ancestors.

Geoffrey Miller has suggested that sexual selection may account for many of the characteristics that distinguish humans from bull seals.[12] He proposes that intelligence, creativity, humour, kindness, generosity may all be ways to achieve status. If, in turn, it was these characteristics that appealed to female choosiness, and led to male success in the Pleistocene mating market, they would have survival value and be part of our genetic makeup today.

Evolutionists give a good account of why human males should have a drive for status that leads to stratification in society. One of the consequences of this stratification is the social gradient in health. But women, too, show a social gradient in health. How does evolution account for social gradients in women?

In some primate species, baboons and macaques, there are also clear social hierarchies in females, and health follows the hierarchy.[13] However, given the role of status competition in human males in producing hierarchies, one would expect hierarchies to be less obvious in human females – at least in the hunter-gatherer state for which we were evolved. As I will explore in more detail in Chapter 6, women do not have the same motivation for social dominance as men: David Buss suggests that women express their dominance in different ways. Men tend to express their dominance as superiority over others; women through actions that are more oriented to the success of the group.[14] Where females competed for male attentions, one would predict that certain traits would become selected for, but these are more likely to be related to signals of reproductive fitness, than status *per se.*

I come back, then, to the fundamental question that this evolutionary account raises: if status hierarchies arose from male competition for resources, why should women show a social gradient in health, as men do? My answer to the question about women is actually fundamental to the understanding of why there should be a gradient in health in men as well as in women. The answer is in two parts. First, the mere existence of hierarchies does not, itself, produce the health gradient. The health gradient arises because of what position in the hierarchy implies in a given society. If resources are unevenly distributed the social gradient in health will be steeper than if they are more equitably allocated. This leads to the second part of the answer. Remember the rather obvious point that we were evolved to be hunter-gatherers. For 2 million years, there were few material goods; the consequences of hierarchies for people were quite different then from what they are today, in modern urban society. The hierarchies in wealth, social resources and access to societal goods that we see around us are far greater than they would have been for our ancestors living on the savannah. These hierarchies in access to resources, including the possibility to lead a flourishing life, will affect women as well as men. Men may have created the hierarchies in society, but women suffer their consequences as well as men. Women are, so to speak, caught in the slipstream of male hierarchies.

Women, therefore, will show a social gradient in health as men do. One can predict, however, that in situations of threats to status, men will be more sensitive than women. We have already seen that the black/white differences in life expectancy in the US are bigger for men than for women. We shall look at this in more detail later in the chapter. As we shall see in Chapter 8, where a whole country such as Russia was under threat after the collapse of communism the effect on men's health was greater than the effect on women's health.

In my view, there are two issues: why do we have hierarchies; and why do hierarchies lead to a gradient in health. The evolutionary perspective gives an account of why sexual selection and male competition should have led to the emergence of hierarchies in males. The account is less clear for females. That there are hierarchies in both men and women in human societies is indisputable, however they arose. This leads to the next question: to what extent will a social hierarchy lead to a social gradient in health. As I have suggested, this will depend on what the hierarchy means for the distribution of goods and opportunities. Here the environment will be crucial.

Not all hierarchies are the same

Hierarchies in males arise from the competition for status; some individuals are more successful than others and have higher status. Troubled by the baboons, I asked: if all societies have hierarchies, will not there always be gradients in health? But hierarchies function in different ways. Consider first, that there are differences among species. It is not sufficient to say that primates have hierarchies, therefore we humans can learn from our 'cousins' – there are differences among primates. Among rhesus macaque monkeys, if the dominant monkey gets a juicy meal, the subordinate may as well eat his heart out for all the chance he has of securing a morsel from the rich man's table. Among chimpanzees, it is quite different. The top chimp will get a succulent monkey to eat. Following suitable supplication from lower orders, he will share it out. Being low status may therefore have a different effect on the well-being of macaques than it does on chimps.

Second, turning to humans, remember the central point: our biological programme shapes the way we react to the environment. The environment will have an impact on how hierarchies function. The implications of saying that we are evolved to be hunter-gatherers and that accumulation of resources is therefore limited, is that one would predict that hierarchies would be relatively shallow in such societies. Two researchers, Erdal and Whiten, reviewed evidence on hunter-gatherer societies and did indeed conclude that they were relatively egalitarian.[15] The way such egalitarianism functions will depend on the environment.

Robert Wright compares two groups of hunter-gatherers: the Native American Shoshone from Nevada and the !Kung San of the Kalahari desert in Africa. Both live in small bands and have simple forms of social organisation. Their groups are too small for much else. The Shoshone, for months at a time, would roam the desert in family groups with a bag and a digging stick, searching for roots and seeds.[16] Their social forms were adapted to the food available in their surroundings: roots and seeds.

The !Kung also live in a desert. One big difference is the existence of giraffes. The Shoshone may have gathered a great deal and hunted the occasional rabbit, but the !Kung hunted giraffes. Without B52 bombers or high-powered rifles, how do you hunt a giraffe? Co-operation with other hunters might be a good start. Going off in a nuclear family group looking for giraffe is a less optimal strategy than co-operating with others. Even if you did hunt and kill a giraffe on your own, what on earth would you do with the meat? After sharing it with your family for a few days, then what? No freezers for storage, should you just let it go to waste? It has been suggested that a good place to store the surplus meat is in some one else's stomach.[17] One giraffe provides enough food for much more than one family. Share it, therefore, with others in the hunter-gatherer band. What comes next is reciprocity. When someone else kills a giraffe, they will share their kill with your family.

Sharing is a good strategy for survival in the environment in which the !Kung live. It makes less sense in the Shoshone environment. Both societies appear rather egalitarian, perhaps because of their small size and lack of complexity. Trappings of wealth and privilege would be difficult to accumulate for nomadic people living in a desert. Even here, though, there are hierarchies. Erdal and Whiten suggest: 'Since respect is still given to leaders in particular situations, the incipient hierarchy is not really reversed but rather prevented from developing beyond those particular situations where leadership is required.'[18]

Change the mix a bit, make the society more complex, and hierarchies emerge more clearly. The //Gana are bushmen nearby to the !Kung San who supplement their hunting and gathering with farming. This is crucial. Where hunting and gathering was the main source of food, sharing was an insurance against an emergency. With farming, emergency shortages occur less often, and one farmer can accumulate wealth and status. It was reported that among //Gana men, a quarter have more than one wife. Some are therefore doing without.[19] The result of this change in the method of subsistence is the emergence of more clear hierarchies.

I conclude from all this that men appear to be evolved to seek status. The effect of competition for status will be the emergence of hierarchies. The form these hierarchies take will depend on environmental conditions. Women are affected by the general stratification of society. To some extent, these effects are the offshoot of male hierarchies.

There is another feature of the competition for status that determines the effect of hierarchies, and that is that men may compete for women's attention by generosity and kindness. Geoffrey Miller suggests that human morality is a product of sexual selection.

> Murder, unkindness, rape, rudeness, failure to help the injured, fraud, racism, war crimes, driving on the wrong side of the road, failing to leave a tip in a restaurant, and cheating at sports. What do they have in common? A moral philosopher might say that they are all examples of immoral behaviour. But they are also things we would not normally brag about on a first date, and things we would not wish an established sexual partner to find out that we had done . . . The philosopher's answer does not identify any selection pressure that could explain the evolution of human morality. Mine does: sexual choice.[20]

Generosity may attract females for at least two reasons. If a man has so much that he can afford to give it away it becomes a complement to conspicuous consumption, à la Veblen. It is a way of signalling to potential mates quite how much command over resources he has – so much that he can afford to share. Generosity itself may also be a desirable quality in a mate and a parent. Robert Frank in his study, *Luxury Fever*, comments that understanding charity's origin as sexual display should not undermine its social status. Frank argues that

> we may have evolved instincts for achieving higher social status through conspicuous display, but as rational and moral beings we can still choose conspicuous charity over conspicuous consumption . . . While designer labels advertise only our wealth, the badges of charity advertise both our wealth and our kindness.[21]

This brief enquiry into the origins of hierarchies suggests that, although hierarchies are widespread, their effects vary. What a hierarchy means for the well-being and health of someone within it will depend on how the environment brings out the features of the motivation for status. It will also depend on the degree of co-operation, and generous sharing behaviour of the sort described by Miller. The baboons may have, at first, given me sleepless nights. An understanding of how evolutionary forces shaped us suggests grounds for optimism that the health gradient can vary, rather than pessimism that it is fixed always and everywhere.

Size matters – or status anxiety

If seeking status is an adaptation, there will likely be psychological mechanisms that go with it such as acute awareness of status, psychological pain in losing status, and concern with others having too much – perceived unfairness. This will lead to concern with relative position. Robert Frank reports on a whole series of experiments that ask people to make a choice between absolute and relative standing.[22]

For example, people are asked to imagine two situations. First, you live in a society where the average income is £100,000 and your income is £125,000. Now consider a new situation. Average incomes are now £200,000 and your income is £175,000. In the two societies, a pound has the same purchasing power. Which situation would you prefer? You are being asked if you would like a higher absolute income at the cost of a worse relative position; or better relative position but worse absolute income. A majority of people opt for the £125,000. They would rather sacrifice material gains for better relative standing.

I wonder with such an experiment whether people are simply unwilling to accept the exercise's premise that a pound would buy as much in the new society where average incomes have doubled. This reflects a concern for positional goods. If average incomes go up, even if the price of carrots and espresso coffee machines stays the same, the apartment with a sea view will surely go up in price if more people are competing for it. Therefore in the lower-income society, with my lower real income, I may be able to buy fewer carrots or coffee machines, but I will have a better shot at the apartment with the view. Not much of a choice really. Go for the high relative standing, with better than average income. How many coffee machines and carrots do I want, after all? If the £125,000 income is enough to get me all the carrots and coffee I need, being in a better relative position means that I have a better chance for positional goods.

Having greater access to positional goods may not be all there is to this experiment. There is likely to be real concern with inequality. In a second type of experiment, the ultimatum bargaining game, there are two players. There is $10 at stake. Player 1 can decide how to divide it. The fair choice would be 50:50 – five dollars each. The most unequal would be $10 for Mr Greedy and none at all for Player 2. Player 2 comes in next. He decides whether to declare the whole thing void, in which case neither player gets anything. If Player 1 offered a 50:50 split, your instinct is correct: Player 2 is likely to say, let's take the $5 each and run. There may be a few people who, when Player 2, would not agree to go ahead unless the payoff was weighted in their direction. Most will accept equity. The interesting part is what happens when Player 1 gets greedy. The more unequal the share he offers, the more likely is 2 to tell him to go jump in the lake; which of course means that neither player gets anything. Player 2 would rather go without altogether than be a bit richer but have to put up with gross inequality.

In one experiment with a group of students, Player 1 offered a 50:50 split, $5 to Player 2, in more than 80 per cent of the cases. The average amount offered was $4.71. This is weighted only slightly in favour of Player 1. The people who played as Player 2 were asked the minimum they would accept to allow the deal to go forward. It averaged out at $2.59. Players were prepared to tolerate a degree of inequality if the absolute reward to them was great enough. But if the inequality increased sufficiently, or the absolute reward went down enough, the game wasn't worth the candle, and they opted for both getting naught.

The result of this game potentially sheds light on a rather crucial issue. The evidence suggests that relative position is important for health and for happiness. Is it simply where you are in the ranking that matters for health, or is it the magnitude of the differences that matters? All societies have rankings, but the magnitude of the difference between ranks varies – whether measured as money or access to social or other resources. This ultimatum bargaining game suggests that the magnitude of inequality matters. A friend sent me an email, wondering if I was a bit healthier, because Bill Gates's fortune had gone down from $70 billion to $45 billion, and my relative position had therefore improved. I may have these figures wrong by a few $billion, but what's $10 billion or so, when it comes to Bill and me?

Why was I not over the moon at the narrowing of the gap between the world's richest man and me? Is it that I am only concerned with rankings, and that if we use wealth as our measure of ranking, my position in the ranking had not changed? I don't think it is that. There has to be more than ranking at stake. My email correspondent had half a point. The magnitude of the inequality is an issue, but Bill Gates is not the relevant comparison. He is on another planet from you and me. The relevant comparison is more likely to be people whose relative wealth or income has more direct impact on us. The ultimatum bargaining game suggests that when we are confronted with inequality in the most direct way, we can tolerate it up to a point, but then we say no more.

Do we only care about inequality when it is of this direct, in-your-face, variety? Or might we care about the degree of inequality in the wider society? If we do, might there be cultural differences in the extent to which we can tolerate inequality in the society around us?

There is some evidence. A group of economists looked at this question by coming back to studying happiness. They asked to what extent a change in income inequality of a whole population might relate to average levels of happiness in a sample of the population.[23] The results support differences between Europe and the US. In Europe, a rise in income inequality was accompanied by a fall in happiness levels; not in the US. As might be expected, in Europe, the subgroup of the population that were most affected by an increase in income inequality was the poor. Their happiness declined more than average when inequality went up. Surprisingly, this was not seen in the US. Changes in income inequality did not affect happiness levels of the poor. The only subgroup of the population whose happiness declined when income inequality increased, were richer people who described themselves as on the left politically.

One study is insufficient. It is, however, reasonable to ask why some countries appear to tolerate greater social and economic inequalities than others. One interpretation of the data above, is that Americans are not unhappy with inequality, *per se*, only with their place in the order. Inequality could be seen as an opportunity for individual A to climb above individual B, rather than a bad thing in itself. Part of my task is to point out that whether the perception of inequality bringing opportunity is correct, inequality itself does have unfortunate consequences. One telling way we see this is with violent behaviour.

Killing for status

As indicated above, my baboon nightmares – that hierarchies are universal and hence unchangeable – were handled by a little understanding and some evidence. A description of hunter-gatherers or primitive agriculturalists may help illuminate our evolutionary past. It can also help in understanding modern urban society, where variations in the effects of the importance of status are still much in evidence. A dramatic demonstration of this point with great relevance for the health gradient comes from studies of violence. They show clearly that the reaction to threats to status depends greatly on circumstances.

I have worked in academic institutions all my life. I have never witnessed an act of physical violence between two academics. I am having trouble remembering if I have even heard a raised voice. About the most violent reaction I can recall is a professor packing up his papers and leaving a meeting in a huff because he thought his ideas were receiving insufficient respect. When one academic threatens another physically, a book gets written about it.[24] Are professors all Mother Teresas, uniquely collegiate and co-operative? Not at all. They can destroy each other's reputations, harbour grudges, and plot and scheme. It is done with the withering epithet, damning with faint praise: ('Among the thirty papers, I have seen this year recycling this same idea, I would definitely rate this one better than average.' 'While somewhat lacking in originality, this proposal's attention to detail is, in parts, commendable.')

Academics are fairly typical of people with resources – psychological, social or material. They are sensitive to threats to their status, but the weapons they use to react to these threats are symbolic rather than actual physical violence. Whereas some may signal their status with conspicuous consumption, the academic jealously signals and guards his status in his own way. What if you do not have these resources? Threats to status are just as important, but the reactions may be more direct.

Consider this family exchange in a poor area of Washington DC between an uncle, Ducky, and his eighteen-year-old nephew, Junior.

> Ducky asked Junior for a loan of a couple of dollars. The holiday spirit
> made Junior feel generous, so he pulled out a fat roll of bills, money he
> had made selling crack. He had intended to give his uncle three or four
> singles, but Ducky tried to snatch the roll from Junior's hand.

> Ducky had barely pulled back his arm when Junior's fists began to fly
> into Ducky's face. Junior was no longer the child Ducky used to push
> around . . . Junior pummelled Ducky until he had to be pulled away.
> As his fists flew his face remained impassive. Afterward, Junior picked
> up the fallen money roll from the floor without comment. He showed
> no sign of anger or satisfaction. Ducky may have been family, but
> trying to take money out of Junior's hand was blatant disrespect. Even
> as a child, Junior had adopted a code of living which dictated that he
> could not let anyone hurt, threaten, or disrespect him, not even
> someone in his family.

This comes from Leon Dash's study of the urban underclass in Washington DC.[25] Junior is the third generation of the family whose fortunes Dash chronicled. This episode captures two crucial elements of what it means to be a young black male in the underclass in American cities: cool pose and obsession with respect. The apparent lack of emotion accompanying Junior's assault of his uncle is the notion of what it means, in this culture, to be a man. 'These youths are obsessed with issues of pride and dignity. Never lose your cool, even when you are fighting. All they have is this cool. Cool is like building a fortress around yourself.'[26]

The salience of respect is described by many observers of minority youth in inner-city communities. 'No small amount of mayhem is committed every year in the name of injured pride.'[27] Status and respect are important to all of us. Most of us can cope with what we see as trivial challenges to our pride. When the clerk in the office is abrupt, when someone jostles you in the street, when someone makes you feel that your job is not as good as theirs, it may be hurtful. It may even induce a touch of existential angst. You may even be prompted to do some of the things we have been looking at: consume a bit more conspicuously, try for higher status at work. But it is not the whole world. When all you have is your self-respect, and your status in the eyes of others, threats to that status may have profound effects. One of those profound effects is murder.

To start with the grim reality: as we saw in Chapter 1, the biggest single factor related to homicide is maleness; the second is youth. Young men kill each other. But not always and everywhere. Young men in the inner cities kill each other. These murders occur under the shadow of status competition.[28] Much has been made of the extreme reaction to perceived slights, threats to status, in addition to murders that occur in the context of competition for scarce resources: sexual, material, territorial.

Why should it be men, young, and inner-city deprived, who react to threats to status with murderous results? If we are all sensitive to status, why does the professor whose ideas have been attacked not do a *High Noon* to his professorial antagonist and fill him full of lead?

Martin Daly and Margo Wilson, from Hamilton Ontario, answer these questions from the perspective of evolutionary psychology.[29] We are shaped by evolution to seek status. How that manifests depends on circumstances. The intensity of competition for scarce resources varies. If it is more intense, our status is more likely to be threatened than when resources are in generous supply. All academics know that the back-biting increases when the pot of grant money shrinks. There is the perception that if he gets a big spoonful from the honey pot, there will be less of it for me.

So it is with homicide in the city. Daly and Wilson show a remarkably strong correlation between degree of income inequality and homicide rates. Countries with higher income inequality have higher homicide rates. Similarly within the US, when comparing states, the higher the income inequality the higher is the homicide rate. It is even seen within the city of Chicago. Daly and Wilson compared seventy-seven Chicago neighbourhoods. There was a remarkably strong correlation between degree of income inequality within a neighbourhood and homicide rates.

This leads Daly and Wilson to argue:

> When rewards are inequitably distributed and those at the bottom of the resource distribution feel they have little to lose by engaging in reckless or dangerous behavior, escalated tactics of social competition, including violent tactics, become attractive. When the perquisites of competitive success are smaller, and even those at the bottom have something to lose, such tactics lose their appeal.[30]

The last sentence sounds as if the high homicide rates could be due to poverty not inequality. In Chicago the very neighbourhoods with high income inequality were those with low median household income. How can Daly and Wilson therefore argue that it is income inequality that is the problem rather than simply lack of material well-being? They solve this conundrum by extending their analyses to Canadian provinces. In Chicago the poorest areas are the most unequal, in terms of income. In Canada it was the opposite. The poorest provinces are the most equal – have the most equal distribution of income. In Canada, government social programmes targeted at the poorest provinces completely reverse the link between inequality and poverty; hence the poorest provinces have the lowest income inequality. Daly and Wilson find that in ten Canadian provinces, as in fifty United States, the greater the inequality the higher is the homicide rate. A major reason for the lower homicide rate in Canada compared to the USA is the lesser degree of income inequality in Canada – partly achieved by government social assistance.

So far, we have a partial explanation. We men may all be driven by the need for status. But aren't resources always scarce? Is that not the fundamental basis of economics? Instead of dying to be invited to the celebrity ball, or to have the home with a view, or to have the lead article in the top scientific journal, why don't we kill to get rid of the competition? There is a small matter of the rules. We don't at least in part because the rule of law does not permit it, and, of course we are aware of the consequences.

Are young men in Chicago not aware of the rule of law and the consequences of their action? Take someone like Junior from Dash's account quoted above. What does he have to look forward to? His grandmother, his mother and several of his uncles have all done time in prison for various infringements. All around him people are dying of homicide, AIDS, and the 'normal' diseases that everyone gets, but at an accelerated rate. Most of the people he knows are dealing in drugs. The figures bear him out. About 30 per cent of black males in Washington DC were charged with selling drugs between the ages of eighteen and twenty-four.[31] There is a clear racial bias here. Nationally, 19 per cent of self-avowed dealers are African–Americans; but 64 per cent of those arrested for drug-dealing are African–Americans. A life expectancy that is drastically foreshortened; little opportunity to take one's place in mainstream society; and greater than evens chance of spending time in prison. How long should he pause to weigh up the consequences of his actions? If he loses everything by one rash action he has perhaps lost a good deal less than a lawyer with her first job in a big city law firm would have to lose, or just about anyone else you can think of in a rich country like the US, Canada or those in Europe.

Daly and Wilson suggest that this realistic appraisal of a blighted future is related to the high homicide rate. The evidence supporting Daly and Wilson is that within Chicago, the areas with the highest homicide rates are those with the highest all-cause mortality.[32] They suggest a direct link. A young man makes a realistic appraisal that the rate of premature death is appallingly high – he sees it in his uncles and aunts, neighbours and acquaintances – and discounts the future appropriately.

What is it about relative position?

I have argued that concern about relative position is built within us. It results in hierarchies. The effect of living in a hierarchical society will depend greatly on the environment which is a feature of that society. It is not difficult to see that some of the characteristics that relate to competition for status, may be harmful for health – aggression is a key example. Some, however, may have positive effects – generosity, kindness, sharing – that achieve status while benefiting others.

The evolutionary account did not do a very good job of shedding light on the reasons for social gradients in women. Women do have social gradients in health. It is possible that the social gradient in women's health is a side-effect of living in a society stratified as a result of men's striving for status.

The fact that hierarchies may arise from striving for status does not tell us why relative position may be important for health and well-being. The next chapter addresses that question. I suggested earlier that there were three ways we could think about social stratification that were relevant for the social gradient in health. The first was absolute level of resources; the second, status, that we have just been considering. The third is power. Power may be one of the reasons why relative position is important. It is to this issue that the next chapter is addressed.

5. WHO'S IN CHARGE?

The success of an economy and of a society cannot be separated from the lives that members of the society are able to lead . . . we not only value living well and satisfactorily, but also appreciate having control over our own lives.

Amartya Sen[1]

Imagine that if you were caught in an earthquake you could simply turn it off. Earthquakes might, then, be part of life's rich tapestry instead of being an uncontrollable stress. Imagine further that your ability to turn it off depended on your place in the social hierarchy. High-status people could turn it off at will; low-status people could not affect it at all; and there were gradations of power over earthquakes from top to bottom of the social ladder. If stress led to illness, such differences in power could have a profound effect on the health gradient. Stress does, and differences in power do. We shall look at both of these in this chapter.

Power is the third of our systems of social classification that convey insights into how position in the social hierarchy translates into differences in risk of becoming ill. The first two were money/material conditions and status/relative position and they may, of course, be linked to power. Happily, earthquakes are rare, but life is full of stresses short of an earthquake, and the power to control them follows the social gradient. Being low in the social hierarchy means having less control over your life. This may play a crucial role in producing the status syndrome. The mind is an important gateway through which the social environment leads to health inequality.

The precipice

On 22 June 1996 the Netherlands played France in the quarter-finals of the European football (soccer) championships, held in England. It was estimated that 9.8 million Dutch people of a total population of 15.5 million – over 60 per cent of the Dutch population – were watching the match on television.

The two teams had fought out a nil–nil draw. They then played thirty minutes of tight, tense, anxiety-producing extra time. Nothing. Fingernails gnawed down to the metacarpals. Now what? Penalty shoot-out. There is nothing more agonising for a committed soccer fan than watching his team in a penalty shoot-out. The teams take it in turns. France then Netherlands. One player, nerves in knots, faces the goalie, strikes, and . . . GOAL!! Then another. A set number of penalty strikes for each team. The tension is unbearable; with the prospect of having your team lose to the French, after all that. There is simply nothing the spectator can do but pray, or burst.

Or drop dead. On this day, Saturday 22 June, forty-one men in Holland dropped dead from a heart attack or stroke.[2] Of course, such deaths occur every day in Holland, why attribute these deaths to a football match? On the average day the week before, twenty-seven men dropped dead from a heart attack or stroke. On this particular Saturday, the death rate went up 50 per cent in men, although not in women. Applying the usual statistical tests, it was possible to draw a connection that was unlikely to be due to the play of chance.

It really did seem likely that the stress of watching this football match triggered heart attacks or strokes in vulnerable men. Sports as a metaphor for life? As former football manager Bill Shankly said: 'it is not as if football is a matter of life and death; it is more important than that'. In an unheroic age, sports bring out passions that can unite or divide us. Canadians, divided by language and geography, feel most Canadian when contemplating their national hockey team. Americans are divided in their sports affiliations along class lines – the smaller the ball, the higher the social rank: golf, tennis, baseball, football and basketball. Sport also divides us along lines of sex. Why did women in Holland not have an increased death rate when the national team lost to the French? Most women would have no difficulty answering that one. They cannot understand how men can get so bound up watching other men in shorts kick a leather ball around. Watching football is not a source of stress for women.

There has been longstanding interest in the question of whether stress itself can precipitate a heart attack. John Hunter, the famous surgeon and anatomist of the eighteenth century, suffered from angina pectoris – coronary heart disease. His angina attacks were brought on by 'agitation of the mind . . . Principally anxiety or anger . . . The most tender passions of the mind did not produce it.' Hunter said that his life was at the mercy of any scoundrel who cared to provoke him. He was reported to have died from an attack provoked by a particularly irritating Hospital Board Meeting in 1793.[3] (I fear attacks of boredom from similar meetings.)

Hunter's opinion that 'stress' could bring on his heart attacks illustrates one of the problems in investigating stress as a trigger of a cardiac event: after a heart attack, in retrospect, anything can look stressful. How many times did the heart-attack victim get angry in traffic, argue with his family, have a fright, without getting a heart attack? When the heart attack comes, the events that happened three times a month for years can get reinterpreted as the trigger that brought on the fateful attack.

The increase in heart-attack rate during a football match played out before a television audience is not subject to the same reporting problem. Here is an uncontrollable stress that affected the men of a whole nation, at the same time, and the death rate went up. In this case an intense stress for men was probably a matter of polite interest for most women. The perception of what constitutes stress in the environment will not be independent of the person appraising it. Women may be immune to death by football-watching. They are not immune to the effects of stress in general, however. Two more sombre examples of the Dutch football effect come from Israel and Athens.

The first Gulf War began on the night of 16 January 1991. As part of their war actions, Iraq tried to bring Israel into the conflict and fired Scud missiles on Tel Aviv on the night of 18 January and the morning of 19 January. The first week of the war led to great anxiety in Israel. Israelis feared the possible effect of non-conventional weapons. There was also the anxiety that Israel would be dragged into the conflict. (As you will remember, the Americans successfully kept Israel out of the war by, among other things, making anti-missile missiles available to them.)

In the first week of the war, the heart-attack rate in Tel Aviv went up in both men and women.[4] The doctors who reported this 'heart break', compared the number of acute admissions to hospital for that week, with the weeks before and after, and with the corresponding week of the previous year. Whatever comparison they chose, they found more acute myocardial infarctions in the missile week than expected. In the Dutch case, the investigators speculated that excess alcohol may have played a role in the increased attack rate. In the Israeli case, they wondered if the donning of gas masks had restricted oxygen supply.

Neither of these was offered as explanations for the increased heart-attack death rate that occurred in Athens.[5] At 11.00pm on 24 February 1981 a major earthquake struck the city. Over the next two days, several more tremors were registered. Despite the considerable strength of the earthquake, there were few human casualties. An earthquake is, nevertheless, terrifying, and the psychological stress it causes can be intense. Over the three days after the first quake hit, the death rate from heart disease shot up by about 50 per cent. The increase was especially marked in people with pre-existing heart disease.

These three events are particularly interesting natural experiments of the effects of acute stress on the risk of heart attacks and cardiac death. In each case, the actual number of excess deaths is small. Most people do not die of fright, even if very frightening things are happening. It is highly likely that those who succumb do so because they had a particular vulnerability. The most likely reason for this vulnerability is pre-existing disease. The people who got the attack were, so to speak, teetering on the brink and the acute stress pushed them over the precipice. To extend the metaphor, might stress also play a role in putting people on a downhill slope? In other words, we should look at the effects of sustained, chronic and long-term stress, in addition to acute stress.

The slope

Sustained, chronic and long-term stress is linked to low control over life circumstances. To see how low control is related to social position, consider the following situation: a threatened factory closure that affects people quite differently depending on their place in the social hierarchy. An uncontrollable stress for the factory hand is a challenge for the CEO.

Maria works in a clothing factory in rural Massachusetts. All the workers feel as though the sword is about to fall. The factory is an anachronism, one of the few clothing manufacturers from the area that have not gone offshore. To cut costs, the work force has already been reduced by 30 per cent and everyone is working harder. Recently, Maria's car was parked illegally and was towed away. The entrepreneurs responsible want $200 to release the car, which she does not have. Without the car she cannot get to work. Without work, the whole shaky enterprise that is life for a woman with a low-paid husband and two young children, is in danger of collapse. Whichever way she turns, Maria cannot seem to make headway. What happens to her seems to be totally outside her control. She has low control over her work. She has low control over her job prospects because of the job insecurity that makes her job vulnerable. Because of financial difficulties she is at the mercy of the unexpected, such as having to find the money to redeem her towed car.

Then it happens. Her husband Paul is laid off. He was working in building maintenance. Maria does not have the whole story. It appears that the contractors for whom Paul works are being sued, and they had not taken out proper professional indemnity insurance. The director has disappeared and Paul and the other men have been summarily fired. To Maria, this is the gross unfairness of the world in operation. Why, because somebody higher up did something wrong, should it fall on Maria and Paul? With all their problems Maria had not expected this. At least he might look after the children, thinks Maria. But Paul becomes depressed and morose and spends a good part of the day drinking. Maria tells herself that she should just accept all this, but she can't. She has to struggle through the days.

Maria and Paul, both initially employed, are not at the bottom of the social gradient, although they could hardly be described as thriving. The events that for them are uncontrollable and stressful have a different impact on someone further up the social hierarchy. In the same factory, same threatened closure, it is a very different situation for someone with the psychological, social and financial resources to deal with it.

Rick owns the business and runs the factory in which Maria works. It is, in the jargon, a small-to-medium-sized enterprise. It is becoming increasingly clear to him that clothing manufacture in Massachusetts has no future. With the cost of salaries in Massachusetts he cannot compete with imported clothes manufactured in Asia. His survival strategy had been to cut back and become increasingly specialised – to move from a range of products to occupying a niche in the market. Even that tactic is no longer working as the range of imported goods improves in quality and competes at lower cost. This is a family business, and the worry of seeing it under threat nags away at him. In the end, he feels he has no choice: close the factory and move offshore, have goods made in Asia and import them. As far as he is concerned, he is just as happy to run an importing business as a manufacturing business. Perhaps more so, as it has the prospect of being more profitable. What he cannot deal with is the uncertainty of the transition. There is also a significant 'but'.

As a benevolent employer, Rick finds it particularly hurtful to lay off loyal employees. The axe dropping on some but not others is creating morale problems on the shop floor. What had been, he likes to think, a factory with a good sense of itself is no longer. The atmosphere has turned sour as the anger and fear of the remaining employees increases: who's next for the chop? 'Why are they angry at me?' Rick thinks to himself. 'It's not my fault. I have always been good to them. When Maria had her car towed I lent her the $200 to retrieve it. There was the time when my foreman, Billy, had his car involved in an accident. The repairers would not fix it until the insurance adjusters had been to view the damage. Billy came to me and asked what he could do. I got on the phone, and told them to let him rent a car while he was waiting. The insurance clerk said she could not authorise that; she would have to consult with her supervisor. So I told Billy, go ahead and do it. I'll bear the cost if they won't. But I knew damn well they would do it in the end. It was just that the little person I spoke to did not have the authority to decide. There was a time when my employees would have thanked me for my generosity. Now, with the unrest in the factory, they say that if I paid them more they would not need to borrow money from me. Can't they understand that if I paid them more, there would be no jobs at all?'

This is a bad time for Rick, but he is helped by having a good support system. His wife, Laura, deputy head in the local school, is secure in her own career and supportive of his concerns. Rick is tempted to give up his community activities with the worry over the business. Laura counsels against it. He needs the diversion from the work situation, and she can see that he benefits from his involvement. Having been long-time members of the community, they have a few close friends and a wide circle of acquaintances, many of whom come from the various communal organisations with which Rick is involved. They are financially secure. Rick could close the business tomorrow and they would have enough to live on. That's not the issue. He does not want to fail, and he has to be careful not to run up large losses.

You get the picture. Are Rick and Maria experiencing stress? They are certainly both experiencing problems that bother them deeply. Is it stress? Start simple and consider first the issue of the car. Maria's car is towed and impounded. It is the last straw. She does not have the money to get it out. What does Rick do? He pays for it. That's what he would do for his own car and he is pleased to do it for Maria. This act of generosity costs Rick next to nothing and gains him a great deal. The pleasure:pain ratio is most definitely plus. He does not miss the $200 and besides, Maria will pay him back, and for this small outlay, he can do good and feel good. Maria will, of course, be grateful to Rick, but his act of generosity only throws into relief the difference between them. It highlights for Maria the precariousness of her own situation and how little control she has over it.

Similarly with the other employee, Billy, whose car was involved in a crash. Billy was stuck, the repairer wouldn't fix the car, and the insurer would not send someone to inspect it. Now what? It is a common situation that we meet several times a month and makes modern life a bit of a trial. But note the difference between Rick and Billy. Rick moves into action. He knows how to operate in the system. He makes the right phone call. He knows what it is reasonable to expect – they should rent a car for Billy at the insurer's expense. He therefore pays for Billy to rent the car. He can charge it to the business.

If all else fails, and the insurer does not cough up the money, it is no tragedy if Rick has to bear the cost himself. How much will it be? The cost of a new suit? Rick has plenty of suits, and Billy has earned it after years of loyal service. If it improves employee relations it is worth it.

The point here is that Rick has the resources to take control of the situation, rather than have events control him. These resources may be knowledge – how to operate the system; financial – he can bear the cost of the solution without pain; psychological – he has the confidence, developed by long experience, to know that he can do what is required and people respond to that confidence, whether it is the clerk in the insurer's office, the repairers, or his employees. These are all resources that to greater or lesser extent Maria and Billy lack.

Take the more serious problem of the precariousness of the business. This causes pain all around, to Rick at the top of the ladder, to Billy half-way down, and to Maria near the bottom. To Rick the big problem is uncertainty. He cannot control the marketplace for his goods. Nor can he control government policy that will decide whether to offer tax breaks to preserve local manufacturing. His desired outcome would be to continue local manufacturing. That would be to preserve the tradition of the family business and his good sense of doing the right thing by the local community. If he has to though, he will switch to being an importer. What gives him the sleepless nights is the uncertainty. In the end, he knows that he will resolve it by going offshore even if there is short-term pain of having to cause mass lay-offs. He knows how to work with a situation and take the decisions that need to be taken. Once he makes the decision to move offshore, much of his worry evaporates.

Whether her problems are caused by Rick, the government, Satan or globalisation matters little to Maria. Something beyond herself is making her life difficult. There is simply nothing she can do about it. The only occupational skill she has is operating a sewing machine. If this factory closes, she is out of a job and she can see no prospect for another. All the other clothes manufacturers departed the scene long since. She is at the mercy of forces over which she has no control. She does not have the psychological resources, the knowledge, or experience simply to start up again in a different way. Nor does she have the financial security to bide her time while she surveys her options.

She does not have the support of a psychologically secure partner, as Rick does, but rather a husband who himself is suffering the result of events over which he had little control. He has no money and no help to offer.

To sum up, we have seen that the events described are particularly stressful when there is low control and little predictability. It is made worse by lack of social support. A further important feature that turns challenge into stress is whether you are going up or down in the world. Maria's potential loss of a job means, as far as she can see, loss of livelihood. To her, it seems that she will go from being a self-respecting person who earns money and pays her way in the world, to someone who will be on welfare. Her husband Paul's reaction to his job loss is to become morose and depressed and to drink heavily. He has lost work, lost money, lost status. The last feature of these stories that has relevance to the degree of stress is the presence of an outlet. Rick has the country club, the golf course, tennis court and communal activities. Maria, with two dependent children and a dependent husband, has access to none of these. The idea of taking out her stress on the golf course is preposterous. Too small a ball for her station in life.

There is a large body of literature supporting the importance of these five characteristics – control, predictability, degree of support, threat to status, and presence of outlets – that modulate the impact of a psychologically threatening stimulus.[6] All five of them are likely to be linked to position in the social hierarchy.

What is stress?

The characteristics I have just listed are highly relevant to the question of what is stress. I long ago stopped counting how many times I have heard critics say: stress for one person is stimulation for another. The clear implication is that you cannot measure stress precisely, and if you cannot measure it, it must not exist. Ergo, let's go and study something else that we can measure. But, I complain, what if stress were a major cause of disease? Surely we cannot just throw up our hands and walk away; we must make it measurable and susceptible to scientific study.

Or there may be a tacit admission that stress exists, but the riposte is:

if you can't stand the heat, get out of the kitchen. No doubt Maria would find such advice a great comfort when she lost her job and her husband started drinking. Understanding that what makes a challenge stressful has to do with the five characteristics I have just described allows us to go beyond simplistic notions of 'stress bad' to studying what it is about a situation that may be harmful.

A second aspect of the 'does stress cause disease' question is how stress gets into the body. How does a threatened factory closure, for example, affect physiology to change disease risk? For insight into what stress does to the body, a look at different animals is helpful. The stress response is similar in many different species. By understanding animal physiological responses to stress, we gain insight into how stress in humans can lead to diabetes and heart disease, for example.

Robert Sapolsky has studied stress in his laboratory in California and on the savannah in East Africa.[7] Let us appeal to him for guidance. Imagine that you are a zebra on the African savannah, desperately trying to evade a lion. You could also be the lion, half starved, desperate for a meal, chasing the zebra. The physiological responses are similar.

For both animals, this crisis requires the immediate mobilization of energy into the bloodstream and its subsequent diversion to exercising muscle; this would be a singularly inauspicious time to be depositing energy into fat cells for a project for next spring. As such, during stress, energy storage is blocked and previously stored energy is liberated into the bloodstream and diverted to muscle. These steps are accomplished by the inhibition of insulin secretion and of parasympathetic tone, and by the activation of the sympathetic nervous system, glucocorticoids, and glucagon (which were named for their ability to mobilize energy by increasing circulating levels of glucose). It is also adaptive to deliver those nutrients to muscle as rapidly as possible, and sympathetic hormones plus glucocorticoids increase heart rate and blood pressure.

During a crisis it is also useful to inhibit any physiological processes that are unessential, wasteful drains on resources. As such, the stress response also involves triaging a variety of functions. Digestion is inhibited (including the inhibition of salivary secretion, accounting for our dry mouths when we are nervous); for the hungry predator, digestion is irrelevant, while for the prey . . . this is no time for the slow and costly process of digestion. Growth, inflammation, and tissue repair are also deferred for later. In addition, reproductive physiology is inhibited; a desperate sprint across the savannah is no time to ovulate. As another feature of the stress response, immune function is inhibited.[8]

What Sapolsky has described is the classic *fight or flight* response. It is the appropriate response of an animal to physical stress or, indeed, threat. There are a large number of neural and hormonal changes in the body. Two of the most important, and most studied, systems are the autonomic nervous system and its associated hormones the catechol amines (adrenaline and noradrenaline if you are in Europe; epinephrine and norepinephrine if you are in North America); and the body system that puts out cortisol – the hypothalamic pituitary adrenal axis.

There are two parts to the autonomic nervous system, the sympathetic and the parasympathetic. If you need to be aroused to meet a challenge, the autonomic nervous system activates the sympathetic part that puts out the catechol amines. Among other actions, these increase heart rate and blood pressure. Ever been to a yoga class? The instructor has every one lie on the floor on their backs and meditate. The result can be quite embarrassing. Yours and everyone else's tummies start to rumble. The room is filled with gurgling. That is your parasympathetic nervous system doing its restorative job. You are not under threat, so it is a good time to attend to relaxed work like digestion.

The other system, the hypothalamic pituitary adrenal axis, puts out particular steroid hormones, the glucocorticoids. It also offers a good example of how the brain communicates with the rest of the body. Higher brain centres send messages to the hypothalamus that the animal is under threat. The hypothalamus, in turn, tells the pituitary gland that it is time to get serious. The pituitary secretes ACTH (adrenocorticotropic hormone), which stimulates the adrenal gland to put out glucocorticoids. If you have chronic arthritis, or asthma, you may well have been prescribed 'steroids' to damp down inflammation. These are the glucocorticoids. Too much of them has a range of effects including too much fat around the abdomen and even diabetes.

I have led a limited life. I have never fled a lion nor chased a zebra for dinner. It does not mean that stress is irrelevant. The challenges I face in life may be more symbolic. I have tried to play my viola in front of other people and could scarcely hold it, so slippery were my hands with cold sweat. I could hardly hear the music for the pounding of my heart. An audience of one is enough for my tennis game to desert me. Peeing on demand at a hospital clinic in Novosibirsk was close to impossible. As humans, this same set of bodily responses that make up the fight or flight response can be stimulated by symbolic threats. You talk to your colleagues about work every day without arousal. If we put you in front of an audience and ask you to say the same things, you could be the zebra fleeing from the lion, or the lion chasing the zebra – your physiological reactions are the same. It is appropriate that they should be. To follow Sapolsky, while you are at the podium behind the microphone, you don't want to be building up body strength or ovulating or digesting a meal. These functions can be delayed for more relaxing moments.

A century ago, the psychologist William James posed the classic question: do you run away from the bear because you are afraid, or are you afraid because you are running away from the bear? My first response when hearing this is that surely I run because I am afraid. I don't find myself running and manifesting other fear reactions, and think: what is this dry mouth and sweaty palms, I must be afraid. There is little doubt, however, that purely psychological stimuli can arouse the physiological stress response, whether or not we experience an emotion such as fear.[9]

My colleague, Andrew Steptoe, tests people's response to stress in the laboratory. One way he elicits the stress response is to ask people to imagine that they are in a department store and have just been nabbed for suspected shoplifting. They have ninety seconds in which to argue their way out of it. Blood pressure zooms, pulses race, glucocorticoids pour out.[10] We all respond to this purely psychological challenge to greater or lesser degree, even though we know we are in a lab, and absolutely nothing depends on the outcome of the speech.

The idea that Sapolsky expresses so eloquently is that the acute stress reaction, fight or flight, is exactly what the body needs in the acute situation of immediate threat. The problem arises if the threat is maintained over time. A rise in catechol amines, and a consequent rise in pulse and blood pressure and diversion of blood away from the intestines, is appropriate to the acute situation. It is not what the body needs day after day. High levels of glucocorticoids raise blood sugar, in part by causing resistance to the action of insulin.[11] Insulin resistance characterises mature-onset diabetes, Non Insulin Dependent Diabetes. Along with this effect on glucose metabolism, we see a pattern of lipid disturbances (changes to fats in the blood). In fact, there is a syndrome in humans, which goes by various names, latterly called the metabolic syndrome, thought to be the result of insulin resistance. It is characterised by central adiposity (fat around the abdomen rather than the hips), low levels of HDL cholesterol (HDL is the 'good' cholesterol), high levels of plasma triglyceride, high levels of blood glucose and insulin in the fasting state, and high blood pressure. This pattern of metabolic change is associated with increased risk of heart disease.

To come back then to acute and chronic stress. Yes, acute stress could cause problems in someone with heart disease. The suggestion of the researchers who reported the increased heart-disease death rate after the Athens earthquake is that the heart deaths occurred in people who had pre-existing heart disease. I would speculate that the people who dropped dead during the Dutch football match with France already had atherosclerotic plaques in their coronary arteries – their arteries were furred up with cholesterol-rich raised areas on the lining of the coronaries. The acute stress may have triggered a disruption of an atherosclerotic plaque and increased clotting tendency of the blood.

The chronic stress idea is that sustained activation of stress mechanisms will lead to the kind of physiological changes that in turn lead to heart disease. There is good evidence from non-human primates that will help understand what we observe in humans.

Rank and stress reactions

I alluded in the previous chapter to the findings from rhesus macaques that low-status monkeys have more heart disease than those of high status. These findings come from a long-term series of studies of atherosclerosis at Bowman Gray University in North Carolina.[12]

(Bowman Gray, incidentally, was the head of Philip Morris, the tobacco giant. I went to a meeting at the university once and was rather put off to find in my room a laudatory portrait of the man who helped sell carcinogens to the world. I was told that it was an imperfectly kept secret that Bowman Gray died of lung cancer.)

A brief pathology lesson to start. Atherosclerosis is the underlying problem in coronary heart disease. It is the name given to furring up of the coronary arteries – the blood vessels that supply blood to the hard-working muscle of the heart. The coronaries have to supply blood, with oxygen and nutrients, to the heart muscle to keep it beating seventy or more times a minute, day and night. If the coronaries are narrowed, chronic heart disease may result. If they get blocked acutely, which usually happens against a background of pre-existing narrowing, you get a heart attack, an acute myocardial infarction. The atherosclerosis usually takes the form of cholesterol-rich plaques. At Bowman Gray, the monkeys in their colony are fed a diet high in saturated fat and cholesterol that encourages build-up of the athero-sclerotic plaques.

But animals are not all equally affected. These animals form themselves into hierarchies. The higher the rank of the animal the less likely is it to develop atherosclerosis, despite, as I have argued, the lack of the usual lifestyle that constitutes risk factors for disease in humans: smoking or variation in diet. One possibility is that there may be a common factor that predisposes animals to being both low rank and to developing atherosclerosis. There might, for example, be a genetic predisposition to being low rank and heart-disease-prone.

This possibility is tested experimentally by varying the ranks. These animals are raised in small groups. In the 'changing ranks' experiment, they take the top two animals from each of a number of groups and put them together. These animals then form themselves into a new hierarchy. Similarly with animals that were previously low rank. In the experiment then, some low-rank animals have become high-rank and some high-rank animals are lower in the hierarchy. It is the new position, not the one they started with, that determines the degree of atherosclerosis that the animals develop. This suggests it is not some inherent predisposition to being lowly that is responsible for the increased risk of heart disease. It is the rank that drives the body's processes, not bodily processes that determine rank. The differences are dramatic. With rhesus macaques, as with humans, males develop much more atherosclerosis than females. A female with her ovaries removed develops as much disease as a male. Making a female subordinate puts her at as much risk of developing atherosclerosis as does removing her ovaries.

There is a fascinating male/female difference in these experiments. When hierarchical positions among females are rearranged, they form into new stable hierarchies, and the low ranks develop more athero- sclerosis. Something different happens with males, however. When the researchers take high-status males from different groups and mix them up, there is jockeying for position. (I think of it like a heads of department meeting at the University. A lot of high-status males fighting for position, recognition and the perquisites that go with rank.) Under these unstable conditions, the high-status monkeys (I'm not sure about the heads of department) develop *more* atherosclerosis. It is a reasonable supposition that this instability, this fighting for position, is stressful. This supposition is supported by repeating the experiment, this time pre-treating the monkeys with a drug that blocks some of the activities of the sympathetic nerves and adrenaline (epinephrine) – a beta-blocker. Once the sympathetic nervous system is blocked, it is the low-status male monkeys that develop more atherosclerosis, despite the instability.[13]

The Bowman Gray studies show that, in animals living under controlled conditions, atherosclerosis follows rank, and stress pathways play an important role. Sapolsky's studies of wild baboons in the Serengeti in East Africa also incriminate stress pathways. If you are a male baboon, you are at the mercy of the baboons above you in the hierarchy. Whether it is a juicy meal, a female in heat, or simply a place to relax, your pleasures are taken – or not – at the sufferance of males above you in the hierarchy. In the baboon troop hierarchical rankings are, in general, quite stable. At times of instability such as when the highest-ranking male gets toppled or a new male joins the troop, there may be good deal of ambiguity as to the outcome of encounters: who dominates whom. Under such unstable conditions, stress hormones rise, particularly if you are a higher-ranking male being challenged by someone below you. He has nothing to lose and suffers less stress than you who have your rank on the line. We saw in the Bowman Gray studies that instability increases presumed stress effects for high-status monkeys. There is a real danger that they will go down in the world.

Sapolsky finds, in general, that all the biological stress markers follow the social hierarchy. He has studied, in particular, the hypothalamic pituitary adrenal axis that is responsible for regulating glucocorticoids. For example, the lower the rank of the baboon, the higher is the level of cortisol early in the morning. You may wonder how Sapolsky determines the cortisol level of a baboon early in the morning. Anaesthetic darts. He creeps up on the target baboon and darts it. He has a few minutes before the blood cortisol level changes. He quickly takes a blood sample and, voilà, he has the basal cortisol level.

He also finds that the lower the baboon's rank, the lower the HDL cholesterol level – a low level being associated with an increased risk of heart disease. The higher the morning cortisol, the lower is the HDL cholesterol. Interestingly, in our Whitehall II study of British civil servants we also found the lower the rank, the lower the HDL cholesterol. All things considered, we thought better of trying to adopt Sapolsky's darting technique for our civil servants. We did, however, find that the metabolic syndrome increased in frequency as the hierarchy was descended: the lower the employment grade, the lower the HDL cholesterol, the higher the plasma triglyceride, the higher the fasting levels of glucose and insulin.[14] All this went along with the central pattern of obesity, which we measured as the ratio of the waist circumference to hips. The lower the grade, the higher the waist:hip ratio. It is important to make the distinction between this central pattern of obesity and simple overweight, where the excess body fat is more widely distributed. Men show little social gradient in obesity – women do – but in both sexes, there is a social gradient in waist:hip ratio. This central adiposity may be the result of a complex series of reactions involving cortisol metabolism.[15] Central obesity occurs in Cushing's Syndrome, which is a disorder characterised by over-secretion of cortisol. In other words, stress pathways may play a part in the development of the pattern of obesity that is linked to heart disease and diabetes.

I find no conflict between attempting to explain the development of disease on the grounds of 'physical' causes, such as diet, as against chronic psychological stress. Yogi Berra, the famous baseball manager, is reported to have said: 'This game is 90 per cent psychological. The other half is physical.' Good on psychology; pity about the mathematics. Despite his difficulty with sums, he may be right. Atherosclerosis in the monkey experiments is induced by feeding them a high-fat diet. Given a high-fat diet, psychological experiences associated with rank play a major part in determining who gets more and who gets less of the disease.

From stress to psychosocial factors in human society

In case it needs re-emphasis, we are not monkeys or even apes. We should not look to them, necessarily, to understand how people behave in the workplace, in the benefits office, on the local council, or the church committee. What these animal studies, from lab and field, give us are biologically plausible ways that social experience can be translated, via biological stress pathways, into disease.

There have been essentially two types of studies of these stress processes in humans: large-scale observational epidemiological studies and small-scale experimental studies. In our large-scale studies, we have bypassed the definitional problem of what is meant by stress. Life is full of challenges for everyone. Despite all the research that has been done on biological stress pathways, it is very difficult to study a large number of people and say who is under stress. If we follow Robert Sapolsky and decide that basal cortisol levels are the best markers of chronic stress, we would have to test people before they wake up, because cortisol levels show diurnal variation. The lowest levels are in the hours before waking. We are now attempting these collections in thousands of people, but it is not a very practical proposition. We do have indicators of activity in biological stress pathways, and we use them, but it is difficult.

Alternatively we could ask people. 'Are you under stress?' 'Who, me? Sure.' If you do that, you find there is a lot of it about. There is a real worry, though, that when people tell you they are under stress, they may be reflecting a general level of anxiety. We are tapping something about people's anxious response to questions rather than their life situation. Parenthetically, it is a good deal more useful to ask people if they are healthy than if they are under stress. People who respond to a question on how healthy they feel by saying 'poor' are correct. This single question is remarkably predictive of subsequent risk of dying.

We tend to avoid the 'stress' questions, then, because we do not want to know if people report themselves as anxious. There is another more theoretical reason: we want to know more about what it is in people's lives that may be causing trouble. This relates to what one might do about the problem if one found it. You might say that from the perspective of a clinician it does not matter much why people are feeling anxious. If giving a pill makes people feel better, why bother where the anxiety comes from: 'But doctor, it feels like I am being whipped with a cat o' nine tails.' 'Never mind where the pain is coming from. Just keep taking the pills.'

This, it will not surprise you to know, is not my perspective. Our aim is to understand what it is in the social environment that may be causing problems in people's lives. Not to give pain killers to take away the pain, but to stop the whipping. We therefore focus on psychosocial factors: psychological factors that are influenced by the social environment.

Work and its shadow

Most people who could work would rather have a job than not. Whether working is, on balance, good or bad for health depends on the nature of the work and on the place of work in the family and social situation. And it depends on whether you have work at all, and the degree of security of your employment. These are all of crucial relevance to the social gradient in health.

For Rick and Maria, their positions in the world were shaped by work – whether they had it or not, the security of their employment, and their status in the labour market. Do we live to work or work to live? You don't have to answer that question to appreciate how central work is in our society, for a number or reasons.[16] First, and most obviously, it provides income and life chances. What is open to Rick in life is quite different from what is open to Maria and Paul.

Second, we are, at least to some extent, what we do. Whether teacher, lawyer, journalist, plumber, clerk or business person, the education and training for occupation makes us part of who we are. My image of myself, and of you, is quite different if we are teachers educating the next generation, or crack dealers doing something else to them.

Third, occupation is a definer of social status. You may be the world's worst parent or spouse, son or brother, but if you are the local doctor, you are somebody in the community. You have something going for you that the street-sweeper does not. A major part of this book is devoted to working out what exactly that status means and why it is related to health. There is no question, however, that one of the measures of status is what job you do. People may also be defined by not having a job. After losing a job, they are initially an un-employed engineer or mechanic or programmer. If unemployment goes on long enough, they are just unemployed.

Fourth, and most obvious, we spend so much time in the work-place that it is a major source of pain and pleasure, demands and rewards, frustrations and fulfilment. With Rick and Maria we dis-cussed their relation to work, but not the nature of work itself. We discussed the wider impact on them of their occupational status and the nature of the labour market, but not what actually happens in the workplace.

The notion of what constitutes stress at work has undergone a revolution. It comes back to the problem of asking people if they are stressed. Ask more successful people if they are stressed at work and they will tell you, in slightly macho fashion, about how many emails they receive a day, how much in demand they are, how many different tasks await their attention, about their deadlines. If you ask about stress, they are unlikely to tell you that work is monotonous, boring, soul-destroying; that they die a little when they come to work each day because their work touches no part of them that is them. But this is the reality of many jobs; and the lower the status, the more likely is it to be so. Ask the people with all the emails which job they would rather be doing, the high-status job with continuous demands, and the

company BMW and the firm's credit card, or the soul-destroying job
with tasks that ask for little use of skills, that are completely determined by others and, oh yes, that offer little in the way of self-
fulfilment, financial rewards or status enhancement. There are not too
many high-status people who would swap their 'stressed' place in the
boardroom for a place on the production line.

We have, therefore, to go beyond the notion of 'stress' at work as
meaning 'having a lot to do'. We need to put some precision into the
concept of the psychosocial work environment. This has been done in
two ways. First, the main issue for a stressful workplace is not simply
the level of psychological demands, but the balance between demands
and control.[17] Second, work will be stressful if there is lack of balance
between effort and rewards.[18]

The demand–control model fits with the stress concepts that we
discussed in the previous section. Everyone has to meet potentially
threatening or challenging circumstances. Whether or not biological
stress pathways are activated has much to do with the degree to which
circumstances are controllable. The man or woman with all the emails,
the city lawyer who works through the night making megabucks for his
client (and himself) has high demands. If he or she has a high degree of
control over work, it is less stressful and will have less impact on health.
Think of your own experiences at work. It is less the busy times that
cause you pain than the times when you feel out of control. High-status
civil servants have a high degree of control over their work. The time
they find the work difficult ('stressful') is when they are treated
irrationally and unreasonably by the politicians, their elected masters.

We hear much about bond traders, wheeling and dealing in the
global financial marketplace, suffering stress and burnout. Yet it is
interesting that in Tom Wolfe's *Bonfire of the Vanities*[19] the chapter that
describes the trading room at Salomon Brothers is entitled 'Masters of
the Universe' – which is how these supposedly stressed types saw
themselves: macho super-heroes running the world. And inordinately
well paid to boot. They thrive on the buzz of the dealing room. In
Wolfe's story, the stress comes to the protagonist not from the
demands of the job so much as from serious threats to his status,
when he is caught out in a chain of deceptions to do with his vigorous
sex life.

After the first Whitehall study of British civil servants, we set up a second study — Whitehall II — including women as well as men. A major focus of Whitehall II has been on the role of work in causing the social gradient in health. In addition to systematic collection and analysis of quantitative data linking work to health, we have also been interviewing civil servants on the nature of their work.

Here is a high-status civil servant, Nigel, in a responsible management position, discussing his job:

> 'It was the best job I ever had in my life. There were 2,000 people and I was responsible for all the personnel aspects, contracts and all the common services, and it really was a superb job. It had every sort of challenge that you could ever wish to meet. A very active job and a lot of stress, but a very enjoyable job indeed and you got a tremendous amount of satisfaction from doing a good job.'

He actually uses the word 'stress', which is precisely why I don't. He uses it in the same sentence as he describes his job as 'very active', 'very enjoyable', offering a 'tremendous amount of satisfaction'. His job is characterised by great demands — personnel aspects, contracts and common services for 2,000 people — but he has a great degree of responsibility and control over the work. It is for this reason that self-reported stress at work is not what we take as the indicator. It is the amount of demand relative to control.

Now contrast that with Marjorie who went to work in the civil service with typing skills but little else.

> 'I went to the typing pool, and sat there typing documents. Which was absolutely soul-destroying . . . the fact that we could eat sweets and smoke was absolute heaven, but we were not allowed to talk.'

The thing that characterises Marjorie's work is not how much demand there is on her, but that she has almost no discretion to decide anything at all: what to do, when to do it, with whom to do it, even whether she can talk.

A large body of evidence now exists that supports the demand/control model: people whose jobs are characterised by high demands and low control have a higher risk of developing coronary heart disease than others in jobs with more control.[20] Our own Whitehall II study in the British civil service showed stronger support for the effects of low control on heart disease than for the adverse effects of high demand.[21] Other studies in the US and Sweden, however, do show that a combination of high demand and low control is harmful to health.[22] We also found a strong relation between low control at work and depressive symptoms.[23]

Having made the point that work casts a long shadow – that who you are in the workplace affects the other aspects of your life – in doing research on this issue, it is also important to ask whether it is the jobs with low control that put people at high risk or whether it is other aspects of people's lives that relate to their status in society. One way of looking at this in the Whitehall II study was to ask whether low control predicted disease within employment grade levels. It did. People at the same level in the occupational hierarchy with differing amounts of control had markedly different rates of disease – low control consistently led to more disease.

But how should we determine who has low control? Should we the observers decide, or let the individual in the job do so him or herself? To put it more generally, which is more important, the self-assessment of a situation or some more objective view of it? Suppose you ask someone if their life is going well and they say 'yes'. You as a researcher look at the person's situation and think that cannot be true. He has a boring, monotonous job in which all the decisions are taken by someone else, he is low-paid, lives in a crime-ridden neighbourhood, has a child who has just been imprisoned for drugs, another who was shot in a drive-by shooting, and he is telling us that life is going well! You think that he doesn't know what it would mean for life to go well. You are going to ignore his judgement and go with yours. You think life is going badly for him. Who is right: him or you? Who is to be the judge?

It is an old question. The argument for going with his assessment is that he is the one to experience it. If chronic activation of stress pathways is what we have in mind, then surely it his perception that counts. The argument for going against his subjective assessment is that he may not be an accurate reporter of his own circumstances. He may think that everybody lives like this. His circumstances are no worse than 'usual'. I have colleagues who rise in the early morning to work. If you ask them if they are getting enough sleep, the accurate response is: 'I don't know.' They only ever get this much sleep. They would not know how it felt to have a different amount.

In the Whitehall II study, we wrestled with this problem in relation to low control at work. We asked whether it was the perception of low control that was important or the 'reality' of being in a job that offered you no freedom of movement. To illustrate, the bane of my life is securing parking for my bicycle at civil-service buildings. It turns out that each building has a place for bikes. The key is getting access. The people who control access always say no the first time. There are rules and these people are at the bottom of the hierarchy. It is not their job to exercise discretion as to whether your suit, tie and meeting papers suggest they are safe in letting you in. After one of these ordeals, finally the doorman shows me to the parking place and says, pointing to two corners of the garage: 'You can leave your bike there, or there, it is completely up to you.' He said it as if he were offering me the choice of an ambassadorship to France or Brazil. My thought at the time was that this man has about as little control over his work as I could imagine. He can say 'no' if people have not got a pass and 'yes' if they do. His tone of voice implied that he was offering me a real choice. Is that what he thinks control is? If he thinks he has control, is that what is important? Or might this be false consciousness? Is the objective nature of the job more important?

It turns out the answer is both. We asked managers to rate jobs for their degree of control, and we asked civil servants themselves to tell us how much control they had. The correlation between them was surprisingly low. It seemed that subjective perception and external ratings of control were capturing something different about the job. Yet these two measures, the one more or less independent of the other, both predicted heart disease.[24] This dilemma about which is more important, self-perception of psychosocial factors or 'objective' reality, has not been solved and will continue. Both seem to play a role.

Work and the hierarchy

Imagine a typical Tuesday morning in a large government department. Marjorie from the typing pool comes to Nigel, who is eleven levels higher than her in the hierarchy and says: 'I've been thinking, Nige. We could save a lot of money if we ordered our supplies over the Internet. What do you think?' I have been trying to imagine such a conversation but my imagination fails me. Even if I rerun the conversation and substitute 'install coffee machines' for 'order supplies', I still cannot manage it. Government departments are extremely hierarchical organisations. Marjorie simply does not talk to Nigel. Nigel is not her boss. Her boss has a boss who has a boss, who . . . ends up with Nigel. If Marjorie has an idea about how the typists could do their job better, she can discuss it with her immediate supervisor. Chances are that this person would feel that she/he does not have the responsibility to do anything quite as revolutionary as make a change to the way the typing pool works. If she thinks it important enough, she may consult her boss who, let us say, thinks it is a wonderful idea. He therefore writes a memo to his superior who is far too busy with other things to give this immediate consideration and there it sits. Marjorie may wonder why she bothered.

It is impossible to imagine working in a large organisation that does not have a hierarchy. It is, however, possible to imagine hierarchies operating in quite different ways. The British civil service is a relatively benign employer in many ways, but it is rigidly hierarchical in job description and practice. One way this plays out is that the lower the grade the less control people have over what they do. Hence Marjorie does what is put in front of her and is not encouraged to do otherwise. The nature of the hierarchy is less control the lower you go. In Whitehall II, we found lower control in lower grades whether we consider people's self-reports or managers' 'objective' assessment of how much control each job entails.

In Whitehall II, this gradient in control over work appears to have strong implications for the gradient in heart disease and mental illness. Statistically, low control was an important contributor to the higher rate of heart disease in the lower grades.[25] We need to be a little careful here. If I am saying that the very nature of low status is low control, how do we know that it is the low control that is responsible for the higher level of disease in the lower grades, not other things?

The answer is slightly tricky statistically but simple enough conceptually. It comes in two parts. First, low-grade people are more likely to smoke and do little exercise and be shorter. Each of these – smoking, no exercise, shortness – predicts heart disease and therefore contributes to the social gradient in disease. Second bit of the argument: after allowing for these effects, low control is still related to heart disease. Statistically, low control makes a substantial independent contribution to the social gradient in heart disease.[26]

The result reported above showed that low control predicted heart disease *and* was an important part of the explanation for the social gradient in heart disease. Another major contributor to ill-health is mental illness. Rather crudely, people often talk about the major psychiatric disorders and the minor ones. The major ones include psychotic disorders such as schizophrenia and bipolar disorder (manic depression). These are potentially catastrophic in people's lives and the lives of those around them. They are, however, of much lower prevalence than the so-called minor disorders, such as anxiety and depression. These 'minor' disorders have a truly important impact on the population.

Let me illustrate what I mean. Suppose we could measure quality of life on a scale from 0, dreadful, to 1, truly wonderful. Suppose schizophrenia reduced the quality of life of the sufferer from 1, the highest to 0.2, pretty awful; and that neurotic depression reduced it to 0.5. If there were 100,000 schizophrenics in a population and 1 million depressives, schizophrenia would be responsible for a loss of 80,000 quality of life points (100,000 × 0.8); depression would be responsible for the loss of 500,000 (1 million × 0.5). If that sounds like some weird calculus of well-being, you could replace the calculation by numbers of days when people were unable to function at full strength, days lost from work, drain on medical care, sale of pills, and come out with similar figures. The 'minor' psychiatric disorders have a major impact on the well-being of the population.

They are also a major cause of lost time from work. Our findings in Whitehall II are therefore of great potential relevance to the whole working population. The lower the level of control over work, the greater is the risk of developing minor psychiatric disorder.[27] Low control was a major part of the explanation of the social gradient in depressive symptoms.[28]

I said that all large organisations have hierarchies. But what if those hierarchies were to operate differently? I would suggest that a hierarchical organisation that gives people lower in the hierarchy more involvement – more use of skills, less feeling of being totally controlled by others – will not have the same extreme gradients in ill-health as those organisations that have a tighter link between low control and low status. There is circumstantial evidence that points in that direction.

A few years ago, there was a large international study of the automobile industry.[29] It turns out that it really is true that the Japanese are unfair to the international competition. They make better cars. Japanese manufacturers produce cars with fewer defects per 100 vehicles than do European or American manufacturers. They are also more efficient: more cars per worker than Europeans or Americans. Why? Because the Japanese are genetically predisposed to be better car makers? Unlikely. Japanese manufacturing plants in Europe or America, that employed local workers but were under Japanese management, were more efficient with fewer defects per car, than local manufacturers. The clear conclusion is that management style matters.

What about the health of workers? The reason I call the evidence circumstantial is that it is based on sickness absence rates, and these may vary internationally for administrative reasons as well as for reasons related to differing rates of illness and injury. Nevertheless, Japanese firms had strikingly lower rates of sickness absence than Europeans or Americans.

There is no question that Japanese organisations are hierarchical. When you visit a Japanese factory, the greater depth of bow that a low-status worker makes to a high-status worker is one indication. But perhaps it really does matter that the head of the factory is in white overalls as are his workers, and there is no executive dining room. Workers in Japanese auto plants had far more hours of training than in European or American plants. There was more job rotation in Japanese firms, so workers spent less time doing the same boring jobs. It may be more illusory than real, but Japanese workers were actively encouraged to make suggestions as to how things could be improved. It is tempting to believe that this different way of operating the hierarchy resulted in better health, lower sickness absence rates, for Japanese workers and higher productivity and higher-quality product for the companies.

We could think of this as a virtuous circle. The iron-rod school of management says: be soft to workers and accept low productivity or crack down hard and force them to give of their best. (Some disgruntled worker put up a poster in one workplace which read: 'The beatings will not stop until morale improves'.) By contrast, the virtuous circle says that there need be no trade-off: health and autonomy of workers and health and economic success of companies are likely to go together, not be in opposition.

Control at work, control at home

Low control at work is an important contributor to disease, but there are ways of depriving people of control other than subjecting them to difficult conditions at work. The Rick and Maria story makes plain that low control over life circumstances is not confined to work. Low control in these other spheres, too, may be important for health.

We examined this issue in the Whitehall II study. Working on the assumption that self-perception was important, we simply asked people how much control they had at home and over life in general. We found that people who reported low control at home had a higher risk of depression. This risk was in addition to the risk of depression associated with low control at work. Particularly striking was the high risk of depression in low-status women who told us they had little control over things at home.[30] Our interpretation was that, for these low-status women, work offers little in the way of psychological reward. The rewards, if any, that their lives offer them come from home. Deprived of control in that sphere, they are particularly prone to depression.

We concluded that low control in the home sphere is particularly salient for women, even women who are employed outside the home. This was given further support in the Whitehall II study. Low control at home predicted heart disease in women, but not men.[31]

Losing jobs, losing control

An efficient way of removing control from people is to deprive them of work altogether. In the account of threatened factory closures affecting Maria and others, her husband Paul had his job taken away from him, against his will. Maria feared the same. Remember the criteria that make an event stressful. For Paul and Maria, Paul's job loss was unpredictable, uncontrollable and entailed loss of status. The only outlet seemingly available to Paul – not a remarkably life-enhancing one – was to drink. Perhaps more importantly, the acute event of job loss is translated into a chronic situation characterised by low control and lowered status and, related to these, worse economic fortunes. Job loss respects social position, and its incidence is greater the lower you are in the hierarchy – another indignity of low status.

The arguments over whether unemployment causes ill-health are typical of those that surround interpretations of the gradient in health. Does unemployment cause illness, or illness lead to unemployment? And if unemployment does cause ill-heath is it due to poverty or something else? These are important scientific questions. The problem is that these scientific questions are heavily bound up with politics. Given that unemployment is seen as related to government policies, the question of whether unemployment causes ill-health goes to the heart of what governments are about.

There were some early studies during the great depression of the 1930s on the health effects of unemployment.[32] At that time, a link between unemployment and poor health would hardly be surprising. In the 1930s unemployment meant extremes of poverty. John Steinbeck's *Grapes of Wrath* captures the great dislocating effect of the poverty associated with mass unemployment and the consequent health effects. It is the kind of poverty that George Orwell described in *The Road to Wigan Pier* and that I quoted in Chapter 3 (p. 64).

Unemployment of the 1980s and 1990s was different. In Western Europe, Britain and North America, 1930s-style poverty was all but gone. Unemployment benefits, while less generous in Britain than many other countries, were sufficient to keep life and limb together. Could unemployment in the 1980s and, indeed, the twenty-first century, be a cause of ill-health?

Let us try a game. I'll give you a statement and you tell me the political persuasion of the person who might have uttered it. The ground rules of the game are simple: there is a consistent finding that unemployed people have worse physical health, mental health and higher mortality than people who remain employed. The statements relate to the interpretation of the finding.

1) Unemployed people have worse health than those employed because people who are sick find it difficult to get and hold a job.

2) Unemployed people have worse health. It is their upbringing and low level of skills and psychological resources that lead to their being both unemployed and sick. Unemployment itself has nothing to do with it.

3) Unemployed people have worse health than employed people because unemployment leads to poverty and poverty leads to poor health.

4) Unemployed people have worse health because unemployment represents loss of a social role and all the things that go with it.

The point of this game is that there is some scientific support for each of these statements. I am not, therefore, casting aspersions at scientists who produce evidence for each of them. The issue is that one or more of these propositions was strongly endorsed by people who had a particular axe to grind.

I did not make up this game of 'guess the political prejudice'. We played it in Britain in the 1980s.[33] Except it wasn't a game. It was all too real. Before you check your answers against mine, let me give you some background. In the mid to late 1970s, Britain had a Labour government that was widely seen as not managing: there was a perception that nothing was working very well. They suffered the indignity of the country's being saved from financial collapse by a loan from the International Monetary Fund; the government's traditional supporters in the unions were annoyed and un-cooperative; business was angry; the general public fed-up. Unemployment had broken the psychological barrier of a million: 1 million people unemployed in a country of 55 million.

Labour struggled on until the election in 1979 and were then booted out. Margaret Thatcher, leader of the Conservatives, came to power with a mandate to change things. She did. She, with the help of the international financial situation, squeezed the economy hard. Unemployment rose from 1 million to well over 3 million. The levels were getting so embarrassingly high that the government made more than twenty changes to the way the unemployment figures were collated. As *The Economist* commented at the time: all but one were in the direction of lowering the apparent figure.

Into this situation come researchers saying that unemployment is bad for health. 'No it's not', says the government. 'Sick people become unemployed. Sickness causes unemployment not the other way around.' A Conservative government minister said that if unemployment was the price that had to be paid to keep inflation down, it was a price worth paying. If the government had accepted that unemployment caused mortality to rise by 20 per cent in the unemployed compared to the employed, the Minister would have been saying, in effect: if killing people is the price we have to pay to keep inflation down, it is a price worth paying. Whatever he might think, no politician is going to admit to that.

Statements 1) and 2) became the mantra of right-wing politicians in Britain in the 1980s. The argument seems to run in reverse order: It is inconceivable that our policies could be killing people; therefore, unemployment cannot be a cause of ill-health. It is not as if there is no scientific evidence supporting statements 1) and 2). There is. Nevertheless, to put it crudely: conclusions determined views of the evidence, rather than views of the evidence determining conclusions. It was fairly clear that views about what was an acceptable conclusion determined judgements about the science. It was not, as one might have hoped, naïvely perhaps, that judgements about the science should influence the conclusions.

From the other point of view, there were people on the left politically who were only too keen to flay a right-wing government with the grim reality that their economic policies were killing people. Which led to proposition 3) above. Many of these people would argue that it is the economic consequences of being unemployed that harm health.

The trouble with all of this is that just because people are right-wing hyenas does not mean they are necessarily wrong; and just because people are left-wing ideologues does not mean they are correct. You can vary that statement any way you like depending on whom you most wish to insult. The point still stands. Although people may have political reasons for holding the views they do, that does not by itself convey much information about the truth of the scientific position they are seeking to argue. It does explain some of their motivation in holding to that position. The study of how society affects health taps into political prejudices. The political arguments tend to get bound up with the scientific ones.

Proposition 4) was less part of the political argument, but there is evidence to support it. We all think our position is the reasonable one scientifically. In fact, I would argue that the evidence shows that 3) and 4) are linked.

In the end, I am pleased to report, the data had an influence on the debate. John Fox was head of a research unit that, in the early 1980s, was examining this issue. He and his colleagues followed a 1 per cent sample of people identified in the national census in Britain in 1971. They showed that people who became unemployed had 20 per cent higher mortality than those who remained employed at the same social-class level. Their critics in government trotted out proposition 1) as a reason to disbelieve a causal link. John Fox describes a crucial meeting in which an economist, who was mounting the government's case that unemployment did not harm health, presented his view on why it was all health selection – proposition 1). Fox came piled high with data to present his case on why the link was causal: unemployment increased mortality. He had worked in government, and the longitudinal study on which he based his research was organised and funded by government. Much hung on the outcome of the debate in addition to getting the science right.

He was so wound up with the tension that he can only dimly describe what happened next at the crunch meeting. A crucial part of Fox's argument was against health selection. He and his colleagues argued that if the unemployed had higher mortality because of the existence of life-threatening illness prior to becoming unemployed this effect should wear off as the sick people died out. It did not.[34] His antagonist did something most unusual in scientific circles. He said publicly: 'I have listened to John Fox's evidence and I have changed my mind; he is right.'

Subsequently, further analyses showed that when there was the huge rise in unemployment in the 1980s, so many people lost their jobs that it was less likely that sick people were selectively chosen for the dole queues. Yet in the 1980s, as in the 1970s, the unemployed had higher mortality than the employed.

Proposition 2) does have validity. The reality of unemployment for Paul, and the risk of it for Maria, are related to their low level of skills. Unemployment rarely strikes randomly. A study in Britain has followed a group of people from their birth in 1958 to the present, gathering data as they went at each stage of the life course. (This is known as the 1958 birth cohort.) Not only do the results fit with common sense, they may be responsible, in part, for these ideas seeming like common sense. Unemployment is more common in people who have experienced unfavourable family circumstances and have less educational attainment.[35] It was precisely these people who had difficulties in the troubled labour market of the 1980s. They spent more time in unemployment. Of course if the population unemployment levels had been low, they would not have spent the same time out of work. There is, therefore, an interaction between susceptibility of the individual and what is happening in the wider environment.

This same 1958 birth cohort was also able to answer the question of whether illness preceded unemployment or the other way round. People who were unemployed became depressed and anxious. This was not simply the result of depressed, anxious people becoming unemployed. You might say it is no surprise that unemployed people become depressed and anxious. A lot of people did a great deal of research and engaged in a huge amount of argument before that simple proposition was accepted as proven.

Accepting then, that unemployment does cause ill-health, it is important to ask if it is due to poverty. Picking up an earlier theme, it is useful to distinguish the two senses of poverty: a lack of basic material conditions for life; and insufficient resources, private or public, to participate fully in society. The first is unlikely to be the sole explanation, as unemployed professionals, who might be expected to have some savings, have worse health than those still employed in the same occupational social class. This is not to say that financial problems are irrelevant. Far from it. Financial strain appears to be the complaint most associated with worse mental health in the unemployed. I would argue that this is consistent with poverty in the second sense – inability to participate fully in society. Whether initially well off, or poorly off, deterioration in economic circumstances will cause real hardship.

This is the link between propositions 3) and 4): diminished economic circumstances make it harder to take your place in society and to have control over your life in the sense of being able to lead the life you most want to lead. It may not only be financial hardship but its anticipation that cause problems. This is shown by the health effects of job insecurity. Maria has not yet lost her job, but she has that itchy feeling on the top of her head that the axe is about to fall on it. She just does not know when.

The thing about job insecurity is the event that has happened is inside Maria's head. To be sure, this is not a delusion from which Maria suffers. The events inside her head are caused by her realistic appraisal of the true situation, to continue the metaphor, of the axe hanging over her. As yet, she still has a job, a wage and the status and structure to her life that work provides. But uncertainty alone, regardless of how justified, has already begun to work its adverse effects on her health.

Assessing the health effects of job insecurity is not straightforward. Ideally, one would like to know how people's health was before they started to feel insecure about their jobs, and then see if it changed consequent on job insecurity. A comparison group would help: a group of workers doing similar jobs who were not made insecure. But how to find people who are about to become insecure? One of my children, when he was aged about five, used to come into our bed at night, saying that he was about to have a frightening dream. Good kid! He had internalised the preventive medicine message from his dad: prevention is better than cure. Most people are not like my son. They don't know when they are about to become frightened of losing their job. If you hear that a factory is about to close, it is too late; the insecurity has already hit.

Inadvertently, the civil service arranged just such an experiment for us. After we started the Whitehall II study, and had already assessed the health status of all participants, the government decided to sell off one department to the private sector. Great anxiety ensued. As luck would have it (for the researchers, not for those worried sick), we had studied these people before the onset of insecurity, during the peak of anxiety as to what would happen, and we then followed them. The health of these insecure participants deteriorated compared to others in departments that were not under threat.[36]

The point about the deterioration of health with job insecurity is that although there may be real worries about financial problems to come, the financial situation has not yet worsened. People's material position has not changed; their expectations have. It is consistent with an effect of unemployment on health acting through proposition 4) above. I told you the other arguments were all 'political' and this would turn out to represent the balanced view. Prejudiced? Me?

The workplace as a model for society

Much of my own thinking about the workplace and its role in generating the social gradient in health has been developed in collaboration with two close colleagues: Tores Theorell in Stockholm and Johannes Siegrist, a German–Swiss sociologist working in Dusseldorf. Theorell comes from a background in psychosomatic medicine, examining in small-scale studies how psychological processes influence stress pathways. He, with Bob Karasek, developed the demand/control model.[37] He has conducted a whole series of influential studies showing how the workplace affects biological function and disease risk. Siegrist, as a sociologist, brings his theoretical perspective to bear on the work that Theorell and I, both physicians, carry out. The three of us differ in training, background, personality, culture, country of origin, language and the fact that the other two are highly accomplished musicians, but it has been a most fruitful and congenial collaboration for nearly two and a half decades. The thinking of each of us has been much influenced by the thinking of the others.

I reported that there was another way of looking at stress in the workplace, in addition to the demand/control model: the balance between efforts and rewards. Siegrist sought to develop a way of looking at work that captured the idea of reciprocity. This is pretty basic to living in society: I do things that benefit others; in return, I receive rewards that benefit me. I do work; you pay me. I give to society; society rewards me for my effort. Matt Ridley wrote a whole book, *The Origin of Virtue*[38], arguing that co-operation and sharing were a basic part of our evolved nature. He was at pains to point out that there was no conflict between selfish genes[39] and unselfish people. Living in society requires co-operation. If living in society is a way of helping genes pass through the generations, then unselfish people are in the interest of selfish genes.

In order for there to be co-operation, there needs to be some sort of reciprocity. The effort–reward model suggests that people's efforts at work should be rewarded in three ways: money, esteem (including self-esteem) and career opportunities. If people's efforts are not appropriately rewarded, they suffer emotional distress with consequent stimulation of biological stress pathways. You can see how this way of looking at work encompasses not only the job but also the opportunities provided by the labour market. In a tight labour market, as in a company with higher positions all held – blocked – by youngish people, the prospects for the career-enhancement aspect of reward will be limited. I described this model at a seminar chaired by the former President of my university. We divided the working population into people with high effort and low rewards, and those with low effort and high rewards, and those in between. 'Low effort and high rewards. That's the University President,' I suggested. 'High effort and low rewards. That's university professors.' 'Absolutely right,' said the President, with a wicked grin. 'This is a well-organised institution.'

This model's relevance to our present concern is not only its theoretical interest. This combination of high efforts and low rewards has been shown to be related to risk of coronary heart disease.[40] We therefore looked at it in the Whitehall II study. A combination of high effort and low rewards predicted incidence of coronary heart disease. Low control also predicted coronary heart disease. The ability of these two measures to predict was independent, each from the other.[41]

Building on these findings, Siegrist looks at the whole field and identifies what he terms two bridge concepts: control and social reward. Each of these can be thought of as acting at three levels: macro, meso/micro and personal. Take control first. At the macro level, there is stratified access to resources and opportunities. At the meso/micro level, there are differential opportunities to exercise autonomy – the workplace being a prime example and, as the Whitehall II study showed, the domestic sphere is another. At the personal level, there is what psychologists call self-efficacy.

Applying the three levels to social rewards: macro – as with control, stratified access to resources and opportunities; meso/micro – balance between cost and gain or, as described above, effort and reward in the workplace; personal – self-esteem.

This is an elaboration of, but entirely consistent with, my hypothesis that what is important is control and opportunities to participate fully in society. The effort/reward model implies that lack of reward means lack of full participation. In the Siegrist model, lack of appropriate reward for effort expended causes emotional distress and activates biological stress pathways, with consequences for disease.

I have been putting out broad hints, and sometimes more than that, that the nature of social relationships may be a buffer against psychological stimuli leading to activation of biological stress pathways. In the Siegrist formulation, they may offer appropriate reward – they are part of reciprocal exchange. It is time to look at social relationships in more detail. Related to this is a question that I have ducked so far, and that is whether the operation of these psychobiological pathways may be sex specific – men and women may behave and react differently. We shall look at this question, too, in the next two chapters.

6. HOME ALONE

But the truth was that he died from solitude, the enemy known to but few on this earth, and whom only the simplest of us are fit to withstand. The brilliant Costaguanero of the boulevards had died from solitude and want of faith in himself and others . . . Solitude from mere outward condition of existence becomes very swiftly a state of soul in which the affectations of irony and scepticism have no place.

Joseph Conrad, *Nostromo*[1]

Conrad's novel, *Nostromo*, is a magisterial tale of revolution and stolen treasure in the Latin-American country of 'Costaguana'. Senses dulled by a surfeit of contemporary action films that involve grotesque, red-blooded violence, you might imagine *Nostromo* to be full of deaths by cutlass and dynamite, cannon and musket. Not in Conrad. Here people die 'from a state of soul in which the affectations of irony and scepticism have no place'. Señor Martin Decoud, a rich romantic young man, finds himself isolated on an island during revolutionary upheaval. He dies of isolation, from lack of irony and scepticism and loss of faith in himself and others. To be true to my profession, medicine, I must confess that had a coroner found the body and heard the story he would have recorded the cause of death as suicide by firearm. I can but wonder how medical science might have been different if doctors recorded cause of death as lack of irony and loss of faith.

Conrad can distinguish causes from consequences even if we in the medical profession get a little confused. The cause of death was isolation. The consequence, the mode by which Decoud shuffled off this mortal coil, was indeed a self-administered shot to the chest from his own gun.

Can isolation really kill people? I am going to show you, in this chapter, that it surely can. Not only because it can cause mental illness, as in the case of Señor Decoud, but because lack of social relationships can increase risk of disease by weakening resistance to disease. So far, we have considered the possibility that people lower in the hierarchy have more disease than those above them because more bad things happen to them: uncontrollable stresses. But disease does not occur solely as the result of exposure to something harmful. We, all of us, are exposed to harmful things – viruses and bacteria, psychological and physical stresses – throughout the day. Mostly, we do not become ill, because our bodies have defence mechanisms – called host resistance. Disease occurs when our bodies lose the battle between 'invader' and resistance. Therefore, anything that weakens host resistance will put us at increased risk of disease. Lack of supportive relations has such an effect or, to put it more positively, positive social relations are a major contributor to host resistance.

In showing the evidence that positive social relations protect people, I have to overcome a different kind of resistance – the scepticism of colleagues who doubt that a psychological phenomenon such as the experience of isolation could increase the risk of a physical illness. I find it interesting that many medical scientists have little difficulty in accepting that biological processes can cause mental states but more difficulty going the other way – accepting that mental states can cause biological phenomena. Such scepticism is surprising given the ample evidence that we reviewed in Chapter 5 of the biological changes that accompany acute and chronic stress (see pp. 115–122). Nevertheless, a common form this scepticism takes is that we know the causes of physical illness. Heart disease, for example, is caused by smoking, diet and sedentary lifestyle acting on genetic predisposition; where do stress and social isolation come into it?

The topic of this chapter is that social relations are not an optional extra, they are crucial to maintaining good health and preventing disease. We need first to look at why social relationships are important, then to understand how they may fit into models of disease causation, and hence may play a role in causing the gradient in health.

A female response to stress

In Chapter 4, I gave an evolutionary account of the male drive to seek status, and commented that evolution would not have designed female hunter-gatherers in the same way. Such sex differences may extend to reactions to stress. As set out in the previous chapter, stress has traditionally been thought of as the fight or flight reaction evoked in response to threat. The model of chronic stress in humans is that the body gets all worked up to fight or flee but does neither and the smouldering physiological reactions that underlie the fight or flight response cause disturbances that lead to disease. Psychologist Shelley Taylor has pointed out that these studies missed half the species. Females don't respond in the same way as males. Observations of everyday life should have taught us that women handle situations differently from men.

Taylor and her colleagues reviewed the literature on stress and concluded that most of it came from studies of males.[2] They proposed that the female response to stress is better characterised as 'tend and befriend' rather than 'fight or flight'. Faced with a predator a female will, of course, show the physiological changes characteristic of the 'fight or flight' response, but she will also demonstrate something else: a tend and befriend response that may overcome the tendency to fight or flee.

Taylor's tend and befriend theory is shaped by an evolutionary perspective.[3] You are, let us say, a female hunter-gatherer on the African plain 100,000 years ago. Chances are you have one or more offspring in tow. Faced with a predator what should you do? Abandon the kids, who you have nurtured at your breast, and run for a tree to save your own life? Is that what the average woman would do now? Of course not. We realise that Lady Macbeth is inhuman and/or mad when she tries to strengthen her husband's weakening resolve to kill the king by saying (Act I, Scene VII):

> I have given suck, and know
> How tender 'tis to love the babe that milks me:
> I would, while it was smiling in my face,
> Have plucked my nipple from his boneless gums, and dash'd the brains
>   out, had I so sworn as you have done to this.

Shakespeare understood how inhuman such action is. The first thought of a woman confronted by a predator would be how to save the child – the 'tend' part of 'tend and befriend'. The problem is that she is quite vulnerable out there on the plain, just her and the infant. She, therefore, bands together with other women and their offspring – there is strength in numbers. This is the 'befriend' part. 'Tend and befriend' is a survival strategy for her and her children.

Tend and befriend will have had survival value to our hunter-gatherer ancestors. A female who, in response to threat, tended to her young and banded together into groups for protection is more likely to have offspring that survive to reproduce. A genetically determined propensity to tend and befriend will be passed on to subsequent generations of females. Therefore, not only the struggle for competition will have survival value, but also co-operation, caring and befriending. Humans may have evolved to have hierarchies as a result of competition, particularly in males, but also may have evolved to care for each other, particularly in females.

When we considered fight or flight as a response to stress, we looked at the argument that what may be a survival strategy as a response to an acute threat may have biological costs as a response to chronic threat. Long-term elevations of stress hormones lead to metabolic disturbances that, in turn, lead to enhanced risk of chronic disease. What about tend and befriend? Here the argument is that the strategy that works well for the acute threat may also work well for the chronic threat. Tending to infants and other people, and befriending, may be good for the health both of the 'befriender' and the 'befriendee'. When Lady Macbeth said that she knows 'how tender 'tis to love the babe that milks me', her emotions are being fuelled by oxytocin, endogenous opioids and perhaps prolactin.

Oxytocin is released during birth and breast-feeding. As a man, I know I am not alone in looking with some envy at the picture of sheer bliss of my wife with a child at the breast. Her blissful feelings probably have a lot to do with release of oxytocin and perhaps prolactin. (Goodness knows what my envious feelings have to do with; not testosterone.) Shelley Taylor reports that when female animals are injected with oxytocin they seek out more social contact with friends and relatives. In humans, women who are breast-feeding have higher levels of oxytocin than other women. These women show less arousal of the sympathetic nervous system and lower activation of the hypothalamic pituitary adrenal axis in response to stress, than other women.[4] There is, therefore, a plausible biological basis for believing that tending and befriending may have important positive health effects. We shall look at the evidence in a moment.

It is tempting to think that men contributed hierarchies and dominance/subordinate relations to the species; and women contributed sharing and co-operating. Tempting as it is, we should not take this to mean simply that men's health is damaged by hierarchies and women's health protected by sharing and co-operation. The sex distinctions are not so sharp. It may be true that hierarchies were originally of men's making, but women are still damaged by them. Women show a social gradient in health as do men. The lower the status, the higher is the mortality and morbidity from a range of health conditions. This is true as well in non-human primates. The Bowman Gray studies of cynomolgus macaques show a clear social gradient in atherosclerosis in female monkeys. The lower the status the higher is the prevalence of atherosclerosis in the coronary arteries.[5]

It may be true, that co-operation is of women's making but men are still protected by it. Befriending is important for men too. Crucially for our inquiry into the health gradient, evidence shows clearly that the degree of social support varies across the social gradient.

In both sexes, then, the balance between hierarchies and co-operation will be important in how individuals in society deal with stress. This, in turn, is likely to have important implications for patterns of illness.

Society is about co-operation

I looked at the *New York Times* on the web yesterday. There were three stories in the National section. The first was about an ex-boyfriend pursuing a legal case to stop his ex-girlfriend having an abortion. The second was a legal case in Florida to do with school vouchers. The third was a criminal investigation about two girls who had been abducted. Are all the stories about lawyers? I wondered.

I moved to the New York Region: three stories about litigation. I was starting to get desperate. There must be some US news story that does not involve lawyers. I scrolled to the Technology section. Relief from litigators there, surely. Don't believe it. Story one involved Microsoft's long-running legal battle about alleged monopolistic practices. Story two was about a legal battle over another software company. Story three, about a national computer system, involved no lawyers. At last! Then I realised it was about Japan. They don't do things with lawyers.

So many lawyers! This profusion goes back a long time. That acute nineteenth-century observer of America, Alexis de Toqueville, wrote: 'There is almost no political question in the US that is not resolved sooner or later as a judicial decision.'[6] Nevertheless, the lawyers have been on the increase in recent years. Between 1900 and 1970, in the US, the number of lawyers per employed person did not change, despite the transformation of America into a complex urban, industrial, trading powerhouse. In the next twenty-five years, though, the ratio of lawyers to everybody else more than doubled.[7] After 1970, the legal profession grew three times faster than other professions. Political scientist Robert Putnam reports in *Bowling Alone* (2000) that

> for the first seven decades of the twentieth century the legal and medical professions grew roughly in tandem, but after 1970 the legal profession grew twice as fast. In 1970 there were 3 percent fewer lawyers than doctors, but by 1995 there were 34 percent more lawyers than doctors.

One interpretation of all this litigation is that it represents a society that decides matters on the basis of the outcome of conflict rather than trust. One looked, in vain, in the newspaper, for stories about consensus. It is tempting to say that if 'society' implies co-operation, there is not much evidence of it in the news. Society implies conflict might be closer to the mark. If you were Britain's former prime minister, Margaret Thatcher, society did not imply anything. Her famous comment was that there is no such thing as society; there are only individuals and families. What a grim view this is: conflict, everyone out for themselves, the successful rise to the top and hence ubiquitous social hierarchies.

Society does entail conflict and struggle for position, but also co-operation. My impressionistic account of the US epidemic of lawyers is consistent with the view that co-operation has been on the wane, allowing conflict a freer reign. Nevertheless, despite the conflict, all that litigation in the US requires respect for the rule of law. It requires co-operation. Everything does. If there is no society, only individuals and families, one wonders which member of Mrs Thatcher's family cleaned the prime-ministerial residence, did the shopping, drove the official car, opened the mail, answered the telephone, looked after the security, kept the diary, replaced a broken fuse . . . None of us could get through the day without co-operation.

Co-operation is essential to society. It is, suggests anthropologist Robin Dunbar, the key evolutionary strategy. Sociality is at the very core of primate existence. Dunbar suggests we evolved to live in groups for three good reasons:

> Protection against predation when the ancestor hominids left the forest for the savannah – in Taylor's terms, tend and befriend.
> Protection against other human groups.
> Becoming nomadic implies greater uncertainty in finding water and food. This leads small groups to form strategic alliances with other groups to share resources. In this way meat today becomes meat tomorrow.[8]

Given these good reasons to live in groups, the question is how we achieve it. In non-human primates, without spoken language, grooming cements social bonds and expresses who is in with whom. But grooming is quite time-consuming and you can do it only to one group member at a time. If you want to interact with every primate in the group, you would have to spend a great deal of time grooming – more so as the group increased in size.

If group sizes were to grow, there had to be another way of communicating with members. Enter language. The evolution of language allowed human groups to get bigger. With language, you can happily communicate quite intimately with three or four in a group rather than the one on one that grooming entails. We use language for all sorts of exalted purposes, scientific advance, technological innovations, culture, complex social arrangements, but we also use it for gossip. Dunbar suggests that next time you go to a restaurant, listen in to what people are talking about. High culture? Scientific advance? They are gossiping; delicious, relaxing, juicy, reassuring gossip. He suggests that gossip is to humans what grooming is to monkeys and apes: it makes our social groups work.

Because we were evolved to live in groups does not, in itself, argue that group living is good for us, including good for health. An adaptation that may have served our ancestors well during the Pleistocene period may not be adaptive to today's radically different circumstances. To pursue an analogy, human physiology may be adapted to a diet alternately abundant and meagre. The metabolic mechanisms that protect the body from the effects of starvation at a time of privation may predispose to diabetes when food supply is abundant.

We cannot, therefore, assume that everything is for the best in this best of all possible worlds, i.e. that we are optimally adapted. Although we may have evolved to live in groups, and hence be protected against predators, it does not follow that living in groups protects against modern-day 'predators' such as the causes of heart disease and mental illness. Whether it does is an empirical question.

An influential paper by epidemiologist John Cassel suggested that the way social relationships protect against illness is by increasing host resistance.[9] Cassel drew on the powerful idea that comes from the study of infectious disease: the outcome of an infection is dependent on a struggle between the infecting organism and the resistance of the host (the individual infected) to that infection. In other words, we cannot simply hold to the view that for each disease there is a single cause. There are a whole array of 'causes' that determine the likelihood of exposure to the infecting organism; and there are causes of host resistance, that determine whether infection leads to disease. To provide a context for understanding the protective effects of social relationships, we need to look more closely at notions of causes and effects as they help us understand health and illness.

Causal thinking –
beyond one cause leads to one effect

On the 26 August 1812, in Tolstoy's account, in the Battle of Borodino in Russia, 100,000 Russian troops fought 120,000 troops of Napoleon's army. At the end of it, the Russian army had been reduced by half and Napoleon's by a quarter, but Napoleon had lost, and the course of history changed. And what was the cause of this cataclysmic loss of life and strategic advantage? On 24 August, Napoleon's valet forgot to bring the emperor his waterproof boots. As a result, Napoleon caught a cold. Napoleon's cold, so the story goes, marred his judgement, and led to the defeat of his army. The forgetfulness of Napoleon's valet led to Russia's survival as a European power, and Napoleon's ruinous retreat from Russia.

That at least is the historical account that Tolstoy quotes. He dismisses it as far too simplistic. Were Napoleon's orders the cause of the carnage at Borodino? This is Tolstoy's view:

> The soldiers of the French army went to kill the Russian soldiers at Borodino not because of Napoleon's orders, but by their own volition. At the sight of an army barring their road to Moscow, the whole army – the French, Italians, Germans, Poles – hungry, ragged, and exhausted by the campaign, felt that the wine was drawn and must be drunk. Had Napoleon then forbidden them to fight the Russians, they would have killed him and would have proceeded to fight the Russians because it was inevitable.[10]

There must, in other words, be a richer, more complex view of causation. Suppose that Napoleon's decision to fight that particular battle had *some* effect in determining that the battle was fought at Borodino, and not elsewhere, on 26 August and not on another day. It was, in a sense, only the proximate cause of death in battle of so many men. A whole set of causal processes determined that the battle would be fought somewhere.

We need to think about illness in the same way. When a person dies, a death certificate is completed which lists cause of death. In the space for 'cause', it does not ask for a judgement call on the failure of memory of Napoleon's valet. It asks for the illness to which the deceased succumbed. If someone died of cancer, the appropriate entry under cause of death might be lung cancer (carcinoma of the trachea, bronchus or lung), not smoking. Statistics on 'cause' of death, therefore, tell us about frequency of different fatal illnesses, not what caused them.

If we move one step further back to look at causes, we might conclude that disordered cellular mechanisms led to the growth and development of the cancer.[11] Such fundamental discoveries of cellular mechanisms lead us to the next causal question: how did these cellular mechanisms come to be disordered? In the case of lung cancer, we know that 95 per cent of lung cancer deaths occur in smokers. Smoking could therefore be usefully considered as *the* cause of lung cancer. From the perspective of prevention, this is reasonable. Eliminate smoking, and you eliminate 95 per cent of lung cancer death. But most smokers don't die of lung cancer. Something must determine whether one smoker will succumb to lung cancer and another not. It is possible, but not proven, that the body may have protective mechanisms to detect and destroy abnormal cells, before they can lead to runaway cancerous growth. In other words, people may have varying levels of resistance to the carcinogenic effects of tobacco smoke. In the case of smoking and lung cancer, this host resistance may not be considered highly relevant because we have our hands on such a powerful causal agent, smoking. In most other chronic diseases, we do not have such a powerful agent. Host resistance might be extremely relevant.

The balance between causal agent and host resistance is well understood for infectious disease. In 1900, in the US for example, the annual death rate from tuberculosis among whites was 200 per 100,000; for black Americans it was twice as high.[12] Why were poor blacks more likely to die of TB than less poor whites? Southerners in the United States believed that blacks were more susceptible to tuberculosis, had lower host resistance, than whites for genetic reasons. Northern commentators were more likely to ascribe the difference 'to the general insalubrity of the sections of the city inhabited by [blacks], the crowded conditions of their dwellings, insufficient nourishment, and the other influences of poverty'.[13] The Southerners might have thought differences were genetic and the Northerners that they were due to malnutrition or other aspects of poverty, but both sets of commentators appeared to subscribe to the notion of differential susceptibility, i.e. it was not simply different rates of exposure to the tubercle bacillus, but different susceptibility to its effects.

It has long been appreciated that the idea that 'agent causes disease' provides an oversimplified picture of the disease process. When tuberculosis was a major cause of death – in that the death certificate read 'tuberculosis' – in Europe and North America, any number of people had been infected with the tubercle bacillus, but they did not die of tuberculosis. Step one was infection with the tubercle bacillus; step two was suffering consequences of that infection. Other factors determined whether an infected person lost the struggle with the tubercle bacillus or won it. Thomas McKeown's argument, which we met in Chapter 1, was that the decline in death rates from tuberculosis in England was the result of improvements in nutrition. Better nutrition meant better host resistance.[14] There may have been other reasons for a lowered host resistance that are related to social conditions. I'll exaggerate to make a point. These social conditions are the cause of death. The tubercle bacillus is the cause of what gets written on the death certificate; which is not the same thing at all. The tubercle bacillus is the equivalent of Napoleon's orders at Borodino – the proximate cause. The social conditions are what brought the armies together in the first place.

Specific causes, agents, are important. Napoleon's orders may have had effect. But so is susceptibility. What matters is their interaction. For US blacks to have twice the death rate from tuberculosis in 1900, they had to have both high exposure to the agent and high susceptibility, or low host resistance, to the effects of the agent. Whether, as Southern commentators believed, genetic susceptibility was part of this lowered host resistance became irrelevant when the environment improved and rates in both groups declined markedly. The likely explanation is that poor social conditions contributed to the increased susceptibility in blacks, in addition to whatever increase in infection there may have been.

Both agent and host are important. I have spent a great deal of time and energy trying to push doctors and governments in the direction of healthy policies on nutrition and alcohol, and I heartily support anti-smoking policies. Alcohol and smoking may be thought of as the agents, the latter-day equivalents of the tubercle bacillus. (Nutrition is more complicated: specific nutrients could be thought of as agents, while nutritional deficiency weakens host resistance.) While concentrating on agents, we must ask also why, when we have taken these factors into account, health and disease follow a social gradient. Host resistance may play a part.

Thinking about disease with causes in mind

In a wonderful short story, 'The Library of Babel', Jorge Luis Borges imagines a library that stretches to eternity.[15] Everything is there. People come to the library to seek understanding, God if you are so inclined, but understanding depends on how the material in the library is organised. There are an infinite number of ways and each constrains what can be learnt. He might easily have been talking about the way we systematise medical knowledge.

As a medical student I learnt about diseases of the heart and vascular system from one set of teachers, about kidney diseases from another, and chest diseases from yet another. Each disease had a different section in the textbook. This was appropriate: medical schools are oriented to treating disease – heart disease requires different treatment from kidney diseases, and hence an appropriate disease classification separates them.

But a system of classifying diseases that is aimed at treating patients is not necessarily the best for understanding causes of disease. For example, a gastroenterologist is confronted with three patients. The first has been feeling increasingly unwell, has headache and fever, and some pain and tenderness of the abdomen. In the second week of his illness he develops diarrhoea and a rash of rose-coloured spots. He has typhoid fever, confirmed by specific diagnostic tests. The second has explosive onset of bloody diarrhoea and is sick as can be – a typical case of bacterial dysentery. The third has increasing jaundice with dark-coloured urine and pale stools and is quite unwell. Tests confirm that he has hepatitis A.

These three patients have diseases that might all be classified as gastroenterological, but different microorganisms are responsible for the pathogenesis (mechanisms leading to disease) and the clinical picture and they require different regimes of treatment. If one takes the view of cause as the specific microorganism then each of these diseases has a distinct cause, as each is 'caused' by a different bug.

There is another interpretation of 'cause'. Each disease can be caused by eating food that has been contaminated. Infected people with hands soiled from their own faeces have handled food and contaminated it. From the viewpoint of prevention, then, these three different diseases have the same cause: eating contaminated food.

As a medical student, this issue of disease classification preoccupied me. I suggested to my surgical teachers that we should classify diseases into those that were failed prevention and those not. I thought that most of surgery was to do with failed prevention. Why would you want to cut things out? If you understood the causes, you would want to prevent the diseases from occurring in the first place. (Needless to say, the surgeons who taught me told me that I would do better to memorise the treatments for cancer than bother about such things.)

The classification issue surfaced again as I pondered why some patients had remarkably thick sets of medical files. They had disease after disease that were apparently unrelated. Some people simply got sick more often. The phrase that brash young medical students used to describe this was 'piss-poor protoplasm'. This summed up the view that some people seemed to have greater susceptibility to any sort of illness. In saying that their protoplasm was poor, we did not make a judgement as to why, whether genetic or environmental, for example. But the picture we saw was not summed up by conventional views of these diseases being separate and distinct entities.

The patron saint of research into stress and illness, Hans Selye, had a formulation that provided an explanation for why some people had greater susceptibility to disease.[16] When he was working as a physician in Montreal, Selye noticed that there were clinical similarities in patients suffering from a variety of illnesses. Regardless of the specific agent causing sickness, there seemed to be something about being sick that led to similar problems. These patients were, according to Selye, suffering from stress. (This did not mean, necessarily, psychological stress, but a bodily state caused by a variety of 'stressors'.) The state of stress, involving particularly the hypothalamic pituitary adrenal axis, may provide a mechanism linking apparently different diseases. Anything that affected the body's stress reactions could, in theory, change susceptibility to a variety of specific diseases.

In introducing this idea, I quoted John Cassel's final major paper, on the contribution of social resources to host resistance,[17] because it gives a possible cause of the general pattern that Selye described – supportive social relationships will reduce the body's stress reactions. A similar conclusion was reached by two other influential epidemiologists, Len Syme and Lisa Berkman. They reviewed the evidence on social class and mortality in a paper they called 'Social Class, Susceptibility and Sickness'.[18] Their point was that people of lower social class had higher rates of most major illnesses. They postulated that social class was related to susceptibility to a range of different illnesses.

Syme taught his students, including me, that there are three types of question in relation to occurrence of illness. First, why do some groups have higher rates of illness than others? Second, why do some individuals have greater risk of illness than others? Third, when an individual gets sick, what illness does he or she get? The answers to these questions will not necessarily be the same.

The distinction between these questions is relevant to the status syndrome. In our findings from the Whitehall study[19,20] we showed a social gradient in mortality for most major causes of death: disease of the cardiovascular, renal, gastrointestinal and respiratory systems, most cancers, accidental and violent deaths. One question is why someone of low status should, when he gets sick, get heart disease. A second question is why a person of low status is more likely to get sick, whatever the specific condition that brings him down. People of lower status in the nineteenth century died of tuberculosis; in the twenty-first, of coronary heart disease. Thus, while the specific pathogens vary, both sets of people had a greater relative susceptibility to getting sick, because they were of low status. A third question is why one individual in a low social position succumbs to illness and another does not – the individual difference question.

'General susceptibility' is a term that is viewed with great suspicion. The Whitehall study was criticised for looking for a general phenomenon, because the magnitude of the social gradient in mortality is not identical across the various categories of illness and injury.[21] To me, what is striking about these gradients is not that there are one or two diseases for which higher social classes are more at risk – breast cancer, leukaemia, malignant melanoma – but that the gradient goes in the same direction for so many. The lower the status the higher the risk. The exceptions are interesting, but so is the rule.

It is not a criticism of this idea of general susceptibility that the magnitude of the gradient varies for different diseases. Remember Syme's different questions. Why do groups, and individuals, differ in their rates of illness, and what determines what illness an individual gets? Lung cancer and chronic bronchitis show steep social gradients because they are so closely linked with smoking and smoking shows a steep social gradient. But smoking cannot account for the social gradient in suicide and other violent deaths, nor for the diseases not related to smoking that show a social gradient. We could go through each disease and ask which specific factor accounts for why that disease shows a gradient. While this is an important part of assembling the causal picture, we are likely to be missing something that way. Simply assuming that the lower the social status, the higher the degree of exposure to a whole range of pathogens, harmful agents, may miss what links these apparently disparate diseases.

To spell it out more explicitly, consider suicide and heart disease. The first approach to explanation seeks out specific causes for each condition. Suicide and heart disease feature in different chapters of the medical textbook, are the province of different medical specialists – psychiatrists and cardiologists – and surely therefore have different specific causes. Both of these 'causes of death' show a social gradient; should we not, therefore, look for the entirely separate causes of these? We could determine, say, that smoking causes the gradient in heart disease and something in the water causes people to take their own lives. The causal question would then be: why do smoking and something in the water both show a social gradient?

The first approach is not wrong; just limited. The second approach to explanation is different, it looks for factors that underlie more than one condition. More than half of suicides are preceded by known mental illness, commonly depression. Depression shows a social gradient – the lower the position in the hierarchy the higher the rate. But depression not only predicts suicide, it predicts heart disease.[22] There may be a common set of causes underlying the social gradient in depression and the social gradient in heart disease.

Our own data from the Whitehall II study suggest that low control in the workplace is a factor common to both increased risk of coronary heart disease and depression.[23,24] Low control at work may also be importantly related to the higher rates of both of these conditions in the lower employment grades.[25,26]

This leads to the conclusion that in addition to looking at specific causes, we need to ask why some groups are at higher risk of disease in general. Social resources and patterns of social relationships play a role in host resistance to disease. These influences follow the social gradient and are important in the social gradient in disease.

Putting the two together: social supports and susceptibility to disease – the case of marriage

For years, if someone gave a paper on social relationships, summarising the effects of marriage (or a stable relationship) on health, they would say: 'marriage is good for men, not so good for women'. The predictable reaction was an ironic laugh of recognition from the women in the audience and embarrassed, slightly guilty, we've-been-found-out type noises from the men. No one doubts the sex difference. And everyone can think of a good reason why it might be true. You probably just did.

There is one slight problem. It is not true. At least, the story is not quite as neat as marriage protecting men but not women. It is worth enquiring into the apparent protective effects of marriage, because marriage is a potentially important source of social support and the research on social supports and health follows in this tradition. Much of the argument as to whether marriage is protective, and whether it is protective for women as well as for men, illuminates the whole study of social relationships and health. Like so much else in studying social patterns of illness, we learn by going back to two great scientists of the nineteenth century.

One was a Frenchman, the sociologist Emile Durkheim, and one an Englishman, the medical statistician William Farr who, among other things, was interested in France. Farr wrote a treatise in 1858 on *The Influence of Marriage on the Mortality of the French People* in which he said:

> The family is the social unit; and it is founded in its perfect state by marriage. The influence of this form of existence is therefore one of the fundamental problems of social science. A remarkable series of observations, extending over the whole of France, enables us to determine for the first time the effect of conjugal condition on the life of a large population . . . If unmarried people suffer from disease in undue proportion, the have-been-married suffer still more . . . This is the general result: Marriage is a healthy estate. The single individual is more likely to be wrecked on his voyage than the lives joined together in matrimony.[27]

All the research since confirms Farr's accuracy and the unfortunate lot of the single individual.

Durkheim's study of suicide was a pioneering work in the study of social integration and health.[28] He teases us by starting out with the observation that more suicides in France in the 1870s occurred among the married than the unmarried, and hence certain authors concluded that the burdens and responsibilities of marriage drove people to the ultimate end of suicide.

But the 'facts' are false. Durkheim points out that these authors make the elementary error of not accounting for the proportions in the population. (To use a contemporary illustration, it would be like saying that more car crashes occur among people with driving licences than among people without.) Once Durkheim takes account of the higher proportion of married people in the population, he shows that married people have a lower rate of suicide than unmarried. He noted that the 'coefficient of preservation' – the protection afforded by marriage – varies between the sexes. In France, marriage protects men more than women. (Is this where the idea that marriage protects men and not women first arose?) He then goes on to point out that in the area of Oldenburg, marriage 'preserved' women from suicide more than it did men. He concludes that the sex enjoying the greatest protection from marriage varies from society to society.

Durkheim's general thesis was that the more integrated the society, the lower the suicide rate. One of his three main propositions was to do with domestic society – the other two were to do with political and religious society. He showed that the protection of married women from suicide was confined to married women with children. This, for Durkheim, was a measure of domestic integration. He was aware, however, that there was another possible interpretation of his findings: selection.

> Not everyone who wants to, gets married; one has little chance of founding a family successfully without certain qualities of health, fortune and morality. People without them . . . are thus involuntarily relegated to the unmarried class which consequently includes the human dregs of the country. The sick, the incurable, the people of too little means or known weakness are found here. Hence, if this part of the population is so far inferior to the other, it naturally proves this inferiority by a higher mortality, a greater criminality, and finally by a stronger suicidal tendency.

Human dregs! This leaves a strong and bitter aftertaste, but this general idea has pervaded the study of marital status ever since. There are two broad camps: social causation – marriage protects; and selection – the sick, or those likely to get sick, are selectively recruited to the unmarried state. The argument of social causation or selection has a familiar form. Selection arguments are that poor health causes low social position; poor health leads to unemployment; poor health causes lack of marriage. The social-causation argument is that the conditions associated with being low status cause ill health, as does unemployment, as does being single, widowed or divorced.

A particularly rich academic put-down of one colleague by another runs: parts of his talk were true and parts were interesting; unfortunately the parts that were true were not interesting and the parts that were interesting were not true. It is as if the selection camp characterises the social-causation argument as interesting but not true; and the social-causation camp refers to selection as true but not interesting. Selection must exist: people who are unhealthy at one time will be more likely to be unhealthy at another. If sickness leads to a greater risk of belonging to group A than group B, then group A will have more sickness. The question is whether selection is all there is. Or having taken account of selection, is there social causation: do low social position, unemployment, and the unmarried state lead to worse health?

It is worth distinguishing two uses of the concept of selection, both of which were in Farr and Durkheim: health selection and social selection. Health selection, as described in the previous two paragraphs, essentially says that sick people find themselves unmarried, and sick people get sick. Therefore, the link between marriage and lack of sickness has nothing to do with the protective effect of marriage. Social selection says not that sick people find themselves unmarried, but that people with a set of social characteristics do. It is these social characteristics, being 'human dregs' in Durkheim's infelicitous phrase, that lead to increased risk of disease. Both forms of selection deny the protective effect of marriage, but the second is consistent with other social causation of illness.

A wealth of international data show consistently that married people have lower mortality than those unmarried. To cite one of scores of examples: Yuanreng Hu and Noreen Goldman at Princeton looked at figures for sixteen developed countries.[29] In all countries, the married had lower mortality than the unmarried. The protection applies to wives as well as husbands. Across all sixteen countries the mortality rate of men who were unmarried was about twice that of married men; for women the mortality rate of the unmarried was about 1.5 times higher.

Goldman considers carefully Durkheim's, and Farr's, selection arguments. On the basis of statistical modelling, she concludes that most of the arguments that attempt to distinguish selection from social causation are specious. Her own conclusion, based on carefully conducted longitudinal studies that link people's marital status to their subsequent mortality, is that, although selection does play a role, there is clear evidence for the protective nature of marriage.[30] Once more: it is not selection or protection that is important, but both.

It seems clear, then. Marriage protects men and women, not just from suicide but from 'all causes' of death. But does it protect men more? Why do I doubt that men are more protected? Consider Alfie and Peter, Clarissa and Sophie. Alfie is married with a family; Peter is single. Clarissa is married with a family; Sophie is single. In a typical US population, Peter the unmarried man is more likely to be out of the labour force than Alfie the married one. Now turn to the women and we find just the opposite. Sophie the unmarried woman is *more likely to be in the labour force* than Clarissa the married one. Why is this sex difference relevant? Because, as we saw in Chapter 5, people not in the labour force have higher mortality than those gainfully employed. Unemployment is bad for health or, if you are a selectionist, ill-health is bad for employment.

Taking this difference between men and women into account leads to the conclusion that marriage protects women as much as it does men. This is the finding of a recent American study.[31] The investigators were puzzled by the question of why many studies show that although women benefit from marriage, men benefit more. They contend that most studies have failed to take into account the socioeconomic circumstances of men and women who were single, widowed, divorced or married. In their study of more than a quarter of a million Americans, aged forty-five and over, their first lot of results was clear. Men, women, black and white, it mattered little: those who were married had less chance of dying over an eleven-year period than those who were not. Unmarried men had about 60 per cent higher mortality than married men. The high risk, compared to the married, extended to each of single, divorced/separated and widowed men. Unmarried women had about 45 per cent higher mortality than married. Again the increase in risk was in all categories of those short of a spouse. Once the analysis took into account labour-force participation the apparently greater protection for men went. Marriage was as protective for women as for men.

Throughout the long period since Farr and Durkheim wrote, married men and married women have had favourable mortality rates compared to unmarried. So found a study in the Netherlands,[32] which trawled through historical data from the middle of the nineteenth century to the 1970s. The magnitude of the difference between the married and unmarried varied, but it was always there for men and for women. By 1970, marriage protected men and women equally. The fact that the strength of the apparent protection of marriage varies over the century suggests that we have to go beyond categories of single, widowed and divorced and look more at the reality of people's lives.

The more one examines these studies, the more one finds that the advantage of being married spreads to protection from a whole range of diseases. A Norwegian study showed that it was true for survival from cancer.[33] The American study showed it was true for mortality regardless of cause, as well as for heart disease and death from causes that are neither heart disease nor cancer. It is also true of mental illness,[34] and self-reported health.[35]

Just as we found that people of lower social position had higher rates of ill-health, mental illness and mortality from a whole range of conditions, so too we find the same generality for marital status. For both men and women, the advantage of being married cuts across all the separate causes of death that reside in different chapters of the medical textbook. The finding stands squarely in the face of conventional views of disease causation.

Being married protects health because of the social support, the tending and befriending, it provides. Wives benefit their men; husbands benefit their women. This protection applies to the major causes of death, because it makes a contribution to enhancing host resistance. If a person's body is better equipped to do battle against potentially disease-causing agents, it may apply across the board to heart disease, cancer, mental illness and other modes of death.

Those who doubt the general susceptibility argument say that higher rates of ill-health are not due to lack of social support but to the rotten life habits of the unmarried: they drink, they smoke, they eat badly, and do other interesting and exciting things that damage their health. As a middle-aged male acquaintance said to me a year or so after his divorce: he spent the first few months finding out what he had been missing out on. Then he realised that there were good reasons why he had been missing out on it.

Adverse health habits are plausible contributors to the health disadvantage of the unmarried. Divorce, widowhood, and indeed permanent single status, may well be accompanied by less healthy lifestyle. This will be part of the reason for the worse health of the unmarried. Those who are uncomfortable with 'common factors' leading to susceptibility would argue that smoking will be responsible for some of the increased mortality, worse diet for some other, alcohol for other and so on. For women, particularly, divorce and widowhood may be accompanied by worse material conditions which may of course play a role in worse health.

To focus only on specific adverse habits misses out the importance for health of the most salient parts of human experience: relations between people. In the previous chapter I argued that the degree of control you have over your life is crucial for health. The evidence on marriage suggests that social relationships represent an important different dimension that is crucial for the maintenance of health. The evidence is strong, but marriage is a crude category, and marriage is but one part of people's social lives.

My colleagues, Mel Bartley and Amanda Sacker, went beyond the simple married/unmarried dichotomy to obtain a fuller picture of women's social circumstances and to examine how they were related to health. They carried out this research in a national sample, the Health Survey for England.[36] They found that a professional single woman had about the same average health status as a married woman with children – they were the healthiest women. A single mother who had never been married was about four times as likely to be in poor health. She lacks emotional and financial support; her health suffers as a result. Being a woman with an unemployed partner is as bad for health as being never married with children.

The group of women with the worst health was the previously married empty nesters. They had lost at least two of their social roles. It is reasonable to speculate that these women lacked social support despite the fact that most of them were employed outside the home.

A careful study such as this though, does not by itself prove the importance of caring for health. We have to go further to look for more direct evidence of the importance of social relationships for health.

Social ties and health

In *Guys and Dolls*, Nathan Detroit, organiser of the floating crap game, has a girlfriend named Adelaide. For fourteen long years Adelaide has been waiting for Nathan to convert their engagement into marriage.

She laments that, being insecure, while waiting around for that band of gold, she could develop a cold.

Frank Loesser, who was responsible for turning Damon Runyon's lovable New York rogues into musical theatre, had a good intuitive grasp of the relation between emotions and physical illness. When I said that marriage seems to protect against a range of physical and mental illnesses, I did not include the common cold. Yet a brilliant series of studies on the common cold by psychologist Sheldon Cohen provides some of the clearest evidence that stress and social relationships are related to illness.

There are certain things about the common cold that everyone knows: one is that when children go off to school for the first time, in the autumn, they come back with a cold. They are exposed to viruses that are new to them, and they become infected. But not all succumb. Some children seem to go through a succession of colds and some very few. Likewise with their parents. The children come home with their infections, and some parents develop their own colds and some not.

With rabies, if you are infected, you die. But most infections are not like that. Infection does not equal disease. Among those exposed, the infection rate could be 100 per cent, but host resistance appears to determine if one person with an infection will get sick and another not.

Sheldon Cohen has studied the factors that influence host resistance to viruses responsible for the common cold. One of his studies relates particularly to the role of social ties in host resistance.[37] Colleagues of mine have volunteered for the type of study that Cohen conducts. You answer an advertisement and agree to some tests and then return to be quarantined for six days. My colleagues said they were given reasonable accommodation and had time to catch up on their reading. The only catch is that you have to let someone put known cold virus into your nose, via nose drops. Over the next five days the closest you can get to someone else is three feet. Then everyone waits to see a) if you were infected and b) if you, like Adelaide, were a person who developed a cold.

In Cohen's study, some people just by chance already had antibodies to the cold viruses used. Among them, the rate of infection was 69 per cent, and the proportion that developed a cold was 25 per cent using an objective measure: nasal mucous was weighed, and the time taken to clear the nose of mucous was recorded. Among people with no antibody evidence of previous infection with the virus, the infection rate was 99 per cent and 58 per cent developed a cold.

This much was to be expected. The striking finding was the link with social ties. Before exposure to the virus, volunteers were given a list of twelve types of social relationship – spouse, parents, parents-in-law, children, other close family members, close neighbours, friends, workmates, schoolmates, fellow volunteers for charity or community work, members of social or recreational groups, and members of religious groups. For each, the study participants were asked if they spoke to someone in that relationship at least once every two weeks. People with few social ties, 1 to 3 of the list, had three times the incidence of a cold compared to those with a diverse set of social relationship, six or more of the above list.

Cohen and his colleagues went through the standard self-criticism to see if something else could have accounted for this dramatic difference in incidence of cold. Susceptibility was related to smoking, to sleep problems, to lack of alcohol (!), and low dietary vitamin C. None of these accounted for the protection from colds afforded by a rich array of social relationships.

This study, then, provides an excellent model for shedding light on the whole discussion of agent, in this case the common-cold virus, and host resistance. Exposure to the agent was universal – everyone had the virus put into their nose. It is differences in host resistance that determine whether being exposed to virus leads to illness. Differences in host resistance are, in turn, related to richness of social ties.

Social relationships – a matter of life and death

If the worst havoc that lack of social ties could cause was an increased risk of a cold, it might be a nuisance but no worse than that. But the damage is a good deal worse. Isolation kills – not only in the form of Decoud in *Nostromo* going crazy on an island – but also by increase in risk of dying from a wide variety of causes.[38]

Sapolsky's stress model based on the study of baboons and other animals, which we looked at in Chapter 5, suggested that one of the important moderators of stress was the availability of support. Rick and Maria (See pp. 110–14) were both undergoing a period of acute uncertainty because of the impending closure of the clothing factory that Rick ran, and in which Maria worked. Rick's problems were made easier by the support of a secure relationship with his wife and a circle of friends, acquaintances, clubs and organisations. Maria was too ground-down by the demands of everyday life to enjoy the luxury of such a supportive network. Her husband's job loss and depressed behaviour meant that not only did he fail to give support, but he was a further burden.

It is entirely plausible that such lack of support could make Maria unhappy and less able to cope. She is also more likely to die. Lisa Berkman's early study was carried out in Alameda County, California.[39] Similar to Cohen's study, she found that people who participated in social networks had lower mortality than those who did not. As with the studies on marriage, it is possible that ill-health could lead to lack of participation rather than the reverse. This was not the case. Since that early study, a large literature has documented the protective effects of social relationships on health.

Berkman suggests that there are four primary pathways by which participation in social networks affect health:

(1) provision of social support;
(2) social influence;
(3) social engagement and attachment;
(4) access to resources and material goods.

Two primary pathways by which these can influence health are through their effect on psychological mechanisms and stress pathways, and through their effects on health behaviours.

The conclusion seems clear that social supports protect against a range of specific conditions. The question that then arises is whether disrupted or disordered social relationships may contribute to the social gradient in health.

Social participation and the social gradient

Recently I interviewed one of my relatives about what it was like growing up in poor areas of the East End of London in the earlier years of the twentieth century. Was living in poverty in the ghetto the idyll I imagined it to be: a close-knit community with lots of interaction and support?

> Happy childhood? Not on your nelly. Mother showed love as she could, but she was too busy. One of my older sisters was very loving, but I was bullied by my brothers, and there was no one to ask for help with homework. I cannot now think of nice times. I wasn't happy and can't think when it might have got better. What I remember is the shame of being sent to the shop on a Friday and having to ask for weekend food on credit; and turning up to a new school with low self-esteem.

No misty-eyed nostalgia there. Poverty is destructive and it does nothing for supportive social relationships. In fact, like so many other aspects of life that we have studied, the pattern of social relationships follows a social gradient. In the Whitehall II study every type of social contact was more frequent as the social hierarchy was ascended, bar one: contact with family. People lower in the hierarchy had more contact with family but less with friends and with work colleagues and were less likely to be members of formal organisations. Similar findings have been reported from the US.[40]

If we turn from social networks – the degree of participation with others – to supports, we find a similar pattern. For example, a national study in Britain asked people if they had adequate social supports. The percentage of people who reported severe lack of social support was then tabulated by social class: I being the highest class; V the lowest. Ten per cent of men in class I reported severe lack of social support, rising to 12 per cent in class II, and continuously up to 26 per cent in class V. Women were less likely to report severe lack of social support than men, but they, too, showed a social gradient: 6 per cent in class I rising to 15 per cent in class V.[41]

The previous chapter focused on the strong links to ill-health of lack of control over one's life. Lack of control is closely linked to place in the hierarchy. Although I have argued that hierarchies in society appear to emerge from the competition among males for status and hence access to resources, hierarchies affect everybody: female as well as male. This chapter has focused on another crucial feature of society: supportive social relationships. These may emerge from females' propensity to 'tend and befriend' in response to threat but, as with hierarchies and control, they too affect everybody: male as well as female. Lack of supportive social relations appears to act by weakening host resistance and is linked to increased risk of a range of illnesses and causes of death. Adding insult to injury, supportive relations are less common as the social hierarchy is descended.

One reason for different levels of friendships may be individual differences in ease of making friends. We should not, however, think of differences in strength of social ties as simply the result of personality quirks. They are related to the structure of society. Societies may vary in the degree to which they encourage the type of relationship that is likely to be protective against illness. This is the theme of the next chapter.

7. TRUSTING TOGETHER

[*Mrs Munt comments to her niece on the foolhardiness of leaving a lower-class stranger alone in the drawing room*] *'Your drawing-room is full of very tempting little things.'*

'Yes, I think the apostle spoons could have gone as rent,' said Margaret. Seeing that her aunt did not understand, she added: 'You remember "rent". It was one of father's words – rent to the ideal, to his own faith in human nature. You remember how he would trust strangers, and if they fooled him he would say: "It's better to be fooled than to be suspicious" – that the confidence trick is the work of man, but the want-of-confidence trick is the work of the devil.'

Mrs Munt longed to add: 'It was lucky that your father married a wife with money.'

E. M. Forster, *Howard's End*[1]

Hostility is bad for you; not only other people's, your own. Peered at through my particular spectacles, I know it is bad, because hostile people are at greater risk of heart disease than non-hostile people.[2] Like most answers, that leads to a question: why are some people more hostile than others? If hostility were part of personality, then some of the differences among individuals would be the result of individual differences in genetic predisposition.

That cannot be all there is to it. The average level of hostility varies from place to place. A survey in ten US cities measured average hostility scores of residents. I suggest that you will have little difficulty in ranking the cities from low to high hostility. Here are a few of them: Honolulu, Seattle, Chicago, New York. You were correct. I listed them in order from low hostility to high. The unfortunate prize for the most hostile city went to Philadelphia.[3] Redford Williams, who conducted the survey, is still waiting for the Philadelphians to simmer down.[4]

If one thought that each person had a fixed amount of hostility that was a stable trait, this survey would pose a problem. How would you explain high hostility rates in New York and low in Seattle: selective migration? For example, hostile people saying: 'I want to be where I feel most comfortable' and taking themselves off to New York where they can snarl and snap to their heart's content? Surely not. That possibility could easily be answered by looking at hostility levels in people who did not migrate. Not a betting man, I am willing to bet that it would show that the effect is not confined to migrants.

Common sense and casual observation tells us that places are different: New York has an adrenaline buzz, Seattle is laid back; some places are friendly, trusting and safe, and others threatening. But a city cannot be laid back or hostile; people in those places can be. People's characteristics vary by where they find themselves. If you are surrounded by hostile people, it is perhaps no surprise that your sunny disposition changes. The fifth time you are jostled out of your place in line, you start to display adaptive behaviour. If put in an environment where the drivers stop at pedestrian crossings, most pedestrians, eventually, will let their guards down and start to trust drivers.

Thus characteristics of individuals, repeated time after time, become characteristics of places. Social ties may be a property of an individual, in that an agreeable individual may find it easy to form friendships. But it can also be a property of a place, if places differ systematically in degrees of social support and social connectedness, just as they differ in degrees of hostility.

In this chapter we shall examine how degrees of social connectedness may vary among societies and hence contribute to differences in health. Raising our gaze to look at whole societies is important. As individuals we are concerned with what we can do for own health. But we are also members of a society. If we want better health, the answer might be not only to look to ourselves but to the society in which we live out our lives. I have been building the case that hierarchies are a pervasive feature of society but their effects vary with consequent variations in the social gradient in health. Co-operation, reciprocity and trust are also fundamental features of society. To put it at its most simple: if hierarchies are bad for health and co-operation and trust good for health, the level of health that we as individuals experience may depend on the balance between hierarchy and co-operation and trust of a society.

A second, related, reason for looking at health of whole societies is that it bypasses the problem of individual differences. For example, in the previous chapter I showed that people with high social supports have better health than people with low social supports. I confronted the argument that health might lead to low social supports, or being not married; i.e. the causal direction might be the 'other' way: from health to low social supports. Similarly, people with a particular personality type could be predisposed to ill-health and to difficulty with relationships; in this case, again, social supports are not protective. Such alternative views of the evidence cannot be the explanation if a whole society is protected by higher levels of social connections. It is a good deal less plausible to argue that a low level of health of a whole society led to low levels of social connectedness. Similarly, in the following chapter, we shall look at societies where the overall level of control is low and health suffers.

The evidence suggests that level of co-operation and trust of a society improves health. Co-operation and trust at the level of societies has been called social capital. Robert Putnam, a political scientist at Harvard, defines social capital as 'the connections among individuals – social networks and the norms of reciprocity and trustworthiness that arise from them'.[5] His book, *Bowling Alone*, struck a responsive chord in the American reading public. It charts the decline in social participation in the US in a whole range of spheres, from voting in elections, trusting people on the street, to going bowling alone. One consequence of this decline in social connectedness may be an effect on health. As a relatively recent concept, social capital has attracted criticism.[6] A particular concern is whether studying relations between people may deflect attention from the material causes in society responsible for inequalities in health.[7] It need not. Understanding that economic and social influences may affect health because of the way they affect human relations of trust and reciprocity makes the social causes of ill-health more, not less important.[8]

Social integration and health

Why one individual is hostile and another not is a different question from why the average level of hostility is higher in New York than Seattle. The first may result from genes or particular early childhood experiences; the second will have more to do with the environment. We owe much to Emile Durkheim, father of modern sociology, for these insights. He looked both at individuals and at whole societies. At the individual level, he showed that individuals who are married have lower suicide rates than people who are not married. As I reported in Chapter 6, Durkheim considered the possibility that this apparent advantage when comparing a married individual with an unmarried one could result from other differences between married and un-married individuals. Durkheim, therefore, lifted his focus to examine whole societies. While we have added a few details since Durkheim, his general thesis that the level of integration of a society is related to the level of health of that society remains valid today – except that we now use the phrase social capital. Durkheim's topic of study was suicide. His general conclusions apply to other forms of ill-health.

Social integration, for Durkheim, was made real by examining integrations in three spheres of society: religious, domestic, and political. In each case the more integrated the society, the lower the suicide rate.[9]

His evidence for the first of these was that suicide rates were higher in Protestant countries of Europe than Catholic ones. Within coun-tries, areas of the country with a predominantly Catholic population, had lower suicide rates than areas with Protestant populations. In general, Jews had lower suicide rates than Protestants and, usually, lower than Catholics. He attributed this, in nineteenth-century Europe, to a stronger collective credo, and more unified and strong society, among Catholics and Jews than Protestants.

His evidence for the second of these propositions was that married people are less likely to commit suicide than never-married, widowed or divorced people. He also notes that not only are divorced individuals more likely to commit suicide, but countries with high divorce rates had, in general, higher suicide rates. This sounds like a simple statistical tautology: if there are more divorced individuals, and divorced individuals are more likely to commit suicide, there will be a correlation between a country's divorce rate and their suicide rate. Durkheim reasoned differently. If divorce rate is high, the commitment to marriage may be weaker, and hence the degree of integration of domestic society weaker. He reasoned, therefore, that in countries with high divorce rates, the protective effect of marriage against suicide would be less. This is indeed what his data showed.

In support of the third proposition was the observation that in times of war, the suicide rate goes down – an observation that was true of many countries in nineteenth-century Europe. Durkheim argues that war may bring a sense of collective purpose to civilians. It is not simply that able-bodied men are being killed in battle rather than killing themselves. The suicide rate goes down in women as well.

His central conclusion from this is that societies exhibit collective tendencies that are not simply the sum of the tendencies of the individuals that comprise them. The individuals making up a society change from year to year, yet the number of suicides is the same so long as the society itself does not change. He acknowledges the criticism of his approach that each suicide corresponds to an incident of private life, be it bankruptcy, unhappy marriage, disappointed ambition, poverty, etc. His response was that even if it were true that these incidents of private life were causal in the individual case, we have to account for the remarkable regularity with which they occur, more in some societies than others. As he puts it, this would

> at best change the problem without solving it . . . This regular recurrence of identical events in proportions constant within the same population but very inconstant from one population to another would be inexplicable had not each society definite currents impelling its inhabitants with a definite force to commercial and industrial ventures, to behavior of every sort likely to involve families in trouble, etc.[10]

In the case of suicide the important collective tendency was to do with degree of social integration.

Durkheim has come into severe criticism from evolutionary psychology for taking the position that social factors mould and determine human natures. As Matt Ridley puts it, perhaps with the words baby and bathwater in mind, Durkheim's rejection of all innateness in human

nature 'has been so demolished by Steven Pinker in *The Blank Slate* as to
leave little to say. But as a positive statement of the degree to which
human beings are influenced by social factors, it is undeniable.'[11]
Durkheim's massive contribution was to show the effect of the social
environment on individuals' behaviour, emotions and tendencies.

By pointing to the existence of human universals what evolutionary
psychology has helped us to see is that a phenomenon like social
integration can have predictable effects precisely because humans may
be expected to respond to its lack in predictable ways. There need be
no contradiction in examining the effects of the environment while
acknowledging the evolved nature of humans, or individual differences. As evolutionary psychologist Steven Pinker has written:

> Natural selection tends to make the members of a species alike in their
> adaptive traits, because whichever version of a trait is better than the others
> will be selected and the alternate versions die out. That is why most
> evolutionary psychologists attribute systematic differences among people
> to their *environments* and attribute only random differences to the genes.[12]

Far be it from me to try and make peace between the father of
sociology and the expositors of evolutionary psychology. Nevertheless, we can accept the best of both. Durkheim points to the
salience of the social environment. We do not need to make the
incorrect assumption that the minds of humans were blank slates to be
written on by the environment, to acknowledge the importance of
the environment in accounting for systematic differences in psychological traits and behaviours.

A collective tendency to social integration can affect not only
suicide. Amartya Sen, looking at the improvement in life expectancy
in Britain in the twentieth century, reaches similar conclusions to
Durkheim. War may be dreadful, but it may have positive effects on
social integration and hence on mortality. Sen notes that during the
twentieth century life expectancy improved most, not in decades
where the economy grew fastest, but in the decades that included the
two World Wars.[13] Sen attributes this to the fact that in the face of
adversity the British population bonded together. He cites the fact that
the origins of the welfare state and the National Health Service were

in the 1940s as supportive of his thesis. What Sen describes is certainly consistent with what Robert Putnam would label social capital.

Cultural differences in social integration

If social connectedness is good for health, and it varies systematically among societies, we might expect health differences to follow, as a consequence. Similarly, if there were variations in social connectedness within a society, there would be accompanying differences in health.

Societies do vary in this way. Consider this everyday scene of family bliss. You are in your flat or apartment and your teenage son and friends are playing their music at 'normal' amplitude. Acoustic trauma, hearing damage all round. You are thinking – to the extent that thinking is possible under the insistent 'drum and bass' – do I try to stop it now or wait until the neighbours complain? Comes the inevitable ring on the door. You know what the neighbour is going to say. What are *you* going to say? Do you, like the she-lion, rise to the defence of your young; do you defend your rights as an individual to do whatever you like at home – an Englishman's home is his castle; do you sympathise with the neighbours that their personal space has been invaded and agree to do something about it; do you phone your lawyer, because you know the next step from the neighbour is legal action?

In Tokyo, this scene plays out differently from San Francisco, Dusseldorf and London. T. R. Reid, an American journalist recently moved to Tokyo, was in this situation when a smartly dressed neighbour arrived. After an extended discussion about the weather, and suitable self-effacement, the neighbour points out that the noise is a *meiwaku*.[14] A *meiwaku* is something that causes trouble or shame for other members of the group to which you belong. The neighbour is not complaining because he is inconvenienced; he is pointing out that the Reid family is in danger of bringing shame on the neighbourhood, by turning it into a rowdy place. He has brought shame on the group. He has violated something basic, his responsibility to the group of which he is a member.

A high degree of responsibility to the group, characteristic more of some societies than others, is an important determinant of health and well-being of the people who live in that society. A society with a higher degree of responsibility to the group should, other things being equal, be a healthier society. Japan fits that description.

Japan's health and the rich countries

In Chapter 3, when examining income, I pointed to the fact that among rich countries, gross domestic product per head does not correlate with life expectancy. The US is the richest country, adjusting for purchasing power, and life expectancy in 2000 was 73.9 for men and 79.5 for women. The US trails Japan, the world leader in health, where life expectancy for men was 77.5, and for women was 84.7. I explained that a three-year difference in life expectancy is very large; abolishing coronary heart disease from the whole population would add about three to four years of life expectancy. Another way of looking at the health differences is to ask about the survival chances of an adolescent. An American boy of fifteen has 60 per cent higher chance of dying before his sixtieth birthday than a Japanese boy of fifteen. The chances are 15 per cent versus 9 per cent. For an American girl of fifteen the chances of dying by age sixty, although lower than for her male counterpart are nearly 80 per cent higher than for a Japanese girl.[15] This is a dramatic difference.

Why are the Japanese so healthy?[16] The arguments that I have heard to answer this question include: Japanese genes, Japanese fascination with medical care, errors in filling out death certificates, nutrition, smoking habits, wealth. None, by itself, provides a convincing answer, but they bear some attention.

Japanese genes may be wonderful, but they were not providing much protection from ill-health forty years ago, when Japanese life expectancy for men was twelve years less than it is now, and for Japanese women it was fourteen years less. The environment changed in the forty years, not the genes.

The Japanese are unlikely to be healthy because of their expenditure on medical care. In 1995, the US spent 14.5 per cent of its gross domestic product on medical care. Japan spent 7 per cent, and that's 7 per cent of a smaller gross domestic product. The argument would have to get pretty sophisticated to suggest that Japan's relatively miserly expenditure on health care accounts for its better health.

The argument that Japanese good health is the result of errors in counting has little to recommend it. There has been scepticism over the low coronary heart-disease rates in Japan. Perhaps, it can be argued, when a Japanese person dies suddenly, the cause that gets written on the death certificate is cerebrovascular disease (stroke), whereas in the West it would be coronary heart disease. That could contribute to the apparent deficit in deaths from heart disease in Japan and the excess in deaths from stroke. It could not explain why the Japanese death rate is low, regardless of cause. One set of authors, having flirted with the error hypothesis – the idea that the apparent protection from heart disease of young men in Japan was related to the way diagnosis was assigned[17] – later decided the low rates were real.[18]

The lifestyle hypothesis offers better prospects for providing an explanation. There is every reason to believe that smoking and a raised plasma cholesterol will harm Japanese as they harm other people, and in Japan, the signs for a coming coronary epidemic are alarming. Although the rate has declined a little, more than half of Japanese men are smokers.[19] This is substantially higher than in the US or Britain. As diet changed, plasma cholesterol levels rose until by the 1990s they were close to American levels.[20] With the high-salt diet of Japan, blood-pressure levels are high.

The only problem for prediction of a coming coronary epidemic is that heart-disease rates in Japan, far from rising, have been declining.[21] And declining, I might add, from their already low level. Despite all the apparent Westernisation of diet and lifestyle, despite smoking as if there is no tomorrow, rates of heart disease have been going down.

It is quite possible, for example, that the decline in stroke and stomach cancer both relate to dietary change – reduced consumption of salt and of pickled food. But there must be more going on here. I suggest that it is the cohesive nature of Japanese society that is protecting the Japanese.

I have often had the conversation with colleagues who listen politely, more or less, to my thesis that low control and lack of participation activate stress pathways and lead to the social gradient in health. They then counter with their trump card. What about Japan! Surely that is the most stressful country imaginable. If stress were bad for health, the Japanese would be dropping at a great rate. These

observers see all the signs of cultural hegemony from the West –
McDonalds, Starbucks, baseball, Disney theme parks – and assume
that Japanese must have all the stresses of the West, only more so. I
think they are wrong. What impresses about Japan is not how
Westernised it has become, but how different it has remained.

Observers of the Japanese scene suggest that the key to understanding Japan is 'Asian values', which can be traced back to the
teachings of Confucius. Asian values have come in for something of a
mixed press. Lee Kuan Yu in Singapore has been an enthusiast for
Asian values: loyalty, respect, commitment to the collectivity. People
are impressed by Singapore's remarkable success at transforming itself,
in one generation, from a developing country to a rich, healthy,
industrialised, trading nation. They are also impressed, in a different
way, that this success appears to have been bought at a cost: lack of free
discussion, censorship, heavy-handed policing of minor crimes.

Nevertheless, commitment to the group, loyalty and respect do
appear crucial in understanding quite how different Japan is from
Western countries. Take as one indicator the proportion of the
population in prison. *The Economist* characterises the US as the land
of the not-free.[22] In 2002, for every 100,000 residents of the US, 700
were locked up. This compares with 132 in England & Wales, 102 in
Canada, 85 in France and 48 in Japan. Perhaps the rate of crime is not
fifteen times as high in the US as in Japan, perhaps America is a more
aggressive jailer. The figures suggest that there are real differences.
Table 7.1 shows crime rates per 100,000 of population.[23]

Table 7.1 **Crime rates in the USA and Japan/100,000 people
(1996)**

	United States	Japan
Murder	7.5	1.0
Robbery	256	1.8
Rape	37	1.5
Aggravated assault	440	5.4
Burglary	1099	187

Source: Adapted from Reid (2000).

The Japanese would argue that their low crime rate is a direct result of the cohesive nature of their society. This is not to say that there are not exceptions. People do get murdered, raped, robbed in Japan, but at a far lower rate than in Western societies. Big cities in Japan do not have no-go areas to anything like the extent of big cities in the US. There is evidence that the greater the level of trust between people in society, social capital, the lower the crime rate.[24] If so, we could argue that Japanese society as a whole is characterised by a high degree of trust between people.

The reaction to white-collar crime in Japan is noteworthy. World-weary, we in the West have come to accept the odd business scandal, executives enriching themselves while cheating workers of their pensions (Maxwell in the UK, Enron in the US) as almost part of the system. An interesting feature of Japanese business corruption is that when the perpetrators are exposed, they go down on their knees on television and apologise for the *meiwaku*, for the shame their actions have brought on their company, their political party, their family.

In American and British cultures, we are under onslaught from the cult of the individual. If we believed the advertising rubbish that insults our sensibilities, a combination of a Windows program, Nike sports shoes and the Marlboro man, and you can 'just do' anything you want today. A cartoon (probably *New Yorker*) summed up the 'me' generation with the caption: 'That's enough talking about me, let's talk about you. What do you think of me?'

It is true that the Japanese are more likely to do things in groups. As evidence that the Japanese are less individualistic in their orientation, recall the study that I described earlier, which asked American college students how they rated themselves compared to their peers. There was a self-enhancement bias. Most students thought they were better than most other students. Not the Japanese. When asked what proportion of people were better than themselves, the average score for the group was 50 per cent. This may be because Japanese students have a more accurate perception of where they stand in the scheme of things than American students. Alternatively, it might reflect a dis-inclination of Japanese to mark themselves out as distinctive from the group.

The group orientation relates closely to the way they do business. Ronald Dore, at the London School of Economics, has been a long-time observer of the Japanese scene. He contrasts three models of capitalism: Anglo-Saxon (Anglo-American), Continental European, and Japanese. In characterising relations between management and labour he says:

> There is first the Anglo-Saxon pattern where the adversarial relation is for real: the knives are out. The second is the continental European pattern; the knives are kept in their sheaths while people play poker according to rules which everybody has a hand in working out. The third is the Japanese pattern: the rules are well established and not much changing, the knives are locked away in the family cupboard and it is only when the senior members of the family flagrantly break the rules that people lower down the hierarchy start wondering where they put those knives.[25]

To make the contrast between Anglo-Saxon and Japanese styles of capitalism plain, he highlights three features of the current Anglo-Saxon version. First, responsibility to shareholders does not extend to employees. In times of economic downturn, employees are let go. A labour market in talent means acceptance that there is little reason for loyalty between employee and company, and vice versa. Second, and related, union membership and power have declined. Third, the power has shifted to shareholders. Companies are run to meet the bottom line, which affects share values. The stockmarket plays a central role in the economies of the US and Britain. Corporations are an instrument of profit for their owners.

The Japanese system is quite different. Dore characterises the Japanese corporation as a community of people that breeds community characteristics. Managers are promoted from within, and they conceive of their role more as that of elders of an enterprise community than as agents of principal shareholders. A strikingly different feature of Japanese capitalism is the near irrelevancy of share prices. There is a great deal of cross-ownership of shares – the banks own shares in the large industries, who own shares in the banks. This means that stockmarket speculation has very little impact on the real economy, and takeovers from buying up shares are a rarity.

Much has been made of the fabled Japanese lifetime employment contract – jobs for life. Dore makes the point that contractual jobs for life are a minority. The system functions on trust and social relationships. In practice there is a limited labour market for talent because of the unwritten practice of loyalty to the firm. The Anglo-American practice of recruiting a top manager from one sector to run a corporation in a different sector and paying him large sums to do it, has no parallel in Japan. The corporation inspires loyalty, and employers and employees tend to stay faithful to each other throughout their working lives.

Similarly, much of the relationship between suppliers and purchasers functions on this basis of trust and tradition. These business arrangements are more relational than they are contractual. In a formal sense, Japanese companies are not highly efficient. It is more important to keep people employed in bad times than to be efficient. Without shareholders breathing down their necks every quarter, it is an option for Japanese companies to be in for the long haul. In the 1980s for example, official unemployment in Germany was 6 per cent, in the US it was 7.2 per cent, in Britain 10 per cent, but in Japan it was 2.5 per cent.[26] Even in 2002, with industrial production down nearly 3 per cent and retail sales down 3.5 per cent, unemployment in Japan, though historically high, still stood at 5.4 per cent.[27]

The social solidarity of the company may have much to do with a more compressed dispersion of wages/salaries in Japan than in most other advanced industrial societies. Figures on income inequalities are notoriously inaccurate, and international comparisons have to be made with great caution. Nevertheless, the impression that income inequalities are narrower in Japan than in the rich countries of Europe and North America is borne out by recent figures from the World Bank.[28] One way of making the comparison is to rank households, or individuals, according to their income from the lowest to the highest and then ask what proportion of all income the bottom 20 per cent receive and what proportion do the top 20 per cent enjoy. This is what Table 7.2 shows.

Table 7.2 Share of total household income of bottom and top 20 per cent of households

	Bottom 20 per cent	Top 20 per cent
Japan	10.6	35.7
Sweden	9.6	34.5
Germany	8.2	38.5
Canada	7.5	39.3
United Kingdom	6.6	43.0
US	5.2	46.4

Notes: (1) 'Bottom' and 'top' refer to ranking of households by income: (2) The greater the differential between a pair of figures, the greater the income inequality in that country.

Source: World Bank (2001).

These figures suggest that Dore's classification into three different ways of operating capitalism correspond to three different patterns of income distribution. The Anglo-Saxon model is marked by high degrees of income inequality; the continental European model by moderate degrees; and the Japanese by the lowest. In the US, for example, the bottom 20 per cent receive 5.2 per cent of all income. In Japan, the figure is double at 10.6 per cent. Turning to the top end, in the US the top 20 per cent receive 46.4 per cent of all income; in Japan, 35.7 per cent. If we confine attention to the top 10 per cent, they receive 30.5 per cent of all income in the US, 21.7 per cent in Japan.

Changing place, changing disease rates

Japan, then, is a country with low crime rates, high standards of educational performance, low income inequalities, and a pattern of industrial relations and economic management that indicates a high degree of social cohesion. Just because they don't like to sack people, and have little penchant for taking things that don't belong to them, doesn't necessarily guarantee fewer heart attacks.

As part of an exploration of how Japanese social cohesiveness can affect health, we can ask what happens to the health of Japanese when they leave Japan. One strategy of trying to understand causes of disease, in particular to separate characteristics of individuals from their environment, is to look at the health of migrants. If disease rates change when people migrate, it is a fair bet that the change has something to do with the environment of the new country and the circumstances there in which the migrant finds himself.

A century ago, there was large-scale Japanese migration to Hawaii and to the West Coast of mainland US. The Japanese migrants were largely recruited to be farm labourers. (Migration was stopped in the 1920s by an act of Congress.) Thus, large numbers of men of Japanese ancestry lived in Hawaii and California. In the 1960s, Japan had the highest death rates from stroke in the world, and the lowest death rates from coronary heart disease (CHD) of any industrialised country.[29] This all changed when they left Japan. The further the Japanese migrated across the Pacific, the lower the stroke rates and the higher the rates of CHD.

Enter our old friend, selection. Could migrants somehow be different from non-migrants, hence putting them at higher risk of CHD and lower risk of stroke than those that stayed behind? Unlikely. Migrants are usually healthier than those who stay behind; how could this then account for an increase in heart attacks in those who left? Perhaps migrants are different in other ways. What if there were a genetic predisposition both to migration and to heart disease? For that to work, the genetic predisposition would have to explain not only the fact of migration, but the distance travelled. Those who went to Hawaii had some increase in heart-disease rates; those who went all the way to California had a bigger increase, although their rates did not reach the high levels of white Americans. Hence a genetic explanation, too, is unlikely.

It is relevant that when we came to study this phenomenon in the 1970s, the majority of Japanese-Americans were Nisei, i.e. born in Hawaii or California of parents who were migrants from Japan. They would not have been subject to the same selection as their parents. The Nisei spanned two worlds, the Japaneseness of their parents and the desire to be American. Telling the story from the inside, Hoso-kawa describes going to school to learn about George Washington and coming home to be given two rules for behaviour: misbehaviour means you will be laughed at by others; and such actions will cause disgrace. School said be an American, carve your own course; home told him to conform and not bring shame on the group.[30] As he grew up, he was likely to have eggs and coffee for breakfast, Teryaki and rice for dinner. There was ample reason why his rate of heart disease might have been intermediate between the low rate in Japan and the higher rate of white Americans.

A study was set up, the NiHonSan (Nippon, Honolulu, San Francisco) study of men of Japanese ancestry living in Japan, Hawaii and the San Francisco Bay Area.[31] It confirmed the gradient across the Pacific – higher rates of CHD and lower rates of stroke. An obvious candidate to explain this was the change in diet from the low-fat traditional Japanese diet to a more Westernised high-fat diet. Indeed, the plasma cholesterol levels, which are influenced by the fat content of the diet, were higher among Japanese-Americans than among Japanese in Japan. This was far from a complete explanation, however, as the plasma cholesterol levels in Hawaii and San Francisco were quite similar, but the heart-disease rates were higher in California.[32]

Enter social cohesion. Scott Matsumoto, a Japanese-American sociologist, suggested that the socially cohesive nature of Japanese society protected against stress. He pointed to the lifetime employment patterns, the practice of (male) workers going out together socially after work, and the stable family life as all being stress-reducing devices.[33] We were able to test his proposition by devising measures of acculturation for the Japanese-Americans of California. We showed that the more traditional these men were in their upbringing, and the more they stayed within the ethnic group in California, the lower their heart-disease rates. The more Westernised, the higher the rates.[34] It was consistent with a protective effect of social cohesion on risk of heart disease. By studying these men in detail we were able to ask to what extent westernisation of diet could account for this pattern. We showed that the higher CHD rates among the Westernised Japanese was independent of their plasma cholesterol levels, their blood pressure or their smoking patterns.

The lesson from Japan, and from the studies of Japanese migrants, emphasises the importance of the social environment in influencing disease rates. Social integration, or its lack, does not act by itself. Smoking, diet and other causes may all act to determine whether rates of specific diseases are high or low. The high rate of stroke in Japan, linked to high blood pressure, is likely to have a dietary component. The overall good health of the Japanese, and their corresponding long life expectancy, may well have to do with social cohesiveness.

Having become a rich country is surely helpful to Japan but, as we have seen, the way the wealth is distributed may be more important. It reflects a commitment to relative fairness. Wealth is helpful, but not essential as studies from a few poorer communities show.

Good health at low cost

A factory in Trivandrum in the Indian state of Kerala; rows of workers at their work stations, making cheap cigarettes. There is something unusual about this beehive. In the centre, one man is reading the newspaper. No, not the foreman taking it easy while everyone else works, but an employee paid to read the newspaper aloud to the other factory workers. Can you imagine spending day after day after day, hunched over the same work table, doing your repetitive low-skill manual task? Deadly dull, and contributing nothing to you as a person. Whether simply to relieve the boredom or to bring people more into the mainstream of social and political events, someone is paid to read the paper to his fellow workers. That, to me, is an unusual but compelling measure of social cohesiveness.

Kerala is an interesting state for study. They have had a democratically elected communist government. Whether because of the political complexion of the government, or because of the attitudes of the population that led to the government, they have pursued economic policies that have been seen as anti-market. This may have something to do with the fact that incomes have not grown in Kerala as fast as in some other parts of India.[35] On one level, therefore, Kerala appears to be one of the poorest states of India. Yet if one examines the state's infant mortality rate − a sensitive indicator of poverty − a different picture emerges. In Kerala in 1990, this rate was 17 per 1,000 live births.[36] By contrast, the richest states of India, those with incomes in the top quarter, had infant mortality of 65 per 1,000; the poorest, in the bottom quarter, of 88 per 1,000.

Why do babies die in the first year of life in poor countries? A few will die for the same reasons they do in rich countries: congenital defects, rare inherited diseases, extreme prematurity, for example. As any parent will testify, whose extremely low-birth-weight baby has been saved from certain death by sophisticated neo-natal intensive care, such high-tech medical care makes a difference. In poor countries, far more babies will die from a combination of infections and malnutrition. Obviously, then, a clean water supply and an adequate supply of nutrition would help. But the best single intervention you could probably make is to educate women.

Look at the Kerala figures, in Table 7.3, that compare Kerala with other Indian states. The figures are for 1990.[37]

Table 7.3 Poverty indicators for Kerala and six other Indian states

	Infant mortality per 1,000 births	Female literacy (percentage)	Females married under age eighteen	Villages with medical facilities	Income ($1985)
Kerala	17	66	3	96	1144
Uttar Pradesh	99	15	20	12	959
Gujarat	72	31	4	28	1601
Tamil Nadu	59	36	9	33	1383
Karnataka	70	27	18	13	1255
Madyha Pradesh	111	15	31	6	1105
Rajasthan	84	11	35	17	1142

Source: Measham, Rao, Jamison, Wang, and Singh (1999) and Murthi Guio and Dreze (1995).

Of the five columns in this table, one does not favour Kerala: income is low even by the standard of Indian states. Kerala is well served in that a majority of villages have medical facilities. The other three sets of figures that favour Kerala are striking. Women in Kerala have much greater participation in education than in other Indian states, and are far less likely to be married off at less than eighteen than elsewhere in India. It is not too fanciful to speculate that a mother who is educated and over eighteen, however low her income, is more likely to take the steps needed to prevent her baby from dying. Therefore, there may be a direct connection between mother's education and low infant and child mortality.

Jack Caldwell, an Australian demographer intrigued by such instances of poor countries with good health, put to the test the importance of women's education.[38] He ranked a whole range of countries according to their gross national product per head. He then ranked countries according to their infant mortality rates. As expected, there was a high correlation: in general, the poorer the country the higher the infant mortality rate. He then focused on the exceptions: the countries with better infant mortality than you would predict from their level of income. The best predictor of such good performance was the level of women's education.

It is not difficult to see why there may be a direct causal relation between a mother's education and low infant mortality. But Kerala's paradoxically good health is not confined to infants. Life expectancy at birth is 76 for women and 70 for men.[39] This is a result both of low infant mortality and low mortality in adult life – much lower than in the rest of India. Education of women may be causally important, but may also indicate that women are highly valued. Let me put a suggestion. A society that invests socially in women as well as men is one that is more socially inclusive. Education, important in itself, is also part of social inclusion. Social inclusion will lead to better health. It is part of what Amartya Sen calls the 'support-led' approach to rapid reduction in mortality.

He contrasts two groups of countries that have had recent success in increasing their length and quality of life.[40] There are those with great economic success, such as South Korea and Taiwan, provided that such economic success raises the incomes of the poor and there is significant public expenditure, including public health and health care, education and social security. He calls this 'growth-mediated'. The second route to longer life, for which Kerala is an example, as are China and Sri Lanka, is the 'support-led'.

The support-led process does not operate through fast economic growth, but works through a program of skillful social support of health care, education and other relevant social arrangements.[41]

This may account, too, for the remarkably good health records of Costa Rica and Cuba. When I visited Costa Rica with my teenaged son, I thought I would show him examples of third-world poverty, such as I had seen in India or in the shanty towns of Manila. We saw none. Cuba, of course, has not been well loved by successive US governments, and for a related reason has been the darling of the left. Whether you think Castro a hero or a buffoon, the fact is that Cuba has remarkably good health at low cost – presumably because they fit into the 'support-led' model that Sen describes. (Sen would also argue that democracy is better for health than its lack.)

I am arguing that societies that are socially inclusive – whether they be rich like Japan, or relatively poor like Kerala and Costa Rica – have good health. Where might we find societies where whole swathes of people are relatively socially excluded? Our own back doors perhaps.

Unhealthy places

Calcutta after the rains, ankle-deep in filthy water, awash with sewage, people emerging dripping from the bits of bric-a-brac that pass for housing in the Calcutta shanty, children squatting in the gutter, with a large block of ice, chipping off pieces to add to a drink; sights, sounds, smells – all press in on you. This is an environment of poverty. You have little difficulty imagining it being bad for health. Dirty water and crowded unsanitary housing spell infection and disease. Bad environment – bad health.

Does bad environment mean bad health in rich countries? Drinking the water is safe; sewage does not run in streets; you can buy food in any part of town and expect it not to give you diarrhoea. In the Introduction to this book we went on a 'life-enhancing' metro journey from downtown Washington DC to suburban Maryland. People at the Montgomery County end live twenty years longer, on average, than those at the DC end. That is as dramatic a contrast as I can find in the space of a few miles.

In New York the contrast is nearly as great. Walk from Manhattan's museum district on Fifth Avenue – an impressive piece of expensive real estate – two miles north to Harlem. Go from shops where you can buy a jade vase or a hideously expensive modern painting to those where you might buy a Coke, cigarettes, or a newspaper, a cup of coffee or a doughnut. From the elegant apartments on Fifth Avenue to the slums of Harlem, life expectancy for men drops about fifteen years. Could this astonishing difference be due to the environment? At neither end does the environment resemble Calcutta. At neither end is there raw sewage or people chipping pieces off a dirty block of ice in the gutter. You could buy a hot dog from a street stand and not expect to get food poisoning. But the differences are in the elegant lobbies of the apartment blocks and uniformed doormen at the one end and the graffiti-daubed walls and the broken glass at the other; the well-dressed, purposeful people emerging to go about their day at the one end, and the young men in groups hanging around the street corners at the other. Do graffiti and broken glass on the streets cause disease?

The differences in the USA are more dramatic than others I know about from rich countries, but don't think such geographic differences are confined to America. If we continued our tour from Calcutta via New York and Washington DC to London, we would find dramatic differences. Take the underground train east from the wealthy City of London. Travel six stops. For each stop, life expectancy drops a year.

People die; places do not. One way of thinking about unhealthy places is that they are unhealthy because they are made up of a number of unhealthy people or, if not yet unhealthy, of people who are more likely to become ill. That would be an unhelpful and misleading explanation of why, when the water supply was full of bacteria, people who used that water were more likely to get ill. The illness was the result of the environment. It may be true that if some people in Calcutta drank Perrier, or other designer water, they would be less likely to get ill than those who drank what was available to them, but to blame their ill-health on their reluctance to drink Perrier is as absurd as it sounds. In the case of Calcutta, the environment of the unhealthy place causes the ill-health. But can the same be true of Harlem compared to Fifth Avenue? Here, where the grossest environmental degradations of dirty water and lack of sanitation are not the issue, the social environment is the crucial aspect that can affect health.

Where you are, or who you are?

American cities are not alone in causing illness. A report on social capital in Britain paints a picture of how living in certain neighbourhoods affects people. A young man who had grown up in a problem housing 'estate' (project housing) but had got out tells us what it is like:

> . . . living where people are pissing in the lifts and stuff like that. Living in that sort of environment drags you down sometimes, it's like everything is a drag. And when you come to an area that is nice, it sort of lifts your spirits really. So things like living in certain places can really depress you.
>
> Sometimes . . . it makes you get drawn into that sort of environment. So if you are living in an ugly environment, sometimes you act ugly. Like you don't care about where you're living, throw your rubbish out or whatever.[42]

Ugly environments are upsetting, so is lack of trust. The same youngsters that are pissing in the lifts are doing more. The following is from an older man living in a deprived area of Bolton in the North of England. He might be summarising the decline in social capital for Robert Putnam.

> People don't want to seem to be congregating together today with their neighbours, they just want to mind their own business, and a lot of that is to do with the youngsters that are roaming the street . . . a lot of people are trying to just come home and leave their house . . . worried what they might come home to.[43]

Young men are committing mayhem, leading older residents to be mistrustful of their environment. What about trust among the young men themselves? They considered that anyone who was trusting was ostracised as a fool.

> I trust my work mates more than my close mates. I've experienced what they've done with each other, I've watched as they've slagged each other off to me, and I think, you know, I'll not say anything to

this guy cos he'll go and tell him, so I just keep it hush hush, I don't tell
'em much. I'd never trust anyone else, not in this area . . . A lot are
drug-dealers who would rob you, it's as simple as that, they would do
anything to get in your house. They would backstab you . . . they will
just turn around and rob you.[44]

The feeling that although 'there's a lot of nice people . . . there's more
of them are scumbags' amounted to a reduction in trust, a general
suspicion, which limited interaction between neighbours.

None of us has difficulty in recognising that these accounts
correspond to our own feelings about wandering into a neighbourhood marked by young people running wild, or threatening-looking
young men doing we don't know what on street corners.

The fact that we find ugly and scary environments ugly and scary
does not, by itself, mean that they are damaging health, to the extent of
a fifteen-year drop in life expectancy; but these environments do matter
for health. The scariness may be more important than the ugliness. In
reaching that conclusion the central issue has been to separate the
differences between environments from the differences between people
who live in those environments; separating where you are from who
you are. A deprived area is more likely to have deprived people living
there. The challenge has been to show that the environment matters for
health over and above the characteristics of its residents.

There is no question that the characteristics of people are important,
but these are not intrinsic properties of the individual; much of what
matters for health comes from the environment. For example, in
comparing life expectancy of black and white men in New York, I am
attributing nothing to 'blackness'. In the Bronx in New York, for
example, life expectancy for black men is 65, and for white men 63.
The blacks do extremely badly and the whites do worse.

We saw that in the case of international migrants, such as the
Japanese, when they migrate their rates of disease change. This points
to the importance of environment. It is different, however, when one
examines neighbourhoods within a country. When people leave a poor
neighbourhood, it is usually because their personal circumstances have
changed. If leavers have better health than stayers, one could argue it is
not because they moved to a more salubrious environment but because

they became richer. Going the other way, if enough high-status people move into a deprived inner city area, average health might improve. This may not mean that gentrification, having camembert for sale in the shops and twee coffee houses, improves health, but that average health improves because richer people with their better health have displaced poorer people with their worse health.

In reaching the conclusion that the social environment of areas matters we have to take account of the obvious: rich people live in rich areas, poor people live in poor areas, and the rest of us live somewhere in between. The evidence now shows clearly, that after you take into account personal characteristics of residents, the less deprived the community the better the health of residents.[45] As with so many other things we have seen it shows itself as a gradient. I presented the contrasts between Fifth Avenue and Harlem, between Washington DC and neighbouring Montgomery County because they are so dramatic, but the reality is not only the contrast between rich and poor, but the graded nature of the relation in between.

There appears to be a kind of double jeopardy going on here. If you are lower in status, your health suffers. If, in addition, you live in a more deprived area, your health suffers even more.

This relation between areas and health is important. It suggests that although it may not be the graffiti and broken glass themselves that worsen health, they and the young men hanging around on street corners do mark out characteristics of places that lead to worse health. It is somewhat artificial to try and separate places from people, since part of what makes up a place is the people who live there. We see the same in schools. If a school has a few disruptive pupils, they are unlikely to have too much effect on the learning of the rest. If, however, the school has a high concentration of disruptive pupils, the climate of the school changes. It now becomes likely that the 'normal' child will do worse in such a school than he would have in a school that consisted mainly of non-disruptive children. Other people create the environment.

The social environment can become more than the sum of the individual characteristics of the individuals who live there. To some, this idea sounds spookily as though we were back in the world of miasmas – mysterious somethings in the ether that affected health. How can the whole be more than the sum of the parts? We are used to thinking this way about infectious disease. Take the concept of herd immunity. Suppose you were worried about the safety of whooping-cough vaccine; worried that if your child were immunised she might suffer side-effects, albeit these are highly uncommon. The safest option for your child is for all other children to be immunised. If a sufficiently high proportion of individuals is immune, the person-to-person transmission of infectious disease cannot be sustained. Therefore, although your child was not immune personally, her risk within the community would be low because of herd immunity. Herd immunity is a property of the collective, not simply of the individuals. If this emergent property idea still sounds strange, think of it as a non-linear effect. If the prevalence of immune people rises from 20 per cent to 30 per cent the chance of your child being infected falls a small amount. But when the prevalence of immunity rises above a threshold such that transmission is interrupted, your non-immunised child's chances of being infected fall to zero.

There are some fairly obvious candidates to explain why the areas of our cities might be important for health. If home or workplace is hazardous because of lead paint peeling off walls, unsafe stairs and probability of fires, there will be real health risks. Important as these are, they have very little to do with the dramatically different life expectation in Harlem or Washington compared to uptown or Montgomery County. The major contributors to premature loss of life in the deprived areas are coronary heart disease, violent deaths and the consequences of HIV infection.[46]

A second way areas can be important is in the infrastructure.[47] In parts of Glasgow in Scotland, you could not buy healthy food even if you wanted to. In such areas, there is not enough money in it for the retailers to bother putting in a supermarket, with a rich supply of fresh fruit and vegetables. If there is no public transport, and people do not have cars, their access is limited. The social infrastructure does not allow full participation in society, whether it is healthy food and sports facilities, amenities such as doctor's surgeries and communal facilities, or transport to go somewhere where these things are to be found.

Social capital

There is a third, perhaps more important, way that area can be linked to health: through the degree of social integration, or social capital. The people I quoted earlier from the UK report on social capital have their equivalents from US studies.[48] Differences in social capital can contribute to these differences in health between areas.

One of the researchers to take on this question has been Ichiro Kawachi of Harvard University. He investigated the marked variation in mortality by state in the US. In Chapter 3, we noted that states with greater inequality of income had higher rates of mortality. To ask whether this could be linked to social capital, he had to come up with measures. He used three questions that were included in a general social survey in the US. The first was social mistrust: 'Generally speaking, would you say that most people can be trusted or that you can't be too careful in dealing with people?'; the second was perceived lack of fairness: 'Do you think most people would try to take advantage of you if they got a chance, or would they try to be fair?'; the third, perceived helpfulness: 'Would you say that most of the time people try to be helpful, or are they mostly looking out for themselves?' In addition they assessed level of civic engagement as the per capita number of groups and associations to which residents belonged.[49]

The state score comes from averaging the responses of individuals for that state. This social capital score can then be linked with other characteristics of that state. The dominant finding is that trust and community involvement go down as income inequality rises. The more unequal the income, the less trust, perceived fairness, perceived helpfulness or civic engagement. Putnam raises the question of which came first. Did the lack of social engagement lead to income inequality or the reverse? His answer is that they reinforce each other, and that 'efforts to strengthen social capital should go hand in hand with efforts to increase equality'.[50]

The next step for Kawachi and colleagues was to show, statistically, that the most likely relation among these measures is that income inequality is related to mortality largely because of its relation with social capital. Low social capital seems to provide the pathway by which income inequality is related to mortality. My health is affected not only by my own standing in society, and all that that relates to, but by the characteristics of the individuals who live around me and whether there is a climate of trust, helpfulness and civic engagement engendered by those individuals.

The link with the social gradient is that people are no more randomly assigned to neighbourhoods than they are to levels of social status. Having said that social capital may affect health regardless of whether you are rich, poor, or something in between, the chances of living in an area of low social capital is greater the lower you are in the hierarchy. Just as individual social status is related to richness of social networks, so an extra hazard of being low social status is living in an area characterised by low social capital.

The research summarised in this chapter is radical and far-reaching. Places matter. Not only because of the ravages of an impoverished infrastructure that fails to deliver the material conditions for good health, but because of the social environment. It is not only a bit unfortunate to live in an insalubrious area, but it is bad for health. Although poor people live in poor areas, the evidence points strongly to multiple disadvantages. It is worse for health to be low-status and live in an area characterised by low trust and low social cohesion. Part of the reason for the link with health will be low investment in infrastructure: transport, shops and other amenities. These in turn will affect social participation. 'Social capital' is a useful term to cover lack of the important social relations between people at the level of whole communities. It reminds us how important it is that we lift our focus from the individual to the community.

Societies that are characterised by social cohesion, whether rich like Japan, poor like Kerala, or somewhere in between like Costa Rica, have better health than others with the same wealth but less social cohesion. These are success stories. In the next chapter, we shall take up the question of whole societies that are characterised by low control and low cohesion, where health has suffered badly.

8. THE MISSING MEN OF RUSSIA

A newspaperman had me on the phone a few days ago . . . and he wanted a statement about plant life and the radiation level increasing. And also dioxin and other harmful wastes. He was challenging about it. Well – I agreed it was bad. But in the end I said, 'It's terribly serious, of course, but I think more people die of heartbreak than of radiation.'

Saul Bellow, More Die of Heartbreak[1]

During the communist era Hungarians specialised in anti-Soviet jokes, delivered with a glance over the shoulder. One had Brezhnev, the Soviet leader, surveying the misery of the Russian people and asking the Hungarian prime minister why the Hungarians were so happy.

'It's Eckstein,' he was told.

'Eckstein?'

'Yes. Eckstein is a comedian. He tells jokes and makes Hungarians laugh.'

'Send Eckstein to Moscow,' growled Brezhnev. When Eckstein arrived, Brezhnev told him he would give him some background:

'We have had a socialist paradise in the Soviet Union for thirty years longer than Hungary.' Eckstein interrupted:

'Who is telling the jokes? You or me?'

Now there is a new joke, told by unemployed factory workers in the former communist countries of Eastern Europe: the worst thing about communism is post-communism. It has a grim truth to it. In the 1920s, famine and forced collectivisation of the land of the Kulaks in Russia, Ukraine and Belarus led to an estimated 9 million deaths.[2] In the decade after the collapse of communism, 1989–99, there were an estimated 4 million *excess* deaths, i.e. over and above what would have been expected from the historical trend. What happened to the health of the people of the former Soviet Union when their country and their certainties collapsed was of the same order of magnitude as the ravages of famine or war. Russians were unhealthy under communism; even more so after it.

The dramatic changes in health in the former communist countries of Europe, not just in Russia, are of great importance, not only if you are a Russian, Hungarian or Pole; not only if you are a concerned citizen of the world who worries about the survival of the Siberian leopard, the preservation of Alaskan wilderness or alleviation of world poverty; but also if you are a comfortable resident of Minneapolis, Manchester or Mannheim wondering why your health is not as good as people above you in the hierarchy. Its relevance is that it shines a bright light, from a different angle, on the theory that I am laying out.

I have been constructing the case that the degree to which you have control over your life and your opportunities to participate fully in society are powerful determinants of health, quality and length of life. The unequal distribution of these vital resources for living is an important contributor to the status syndrome. My case draws on evidence from monkeys and apes, from Keralans and Costa Ricans, Japanese and Cubans, US blacks and whites, civil servants and Swedish graduates, Oscar winners and polar explorers. It includes animal experiments, psychological studies in the lab, and large-scale population studies.

In the eyes of some, all this evidence is circumstantial because they see the essence of science as experiments. An experiment would determine whether my theory is correct rather than some of the many competing theories that I have been examining as I laid out the evidence. To see why the usual type of experiment would not solve my problem, but the study of East Europeans might, look at an example that is much simpler than the link to health of control and participation.

Could eating watercress cause leukaemia? Compare people who eat watercress with those who don't. But the watercress eaters may be different in other ways. Perhaps they are English ladies taking tea from silver teapots, eating watercress sandwiches on the manicured lawns of stately homes. Should I compare them with people eating bacon-and-egg sandwiches in the Dog and Duck pub? Too many differences, hard to sort out? Do an experiment. Expose some people to watercress, and have a control group who are not exposed and see who gets leukaemia. Two small problems with this experiment: it is unethical and impractical. If you really thought that watercress causes leukaemia, you would have to expose people to a potential carcinogen for years, and you would have to expose large numbers and make sure they stuck to their diet. If, like me, you did not think watercress caused leukaemia, you wouldn't have an ethical problem but then you wouldn't bother to do such a cumbersome experiment. You would only want to do it if you thought watercress was likely to kill people, but then you wouldn't want to do it. Problem. You could go the other way. If you could find enough watercress eaters, get half to stop and then follow them for long enough to see if the ones who stopped were less likely to develop leukaemia, assuming of course that they stopped in time. Huge numbers, much expense.

If the essence of science is experiments we are in real trouble with understanding causes of disease in human populations. Most of the experiments we would want to do are unethical and impractical. It is quite impossible to conduct a large-scale experiment in which people are deprived of control over their lives and opportunities to participate. This is so, whether the experiment is giving more control or taking it away.

However, an approximation to such experiments has been conducted on a grand scale, and dramatically, in Central and Eastern Europe and the countries of the former Soviet Union. Since World War II, these countries went from cleaning up the debris of the war, to a situation of restriction of freedom to live and to consume, to one where there is food in the shops but only some people can afford to buy it.

Just as we examined societies whose health improvement was impressive, such as Japan, to learn the importance of social cohesion, so we can look at societies that have suffered to try and learn lessons from their experience. Such explorations shed light on the reasons for the social gradients in health. The hypotheses that I have laid out, low control and lack of participation, find ample support in these countries. What may be responsible for the health gradient within a country may be responsible for ill-health of a whole country. Good for my theory; bad for the people who have had their lives blighted.

An Austrian and a Hungarian – an empire divided

Istvan was admitted to hospital in Budapest with a heart attack. He survived the acute attack, was given a cocktail of pharmaceuticals, and had time to reflect. His first reflection was that in a way he was not surprised. At sixty-five, he did not expect to be healthy. Most of the men he knew were not: they were either not alive or not healthy. He had been to a school reunion on his sixtieth birthday. Of the people he had been to school with at age fifteen, about 30 per cent had died before their sixtieth birthday, and several more had died in the few years since.[3] He might have reflected, had he known the figures, that his chance of limping through to retirement in Russia would have been even less. On today's figures, the chance of a fifteen-year-old boy in Russia dying before his sixtieth birthday is 43 per cent – about what it is in Guinea and worse than in the Sudan and Senegal and most countries outside Africa.

Istvan and his companions had spent a good part of the last decades drinking home-brewed palinka (spirits) Two of his drinking companions had had close brushes with death from alcoholic liver disease, but that acted as little deterrent to the rest of them. One had died in strange circumstances after one of their drinking bouts. He fell from a bridge, and it was unclear whether he had committed suicide or fallen in a drunken stupor or a bit of both. He had been depressed.

In addition to the drinking, even Istvan had to admit he was overweight, not to say obese. He had the ample middle-aged midriff that men of his class expected to have at sixty-five. Why would it be any different? Was that not how you were supposed to look at that age, if you survived at all? He had no pretensions to be a television actor or a footballer. He had vaguely heard the idea that smoking was bad for health. As he did not expect to be alive at sixty-five anyway, he couldn't see why he should bother his head with that. After the social and economic changes of 1989, he had even heard people wittering on about the unhealthy Hungarian diet. His thought about that was similar to his thought about smoking. Large proportions of the people he knew were dropping dead before they reached retirement age. What was the point of worrying about whether his goulash had too much fat or salt? If the

Austrians, a little way up the Danube, wanted to worry about it, let them. It was not for him.

It occurred to him to wonder how things might have been different had there still been an Austro-Hungarian empire or if, when the split came, he had ended up on the other side of the border. Suppose he had been Franz, an Austrian in Vienna, rather than Istvan, a Hungarian on the outskirts of Budapest. The most obvious difference between Franz and Istvan is that for Franz at sixty-five, disease would have been much less the norm than for Istvan. By the time of his sixtieth-birthday school reunion, only 12 per cent of Franz's schoolmates would have died, compared to 30 per cent of those of Istvan. (If he had gone further to the West, the figures would have been even more favourable: 10 per cent in the Netherlands, 9 per cent in Sweden; the US lags, as usual, with 15 per cent). There is a two-and-a-half times greater chance of death by age sixty for a man on the Hungarian side of the Austria–Hungary border than on the Austrian side.

It was not always thus. After World War II, health improved steadily for the people of Hungary as it did for those of Austria. For a Hungarian, as for a Czech, a Slovak or a Pole, things got better after the war. The postwar chaos was cleaned up. Under the new communist regimes, in the 1950s and 1960s, people were fed, housed, educated, clothed, employed, and the elderly were looked after. It is not surprising to me that with this set of social arrangements, health should improve. It did.

Figure 8.1 shows life expectancy in Europe from 1970 to 2001 for groups of countries. These are graphs my colleague Martin Bobak and I drew up from statistics reported by the World Health Organization. Here we have done something different with the calculation of life expectancy. We have removed the first fifteen years of life, in order to remove the effect on life expectancy of deaths in infancy and child-hood. Such deaths, although more common in the East than the West, were not where the disadvantage for the East really showed up; it was in mortality at later ages.

The figures are striking. In the 1970s life expectancy was favourable in the European Union (EU) countries, compared to the then communist countries, but the differences were small compared to what happened during the 1980s and 1990s. The European Union

Figure 8.1 Life expectancy at age 15 in Europe for the years 1970–2001

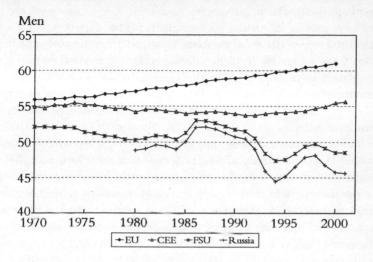

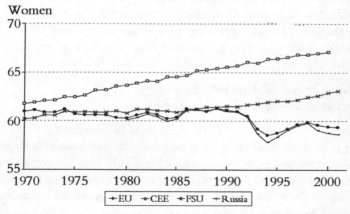

Note: The graphs show life expectancy at age 15 for men (top) and women (bottom) in Europe for the years 1970–2001. EU = the countries that now make up the European Union; CEE = former communist countries of Central and Eastern Europe; FSU = former Soviet Union. Subsequently, figures became available for Russia, the biggest country in the former Soviet Union. Life expectancy at fifteen is not directly affected by infant and child mortality.

Source: Adapted from Marmot and Bobak (2000), data from WHO, Health for All database.

countries had an improvement year on year: life expectancy at fifteen just kept rising. The improvement amounted to five years – which, as we have seen, is substantial. At the same time, life expectancy in CEE stagnated or even declined by about a year, and then slowly picked up after 1990, so that by 2001, the life-expectancy gap between East and West had increased to six years. Women in the East also suffered compared to those in the West although, by the end of the period, the life-expectancy gap was four years – a smaller disadvantage than men experienced.

The former Soviet Union life-expectancy graph looks like a roller-coaster. Life expectancy at fifteen declined in the 1970s and 1980s. Some observers attribute the dramatic improvement in the mid 1980s to the success of President Gorbachev's anti-alcohol campaign. The tragic plunge in life expectancy of about seven years after 1989 has little parallel in modern history. Life expectancy started to pick up in the second half of the 1990s. The decline in 1998 corresponds to the rouble crisis. By the end of this breathless voyage, the difference in life expectancy at fifteen years old between Russia and the EU is a staggering fifteen years for men, eight years for women.

This ghastly natural experiment screams out for explanation.

Where have all the young (and not-so-young) men gone?

Amartya Sen devised a very simple way of demonstrating that some countries of the world treat women badly.[4] In populations with good health, there are more women than men. Women are the stronger part of the species biologically. Hence in Europe and North America the ratio of women to men is about 1.05. In countries of Asia and North Africa, however, the ratio can be much lower: 0.95 in Egypt, 0.94 in Bangladesh and China, and 0.9 in Pakistan. He calls this 'the missing women'.

In Central and Eastern Europe, we have the opposite problem: missing men.[5] The life-expectancy gap across Europe is greater for men than women. Therefore, the disadvantage in the East can be shown by looking at the ratio of men to women for different countries. The peak age of mortality disadvantage in East versus West was middle age, so we simply plotted the ratio of men to women in the age range 45–64. These figures are shown in Figure 8.2. The first dramatic contrast is: no overlap between East and West. All the countries of Western Europe have more men per 100 women than do the countries of the East. For example, in Germany for every 100 women aged 45–64, there are nearly 100 men. In Russia the figure is 84 men for every 100 women.

Figure 8.2 Ratio of men to women aged 45–64 in countries of Western and Eastern Europe

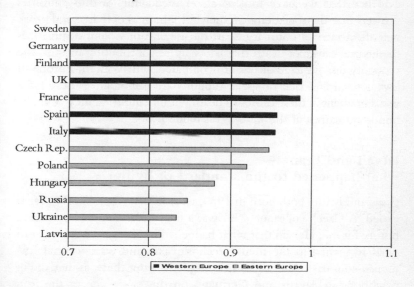

Source: Marmot and Bobak (2000).

In a survey we did in Russia of women aged 45–64, a quarter were widowed. This figure was twice as high as in Poland, which in turn was higher than in Western countries. The toll of premature mortality affecting primarily middle-aged men cannot be exaggerated.

Saul Bellow's character, a scientist, says that more people die of heartbreak than radiation. He could certainly have been referring to the Ukraine and Russia. Chernobyl was a calamity – the release of radiation from a nuclear reactor. It devastated the local town, and a deadly cloud drifted across Western Europe. Yet the disease and suffering it may have caused pales alongside the medical causes of the premature loss of life in Ukraine, Russia and other countries, such as Lithuania, Estonia and the Central Asian countries that made up the former Soviet Union. About half the difference in life expectancy between all the Eastern countries and Western Europe is due to cardiovascular disease, and another 20 per cent is the result of accidents and violence.

Coronary heart disease and violent deaths are both 'causes of death' that, within countries, are closely linked with the social gradient. The evidence that we have looked at on inequalities within countries showed that the social environment in which people live and work will affect rates of coronary heart disease and of violent deaths. It is these same causes of death that show up as contributing most to the mortality disadvantage of Eastern compared with Western Europe. If low control and lack of social supports are important causes of the social gradient in these causes of death within countries, they could be important causes of the East–West difference.

Istvan and Franz –
what happened to the standard of living?

Franz and Istvan, both born in 1930, were fifteen when World War II ended. A Czech colleague who was a little older summed up recent history for me. He said that what happened in Hungary was similar to what happened in the then Czechoslovakia and other central European countries. After the war, things got better there, as they did in neighbouring Austria and Germany on the other side of the iron curtain. As described above, basic needs were met. Despite being relatively poor in monetary terms, conditions improved so that good nutrition and education led to low infant mortality. Housing often came with jobs that were stable and guaranteed. Older people were looked after. There was Stalinist political repression, but that mostly affected the elites.

He said that he remembered the year in the 1960s when gross national product stopped rising. Istvan in Hungary, or Marek in Czechoslovakia, could watch Austrian or German television and see what they were missing. Vienna may be only a couple of hundred kilometres up the

Danube from Budapest, but the living standards of the Austrians might have been from another planet. Istvan's chance of running a car that did not break down, having the 'usual' panoply of consumer goods, having a holiday on the Italian Riviera, seemed to be about the same as Hungary winning the World Cup – a bit less, actually.

The feeling swelled up that if communist governments had been delivering the goods after the war, they were no longer. Hungary had had their revolution against the Russians in 1956 and another was not in prospect – hence no change was on the horizon. In Czechoslovakia, the dissatisfaction with what people had rose. The demand for more – more freedom, more democracy, higher standard of living – culminated in the Prague Spring of 1968, an open surge of dissatisfaction with the way things were and of optimism that they would change under Czech leader Dubcek. This uprising, in turn, led to the Russian tanks and Soviet domination which lasted until communism collapsed in 1989.

When my Czech colleague heard us discussing imbalance between efforts and reward as a cause of heart disease, he sprang to his feet. 'That exactly described our situation post-1968,' he cried. It did not matter how much effort people put into things, there was always the feeling that the wrong people were rewarded.

If most Hungarians were equally poorly off during the communist period, there is an interesting scientific opportunity. If there were inequalities in health despite relatively narrow spread of income this might give us a further clue as to which aspects of social position were most important in generating health inequalities. We have noted in the West that, in general, poorer people have had less education, have worse jobs, and live in less attractive neighbourhoods. It is therefore difficult to distinguish the effect of income from those of other characteristics that mark out social status. In the communist countries of Europe, identifying social status was much less straightforward. These different measures of status did not correlate so highly. Heroes of socialist labour might have been bricklayers or factory workers. But this was propaganda. That did not, of course, mean that all bricklayers felt themselves superior to doctors and engineers.

Such data as we have from that time suggests that there were differences in mortality according to people's education. In a study we did in the Czech Republic right after the Velvet Revolution of 1989, we showed that people of low education had higher heart-disease risk than those of higher – very similar to results from Western countries. Interestingly, markers of material well-being were not related to heart-disease risk. The relation with social status was with education.[6]

Istvan was poor during the communist period in that he had few consumer goods, but so was everybody else. There were more consumer goods in Hungary than in some of the other communist countries, but nothing like the amount in Austria, a few kilometres away. Things changed after the collapse of communism. Istvan had had a boring low-paid job ('they pretend to pay us and we pretend to work') in a state-run enterprise. With the economy of Hungary having to cope with dramatic adjustment to the global market economy, there was a big shakedown and Istvan found himself out of work and in serious financial difficulties. He found work, first as a waiter and then part-time as an attendant in a parking lot.

Istvan was not alone in feeling poorer. Gross national product per capita declined in Hungary by more than 10 per cent between 1989 and 1997. It was worse in other countries. In Russia the decline was greater than 40 per cent; in Turkmenistan greater than 50 per cent; and in the Ukraine greater than 60 per cent.[7] By contrast, the economic outlook was a little better in Poland and the Czech Republic with small increases in GNP over the period.

It was not only feeling poor that bothered Istvan but the big changes that were happening around him. Now there were desirable consumer goods in the shops, but Istvan could not afford them. Before he had enough money but there was nothing to do with it, now there was lots to do with it, but no money to do it with. As far as Istvan could see, they were becoming a society of haves and have-nots: better things to have, but only some could have them.

In Russia, the newly rich that have benefited from the change are known as 'new Russians'. They build country dachas that look like housing out of a new development in an American suburb. A store I visited in Novosibirsk in Siberia was selling international-brand running shoes for hundreds of dollars. How could a doctor making $70 a month buy a pair of running shoes that cost $190, I wanted to know. The answer is that they cannot. These are for new Russians.

The figures on income inequality bear out Istvan's impression of growing disparities. What little information we have on how income was distributed during the communist time suggests relatively narrow income distribution. Figures for income inequality in the early years after communism collapsed showed that income inequalities were relatively narrow, but increased rapidly. The Gini coefficient is a commonly used measure of income inequality. A Gini of 0 means that everyone has the same income; a Gini of 100 means maximum inequality: the higher the Gini the greater the inequality. Figures from UNICEF show that in 1996 the average Gini for rich OECD countries was 33. Hungary went from a Gini of 21 in 1989 to 33 in 1996; the Czech Republic went from 19 to 28; Poland from 25 to 29; Lithuania from 28 to 35; Russia from 26 to a massive 48.

This situation is quite alarming. At the same time as gross national product was plummeting all across the former Soviet Union, income inequality was growing rapidly. Some people were getting rich, but it was having very little benefit for the rest of the society. By using health as our social accountant, our marker of well-being, we can see clearly that the effect was negative. When we compared countries of Central and Eastern Europe, the greater the increase in income inequality between 1989 and 1996, the greater the increase in mortality rates.[8]

The health picture in Central and Eastern Europe and in the countries of the former Soviet Union confirms the conclusions we reached in Chapters 3 and 4 about the degree to which income is important for health and the role of relative position. Infant and child mortality are the health indicators that are most sensitive to material deprivation. These were preserved, at low levels, to a remarkable degree during the communist period. They were, indeed, much lower than would have been predicted from the level of gross national product in those countries.

The benchmark, as usual, is Japan, where the chance that a male baby will die before the age of five is 5 per 1,000, and of a female baby dying is 4 per 1,000; in Sweden the figures are 5 and 3. At the other end of the spectrum there is Sierra Leone, where the chance of death before age five is 292 per 1,000 for boys and 265 for girls. On this spectrum, Hungary looks a good deal more like Sweden or Japan than it does like Africa, with figures of 11 and 8 per 1,000. In Russia, the corresponding figures were 23 for boys and 17 for girls.

The low infant and child mortality is a powerful argument that poverty, defined as lack of material conditions for good health, is not the explanation of the health crisis in Central and Eastern European countries. These countries and those in the former Soviet Union therefore illustrate a unique phenomenon. In childhood their health records look close to, albeit not quite as good as, those of the prosperous West. Yet for adult men, their health records look as bad as, or worse than, those of many poor countries. There is a vitally important difference. The health problems in 'eastern' Europe are not those we associate with third world-style material deprivation. In the poor countries of Africa, people are dying of tuberculosis, AIDS and other infectious diseases. In these Eastern European countries, they are dying of heart disease and violent deaths.

These causes of death are important contributors to the status syndrome in Western countries. It adds fuel to my argument that examining the determinants of the health crisis in Eastern Europe will help understand the social gradient in health within Western countries as well as within these Eastern ones.

To understand how the cataclysmic social and economic changes affected health in these countries, let us look in more detail at lives on both sides of the Austrian–Hungarian border

Istvan – him, indoors

At the time of his heart attack, Istvan was living alone. He and his wife, Vera, had had marital troubles since the 1980s, when it seemed that their dire situation would last forever. After a day at his low-paid job he indulged in one of two activities; getting jealous watching Austrian television; or, disgruntled and unhappy, drinking with other disgruntled men.

Meanwhile, Istvan's wife Vera was keeping it together, with a struggle. She worked as a clerk in the state bank. She was a good deal busier after work. To get what she needed for her family to function she worked her networks. Whether it was a doctor's appointment at the clinic, getting the car fixed, having her application for a new flat processed, or simply obtaining some fresh fruit, she could achieve none of this without operating her informal networks. When she returned to their flat, she cared for their children, cooked, cleaned and kept the family functional. She was usually at this activity when Istvan went out for his regular drinking sessions.

After the communist government collapsed in 1989, when Istvan lost his job, Vera's patience ran out. It was enough that she was the sole breadwinner, the sole keeper of the family, and lacking in companionship from her spouse. Istvan was one more problem that she could happily do without. She kicked him out. Eventually he found part-time work as a security guard on a parking station, and found himself sleeping on the couch in a one-bedroom flat that belonged to a female companion. In his suburb, on the outskirts of Budapest, unemployment was high and crime was rife.

The contrast with Franz across the border in Austria was sharp. Starting in the 1960s, and increasing until the present, Franz had a reliable German car, foreign consumer goods, and travelled abroad on holidays. Imported fruit and vegetables meant that he could eat healthily all year round. Franz, despite himself, became health-conscious. There were some early sightings of joggers, a few sports clubs, and before he knew where he was, Franz was surrounded by people who seemed to care about their appearance and health.

Franz took planned retirement at sixty-five from his firm, and he and his wife looked forward to life on a comfortable pension, holidays with the grandchildren. When a visiting American cousin asked about his private store of wealth, Franz told him of his modest accumulation. The American asked how he could cope with unexpected shocks. Franz was mystified. He had a guaranteed pension. If he got sick, he would be looked after by the social-security health system. His house was paid for. No one would sue him for anything. His children had been to university and were now financially independent. What shocks?

Him alone

I asked, where have all the young men gone? Strictly, I should have lamented: where have all the unmarried men gone? It is they who were most affected by the mortality rise of the 1970s and 1980s in Central and Eastern European countries. It wasn't that being unmarried dropped out of fashion, unmarried men dropped out of existence. They died.

A riveting feature of the rise in mortality that affected middle-aged men in Central and Eastern European countries was that it most affected men who were single, widowed or divorced. In Chapter 6, we reviewed the evidence that marriage protects men and women. It reduces their risk of developing major disease and of premature death. I pointed to this as an example of the protective effect of social supports. Some, but not all, studies showed men to be more protected by marriage than women. The relative protection depended on circumstances. In Hungary, Poland and the Czech Republic, as in Western countries, married men have always had lower mortality than men who are single, widowed or divorced. Married women have had lower mortality than unmarried. However, as mortality rose through the 1970s, and 1980s and past the economic transition of 1989, the mortality of unmarried men rose faster than that of married. In other words, the advantage of being married increased among men. Married women had always had the mortality advantage over unmarried, but, in contrast to the men, the magnitude of that advantage did not increase.

Istvan is typical. Istvan's wife Vera had her social networks. They were her survival mechanism. When Istvan lost his marriage and family, he became socially isolated. When he lost his job, Istvan lost a role and a connection with the wider world. Our study of heart attacks in the Czech Republic confirms that men with fewer social supports have higher risk of heart attack.[9]

One of my key hypotheses was that lack of opportunity for full social participation was important for health and would be important in generating the social gradient in health within countries. It also appears to be playing an important role in generating the health disadvantage of the countries of Central and Eastern Europe.

One way of depriving people of full social participation is by depriving them of a social role and isolating them socially. Another is to deprive them of the 'necessaries' in the Adam Smith sense of 'whatever the custom of the country renders it indecent for creditable people in the lowest order to be without'. I have suggested that lack of material possessions may be important for health, *in people above the poverty threshold*, not because it deprived people of the means for the support of life, but because it reduced social participation.

Our studies in Hungary and Poland provide strong evidence in support of this Adam Smith concept of necessaries.[10] We asked people which of a number of material possessions they had in their household. We then grouped these into three categories. First, basic items: without these, life would physically be a great deal harder. In this category, we placed washing machine, refrigerator, freezer, microwave and telephone. Second, socially oriented items: objects that were not quite as basic for living, but did help with keeping in touch with the world: a colour television, radio/cassette recorder, stereo system, motorcycle, car, car radio. Third, luxury items: my teenage son may have thought that cable television was a basic necessity, but we still put it in the luxury category along with satellite TV, video recorder, video camera, CD player, personal computer, dishwasher, garden, dacha (holiday home).

Each group of items showed a strong relationship to health. The more basic items, the better the health; and similarly for socially oriented items, and for luxury items. The more socially oriented and luxury items they have, the more people are participating in society without shame, and the more they benefit from what the society has to offer materially.

This approach to what material possessions mean harks back to the discussion on conspicuous consumption – goods signal something to the outside world. In addition, having a car may be more than a signal to others, it might crucially relate to feelings about yourself. Studies in Britain have shown that people who have access to a car have lower mortality rates than those who do not.[11] Similarly, people who own their own home have lower mortality rates than those who do not. This prediction of mortality is in addition to measures of their socioeconomic position, based on occupation. These associations have been interpreted as wealth measures being good for health. There is another interpretation that is closer to the perspective of our studies in Central and Eastern Europe.

A study in Glasgow, drawing on the work of Antony Giddens,[12] suggested that cars and houses may contribute to what he terms 'ontological security', which is:[13]

'The confidence that most human beings have in the continuity of their self identity and the constancy of their social and material environments. Basic to a feeling of ontological security is a sense of the reliability of persons and things.'[14] For Giddens, ontological security is about continuity and having trust in the world. It is a deep concept about people having confidence in the social order, in their place in society, in their won right to be themselves, and a belief that their self-realisation can be achieved.[15]

Trust, continuity: ontological security appears to be the individual equivalent of social capital. In their Glasgow studies, Rosemary Hiscock and colleagues suggest that having a car and owning a home confer the psychosocial benefits of protection, autonomy and prestige. These are linked. A feeling of protection helps to foster autonomy, which in turn will relate to better health. Perhaps the Hungarians and Poles who have more 'things' gain thereby an enhanced sense of ontological security. At a more prosaic level, the society is working better for them than for those who want these things, now that they are available, but cannot have them.

I said that there were two psychosocial features that may account for poor health in Central and Eastern Europe: social participation and control. The discussion on ontological security suggests the link. Being a full participant in society does give one autonomy and a sense of control over one's life.

Control

When, in the 1980s, I used to meet colleagues from communist countries in Europe, they used the term 'command economy' to describe their own economic system as opposed to the market-based system of the West. The very term 'command economy' makes clear that the individual consumer or worker is not sovereign. In the West, I fear we exaggerate the degree of autonomy the market confers. Little money means little choice. But whatever the defects of the market-based system – and the degree of inequality that gives rise to the social gradient in health is a major one – it allows a good deal more personal freedom than did the command economies of communist Europe.

Istvan's history demonstrates that lives under the communist system were characterised by low control. When Istvan's life situation deteriorated after the collapse of communism, in a real sense, his power to affect what happened in his life was quite limited. There is direct evidence that lack of control is important for health. The evidence that we shall look at shows that this damaged health in Eastern Europe along with other reasons why Istvan's health was bad. His friends were dropping with chronic liver disease, he was over-weight, unfit, a smoker, and his diet was a health educator's night-mare.

Doing cross-cultural research is not straightforward. There are conceptual as well as linguistic differences between cultures. The 'same' question in two different cultures may be interpreted in two different ways. When we went to look at the question of low control at work in our study of heart attacks in the Czech Republic, in one sense, we did everything wrong. We simply took a questionnaire on people's descriptions of their work that we had used in the Whitehall II study of British civil servants, translated into Czech, and adminis-tered it. Good research practice dictates that a questionnaire should be piloted in the new culture, then back translated into English to check on the translation, and then validated – to show that it means what we think it means. We did none of that initially and yet, to our surprise, in a representative sample of men in the Czech Republic, as in British civil servants, the less the control men had over their work conditions the greater their risk of coronary heart disease.[16] Men with least control had twice the risk of heart attacks of men with most control. Careful analysis showed that this could not be attributed to more smoking, higher plasma cholesterol, higher blood pressure, or greater obesity in the men with low control.

It is not only in the sphere of work that Istvan had low control but everywhere he looked. In order to study this we needed measures of degree of control. Based on the rich psychological literature on control and self-efficacy, we developed some simple measures. Richard Rose, a political scientist from Glasgow has been conducting a series of studies in Russia and elsewhere on people's attitudes to the social and political changes. We added a few questions to these surveys: on health and on perceived control. The control questions asked people about the degree of control they felt they had at home, about whether what happened to them was beyond their control, whether they expected positive experiences to outnumber negative in the future, fair treatment, whether in the past ten years they could predict the changes that happened to them; whether they were still trying to make improvements in their life. There were also three questions on the degree to which people felt they could themselves control their risk of getting ill.

These nine questions on control were combined into two simple measures: control over life and control over health. In Russia, the results were clear: the more control people had the better their health. Allowing for the effects of alcohol consumption and smoking made little difference to the protective effect on health of high control.[17]

We then extended our study to seven countries: Russia, Estonia, Lithuania, Latvia, Czech Republic, Hungary and Poland.[18] In each country, people who reported less control over their lives had worse health. Further, the greater the degree of inequality of material deprivation and of income, the worse the health. We found that the link between income inequality and poor health was low control. The study suggested a causal chain: the greater the degree of inequality, the less control people had over their lives; the less control, the worse their health. Self-reported health is a useful measure because it tells us something important about how people feel as well as being a predictor of subsequent risk of death. Nevertheless, a study that uses self-reported health and how much control you think you have is subject to the criticism that we are simply tapping into a general sense of things not being right. As one way of checking that there was more than general negativity at play here, we looked at average control scores for each of the seven populations. The Russians reported least control, the Czechs the most. This was linked to the country's mortality rate. The lower the control reported by the population sample that we interviewed, the higher the mortality for that population.

Capitalism? Social capitalism might help

Lack of control, lack of full social participation including low social supports – the experience of people in the East bears out what we have learnt in the West. Deny people these vital resources for living and health suffers. These are affected by what happens in society. Istvan's social supports changed – his wife tossed him out – when the country's economic and social circumstances changed.

I have used Istvan's story to illustrate what was happening in the society as a whole. The contrast with Japan is striking. Japan is a society marked by a high degree of social cohesion. Paradoxically for countries that were supposedly built on socialist principles, what was lacking in Central and Eastern Europe was social cohesion. Gorbachev, in his speech to the Central Committee of the Communist Party in 1987, said that the failure of the economy of the Soviet Union was due to 'unresolved problems piling up' which 'seriously affected the economy and the social and spiritual spheres'. He described a country in which:

> elements of social corrosion which emerged in the last few years had a negative effect on society's morale . . . interest in the affairs of society slackened, manifestations of callousness and skepticism appeared . . . The spread of alcohol and drug abuse and the rise in crime became indicators of the decline in social mores.
>
> Disregard for laws, distortion of reports, bribe taking and the encouragement of toadyism and adulation, had a deleterious influence on the moral atmosphere in society. Real care for people, for the conditions of their life and work and for social well-being, were often replaced with political flirtation.[19]

Gorbachev has provided an excellent description of a decline in social capital. And it got worse post-1989.

Richard Rose, the political scientist with whom we collaborate, described the Soviet Union as an hourglass society. At the top was the heavy superstructure of the state; at the bottom were individuals and families. What was missing was the layer in between: the informal networks of friends, neighbourhood associations, clubs, churches and societies. When the superstructure crumbled post-1989 and the formal institutions of the state were under threat, people who had to rely on these institutions were in trouble. In our survey of health among Russians, we asked whom people could rely on in times of trouble.[20] If they responded that they would rely on informal institutions, we found their health to be better than if they had to rely on formal networks.[21]

Andrea Cornia, now professor of economics at the University of Florence, has been studying the mortality crisis in what he terms the Transitional Economies of Central and Eastern Europe.[22] He considers a variety of explanations for the dramatic changes in mortality that happened in the 1980s and 1990s. One intriguing hypothesis is that we are looking in the wrong place for explanations. Given what happened in the period leading up to and following the 'Velvet Revolution' (as the Czechs describe their big change) of 1989, it is tempting to attribute the mortality changes to the social and economic changes that happened then. Cornia does as do I. But when were the people dying in 1990 born? Someone who was fifty in 1992 was born in 1942. The years 1942–4 were shockingly difficult in Russia. People born in those years had a greater risk of dying between the ages of forty and fifty than people born in the previous three years, but the increase was small compared to the actual increased risk of death that occurred in Russia after 1989. Far more likely, concludes Cornia, is that the mortality increase is the result of influences with a short latency period.

Cornia thinks that the social changes that lead to stress are prime candidates to explain the mortality increase. Among these he lists the general sense of personal insecurity attendant on the rise in crime rate and murder rate, growing family instability as shown by decline in marriage and rise in divorces, unemployment and rapid labour turnover, job insecurity and growing social stratification. These link together.

> For instance, the faster than average rise in unemployment recorded between 1992 and 1994 in the Northern part of Russia caused high labour turnover, the spread of an unregulated grey economy, an increase in migration under difficult circumstances and a rise in family instability.[23]

To test this thesis in relation to mortality in Russia, he constructed a stress index composed of changes in unemployment, labour turnover, and changes in marriage and divorce. He then looked at changes in mortality in twelve regions of Russia. The relation was clear: the higher the stress index the greater the increase in mortality. The North was particularly hard hit by these stressful changes and had a big increase in mortality from 1989 to 1993. The areas least affected by the stress changes included Caucasus, Volga-Vyatsk and Central Black Soil. They had the smallest mortality increases.

Cornia's approach links the rapid changes which we might loosely describe as a decline in social capital with stress related to problems with work, rapid changes in family and working life and the rise in insecurity.

The other manifestation of a decline in social capital is a weakening of reciprocal relations. This is fundamental to the idea of imbalance between efforts and rewards which is, in Whitehall and elsewhere, linked to increased risk of heart disease. Basic to social capital is the idea that there is reciprocity of exchange. My efforts are appropriately rewarded, as are yours. I do things because they are the right things to do, but I expect the same in return. My efforts should be rewarded in an appropriate fashion. We used measures of effort/reward imbalance in the workplace in our studies in Poland, the Czech Republic, Lithuania and Hungary.[24] This study confirmed the importance for poor health of low control at work and generally. In addition, people whose work was characterised by a high degree of imbalance between effort and reward had a 60 per cent greater chance of being in poor health than those with an appropriate balance.

The deadly drink, or smoke, or fat, or medical care

Two Russians are sitting, pouring glasses of vodka and drinking in silence. After three or four of these one Russian says: 'So, Tovarich, how are you?' The other replies gruffly: 'Did you come to drink, or to make a speech?' The Russians take their drinking seriously.

My colleagues and I are examining the role of alcohol, diet and psychosocial factors in causing ill-health in a collaborative study in the Siberian city of Novosibirsk. We surveyed men aged from 25 to 64. The pattern of drinking there is similar to the rest of the Russian Federation but different from the French and Italian pattern of regular daily drinking. In Novosibirsk, 70 per cent of men drank less often than once a week, but the typical amount drunk per drinking occasion exceeded 80g alcohol for more than half the population; more than 120g for a third. Eighty grammes of pure alcohol is equivalent to about 250ml of vodka – a small bottle. A third of men, at a typical drinking session, will consume about twelve shots of vodka.

The question is whether this mode of alcohol consumption is as destructive as it looks. Certainly, many have speculated that alcohol has played an important role in the Russian mortality crisis. In the mid 1980s, as part of his attempt to improve the moral fibre of the Russians, Gorbachev launched an anti-alcohol campaign. During this period if you were in Moscow at an official gathering, your hosts embarrassedly proposed toasts with caviar and mineral water. There was during that time a temporary halt in the decline in life expectancy, which some observers attribute to a reduction in alcohol consumption.

About 20 per cent of the increasing mortality gap between East and West has been the result of an increase in accidental and violent deaths. There is little difficulty in imagining how heavy drinking could be playing a part in these. Similarly in Hungary, particularly, there has been a steady increase in mortality from cirrhosis of the liver. The drinking of Istvan and his friends will have contributed to that.

The problem comes with coronary heart disease – the major contribution to the mortality disadvantage in the East. As anybody in the Western world who has read a newspaper now knows, alcohol protects from coronary heart disease. The low rates of heart disease in France, despite avid enthusiasm for butter, cream, meat and cheese, have been attributed to their equally avid enthusiasm for alcohol. If the Russians and Hungarians and others are drinking in excess, how come their rates of coronary heart disease are still high? The answer could lie in the type of alcohol: vodka could be less protective than wine. The answer could also lie in the pattern of drinking: wine drinkers, the French being the archetypes, typically drink daily, with meals, whereas the Russians drink infrequently, to get drunk.

Our own view is that the pattern of drinking is more likely to be important for protection from heart disease than the beverage type. Martin Bobak, my Czech colleague, pointed out that the Czechs drink beer like the French drink wine. They get as emotional about their Pilsner as the French do about their Bordeaux. The pattern of beer-drinking in the Czech Republic is regular daily drinking with meals. If it were pattern of drinking that was important for coronary protection rather than beverage type, Czech beer drinkers should be as protected from heart disease compared to Czech non-drinkers as French wine drinkers are compared to French non-drinkers. That is exactly what we found in our study of heart attacks in the Czech Republic. Lower rates of coronary heart disease in Czechs who were regular beer drinkers compared to non-drinkers.[25]

It seems likely then that the Russian pattern of drinking confers no protection from heart disease. Might it be damaging? Well, yes, it might. In Novosibirsk, we found no increase in heart-disease mortality in the men who binged once or twice a month – although there was the expected increase in accidental and violent deaths. In a small subgroup who drank up to half a litre of vodka at least three times a week there was a clear increase in mortality from heart disease. This frequent heavy drinking was, however, confined to about 4 per cent of men in our study. Although such drinkers might have been otherwise engaged when we invited them to take part and therefore not have been in the study, we estimated that the contribution of such extreme intakes to the total problem of heart disease in these populations is relatively small.[26]

There are therefore two questions. The first assumes that alcohol plays a definite role in the mortality problems of Eastern Europe. It asks what drives people to such destructive patterns of drinking. To what extent can these drinking patterns be attributed to the type of stress that we have been discussing and is well summarised by the work of Andrea Cornia? The second question asks what else is influencing the Russian mortality pattern, in addition to a destructive pattern of drinking. This chapter has set out my views of the answer to this second question.

As with discussing the social gradient within countries, there are many observers who wonder why we feel the need to pay attention to psychosocial factors when we can blame smoking or too much saturated fat, or inadequate medical care.

A useful reminder: the importance of one set of factors, the social and psychological factors, does not negate the importance of others. A Hungarian who smokes is at greater risk of heart disease than a Hungarian who does not. Smoking will be bad for the health of a Pole or a Russian as it is bad for the health of an American or Swiss. But the evidence that we can account for the 4 million extra deaths in Russia from 1989 to 1999 on the basis of smoking does not exist.

Similarly, diet is likely to be important. In the early 1990s I was taken to a restaurant in Prague and my host offered to translate the menu. 'The first dish is pork,' he said, 'then beef, pork, beef, pork, beef and pork.' The 'salad' turned out to be pickled cucumbers. These days a vegetarian has a slightly greater chance of dining out without suffering caloric deficiency. Nevertheless, the evidence shows that intake of antioxidant vitamins is low in Eastern European countries. In the West, particularly, we have become accustomed to expect shops to sell mangoes and pineapples in the depths of a northern winter. We have reduced the seasonal differences in intake of fruit and vegetables. Such seasonal differences in intake continue to be notable in Eastern countries. These may well contribute to increased risk of cardiovascular disease.

Could inadequacies of medical care be responsible for the mortality problem in the East? This is a big question. There is evidence that the quality of care for heart attacks is less satisfactory in many of the Eastern European countries.[27] This could, of course, contribute to the differences in heart-disease mortality, although less plausibly to the differences in violent deaths. One approach to this question is to classify diagnoses at death into those diseases that are amenable to medical intervention and those that are not. We have, thereby, calculated that some 10–20 per cent of the East–West gap could be attributed to differences in medical care. After 1989, improved cardiac care in the Czech Republic may have contributed to its relatively favourable mortality trend.[28]

My view is that if you become ill, the last thing you want is inadequate medical care. But what you really want is for the set of conditions to obtain that make it less likely you become ill in the first place.

Not selection

At various points in my investigations of how the conditions in which people live and work affect their chance of illness and their quality and length of life, the question of selection has been nipping at my heels like an annoying terrier that won't give up. Why could it not be that high-status people are high status because they have less illness, not the reverse? Why could it not be that socially isolated people are isolated because of their tendency to illness, not the reverse? Perhaps people who are likely to become ill choose jobs that offer little opportunity for control.

One big scientific plus of looking at what happens to health when whole countries undergo changes that lead to less control, to breakdown in social capital, and to reduced opportunities to participate in society, is that the selection argument becomes less plausible. Russian society did not collapse after the fall of communism because people fell ill. People fell ill because of the social and economic changes. Unemployment rates did not rise because increasing numbers of people were too ill to work. Illness rates went up because of the rise in unemployment. Crime rates did not go up because ordinary residents were suffering from insecurity that contributed to illness. Insecurity was a result of the rise in crime. Increased illness did not lead to the rise in divorce rates, but the rise in divorce may well have led to increased illness. The key themes that I have been developing to explain the social gradient in health appear to be affecting the health of whole societies. Plausibly, the same set of factors responsible for the East–West gap in mortality is responsible for the social gradient in health within society.

9. THE TRAVAILS OF THE FATHERS
. . . AND MOTHERS

You and I will sit at a table, each with a pile of paper and pencil. Now we both have an equal opportunity to write a play.

George Bernard Shaw[1]

One advantage of having three children is that I had the excuse to read *The Phantom Tollbooth* three times. Milo, a young boy, is travelling on the open road from Dictionopolis.

Milo turned around and found himself staring at two very neatly polished brown shoes, for standing directly in front of him (if you can use the word 'standing' for anyone suspended in mid-air) was another boy just about his age, whose feet were easily three feet off the ground.

'How do you manage to stand up there?' asked Milo.

'I was about to ask you a similar question,' answered the boy, 'for you must be much older than you look to be standing on the ground.'

'What do you mean?' Milo asked.

'Well,' said the boy, 'in my family everyone is born in the air, with his head at exactly the height it's going to be when he's an adult, and then we all grow toward the ground. When we're fully grown up or, as you can see, grown down, our feet finally touch. Of course, there are a few of us whose feet never reach the ground no matter how old we get, but I suppose it's the same in every family . . . You certainly must be very old to have reached the ground already.'

'Oh no,' said Milo seriously. 'In my family we all start on the ground and grow up, and we never know how far until we actually get there.'

'What a silly system.' The boy laughed. 'Then your head keeps changing its height and you always see things in a different way? Why, when you're fifteen things won't look at all the way they did when you

were ten, and at twenty everything will change again . . . We always
see things from the same angle.'[2]

Everyone in the Boy's world, child or adult, has his or her head at the
same height. I showed at the beginning of this book that height was
related to status: the higher you are, the higher you go. Reading *The
Phantom Tollbooth* we could take height as a metaphor for status. We
could describe the Boy's scheme of things as equality of outcome.
Everyone, children and adults, is the same status, has the same view of
the world, and the world of them. In Milo's (our) world, we know
how we start out, but not how far we will go. 'We all start on the
ground and grow up, and we never know how far until we actually
get there.' Milo did not add, but I will: it will depend on what happens
to us along the way, on the journey from infancy to childhood to
adulthood.

We can distinguish two important approaches to equality. In the
case of the Boy with his head at adult height, we might say that there is
equality of outcome: everyone achieves the same status. For some
social critics, such an idea will be anathema. Equality of outcome? Not
only a depressing thought, they will say, but a deadening one.
Uniformity means lack of enterprise. Not only is it not achievable,
they will say, but it is not desirable. They might suggest that what is
required is equality of opportunity. If there were equality of opportunity, all the Milos would have the opportunity for achievement of
maximal adult height. The fact that some did not suggests that they did
not make appropriate use of their opportunities.

Opportunity translates into social mobility, climbing out of one's
class origins. Throughout the Western world, there has been impressive
social mobility. Even in class-ridden Britain, the son of a purveyor of
garden gnomes, John Major, not university educated, became prime
minister. Margaret Thatcher, famously a grocer's daughter, read science
at Oxford University, and went via elocution lessons and the prime
ministership to being Baroness Thatcher. Who you are is no longer a bar
to what your children can be. That's the good news.

The sober news is that who you are still matters enormously to your
children's life chances. This chapter is about the fact that our present
set of social arrangements does not deliver either equality of outcome

or equality of opportunity to children. The factors responsible for the status syndrome, the social gradient in health, affect not only us, as adults, but have an effect on our children and shape their life chances and hence their health. A second, related point is that, important as the social environment in which adults live and work may be for health, people do not enter adulthood in an equal state of readiness to meet the challenges of work and life. They bring baggage with them from earlier life that both determines where they end up and the way they respond to environmental challenges.

A legacy for our children?

Do you have an eye to posterity? Ignore the giants who leave great works or achievements by which to be remembered. For everybody else, our main legacy is our children. We are, of course, programmed by evolution to want our children to survive and breed. If our ancestors had not bred, we wouldn't exist. Most of us probably want our children not only to breed but to have good lives. My contention is that whatever it is we mean by the 'good life' it is likely to include, or at least have an effect on, health.

You are, let us say, a parent. What is it about you or the circumstances in which you live and work that might affect your child's chances of good health as he or she grows up? We have been reviewing ample evidence that there is a social gradient in health among adults – the result of the circumstances in which you live and work. Do these circumstances pass on their effects to your children? Will their health be affected by you, or by where they end up later in life? And to what extent is where they end up related to your position in the social hierarchy?

There are a number of ways that what happens to you could affect what happens to your children: your socioeconomic position, in-cluding education and income, the community in which you live, your family life, health behaviours such as diet and smoking, and genetic inheritance. Some of these will be out of your control and related to the society at one end or to biological inheritance at the other. Some will be more closely related to the degree of control you have over your life and degree of social participation.

The social gradient in parents affects children's education

To start, let us look at education and the set of competencies such as literacy and numerical skills that we hope it delivers. This is a good place to start because we know that, in general, the better the educational achievement the greater the range of life chances. To borrow a concept from economists, the returns to education are considerable: more education leads to higher income in adulthood and higher socioeconomic position. This, in turn, leads to better health. As we have seen throughout this book, education is worthy of attention.

If you want your children to be well educated, you should make sure they go to a good school, surely. Not quite. In fact among all the influences on children's educational performance, the school may not be the most important. This is shown by an annual ritual that takes place at the breakfast tables of the newspaper-reading public.

In Britain, we are obsessed with league tables. (These are akin to the rankings of sports teams according to matches won, drawn and lost.) They are supposed to be useful as an instrument of management. They may well be, provided they are used and interpreted properly. We now have a league table for schools. Every school in the country is rated on the examination performance of its students. The results are published in the newspapers with some fanfare. Middle-class parents pore over them to see how the likely schools for their progeny fare. There is one huge catch. The league tables are nearly totally useless as a measure of the school's contribution to educational performance. Schools may be performing excellently or poorly, but the league tables don't tell us that. Mostly they tell us about the abilities of the children who are admitted.

In fact, the league tables for school performance are a remarkably good indicator of deprivation of the area in which the school is located. The more deprived the area the worse the average school performance. If you look up a school to see how it is performing, you are actually reading off an exquisitely sensitive indicator of deprivation. The league table is telling us something, but if it is so closely linked with deprivation, it may not be telling us much about schools.

This is how it works. All British students take a national examination at age sixteen, the GCSEs. One standard measure of success is the percentage of children sitting the exams who pass five or more GCSEs at C grade or above. To put you in the picture, there is nothing special about five Cs. The best children might expect ten or eleven A *s. Five Cs is decidedly ordinary. A few years ago, medical sociologist David Blane and social medicine pioneer Jerry Morris went through an interesting exercise. They summed the results for each of 105 areas of England and Wales. They then compared the average percentage of children having five or more passes at A* to C with a measure of deprivation of the area. So close was the link between school performance and deprivation that they looked as though they were simply alternative measures of the same thing.[3] Pass rates of children, by themselves, tell almost nothing of how well schools are performing. They are remarkably sensitive as a measure of the average level of deprivation of the area in which the school is located. The relation is continuous, as with the health gradient. It is not only that schools in slum areas do badly, but the more affluent the area the better the pass rate.

Why the close link between educational performance and deprivation, throughout the whole range of deprivation from most to least deprived? The quality of the school will be only one input to the performance in the league table of examination results. Other influences on children's performance will be crucial. First, think of yourself, your family, and the characteristics of both, and then ask how they might affect your child's educational performance. Second, ask if you lived in a different area, but with the same family characteristics that you have now, would that make a difference? Third, ask if given all that, the characteristics of the school matter. The answer appears to be that all three matter and the effects are substantial.

Doug Willms in Canada has been investigating literacy and other performance measures in international studies. Literacy describes an individual's ability to 'use printed and written information to function in society, to achieve one's goals, and to develop one's knowledge and potential'. It matters for economic success, health and well-being.[4]

Figure 9.1 shows the relation between literacy scores of people aged 16 to 25 and parents' education. (The literacy score is the average score on three tests: prose, document and quantitative.) In Sweden, in Canada and in the US, the higher parents' education, the higher the literacy scores of these young people. But the differences among these countries are striking. Look at the three graphs and ask yourself where, if you had low education, your children would be best off, using literacy as the measure. It's a no-brainer: Sweden, then Canada and lastly, US. The slopes linking parents' education to literacy are different. What this means is that at high levels of parental education, literacy levels of offspring differ the least. Americans, Canadians and Swedes with highly educated parents perform equally well on a standard literacy test. As we move down the slope of the line linking parents to their children's literacy, the more the gap between countries opens up. The less educated the parents, the more advantage accrues to the Swedes. Among parents with the least education, the disadvantage of being in the US is substantial.[5]

Figure 9.1 Literacy scores of people aged 16–25 according to level of education of their parents in US, Canada and Sweden

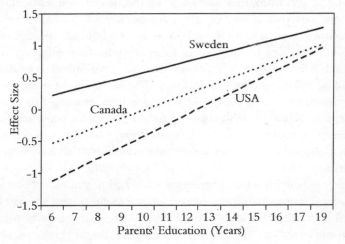

Note: The figures show performance on a standard literacy test. The scores are measured in standard deviation units. One additional year of schooling would raise literacy by 0.15 units.

Source: Adapted from Willms (1999a).

To help interpret figure 9.1: the units are standard deviation units. And that means? A difference of 0.15 standard deviation units corresponds approximately to the effect on literacy of one additional year of schooling. This figure is arrived at by averaging results across all the countries that took part in the international study of literacy from which these results come. At the low end, then, a difference of 1.5 standard deviation units between the US and Sweden is the size of difference that could arise if the Americans had ten fewer years of schooling *and* if schooling had the same effect in each country. Americans at the lower end don't have ten fewer years of schooling. Which means that there are other influences affecting literacy levels.

I find these international results profoundly important and, depending on your perspective, either profoundly encouraging or depressing. My optimism and pessimism relate to the first two of the three questions above: your characteristics affect the literacy scores of your children; but the degree of that effect depends on where you happen to live. If you live in Sweden, your own educational level has less effect on your children's literacy than if you live in the US. The glass is half full if you think that Sweden is a good model. It is half empty if you are happy with the American arrangements.

Before we go on to try to understand what is behind these figures, it is worth dwelling for a moment more on why they might provide grounds for optimism. Just suppose that literacy is linked to health. It could be linked in a direct causal way. The definition of literacy used was ability to 'use printed and written information to function in society, to achieve one's goals, and to develop one's knowledge and potential'. People with higher levels of literacy may, as a direct result of that improved ability, experience the conditions that lead to better health.

Alternatively, the link between literacy and health might be more indirect. Literacy may be a marker of how investments of material, social and cultural resources made by the previous generation have been converted into benefits for the new generation. Health may be a similar marker. I argued that social gradients in health are not fixed when we compare societies. This suggests that they can be changed. The gradients in literacy hold a similar message. They can be changed.

A social gradient in literacy is rather an abstract construct for an individual to comprehend. You don't go home saying: wonderful, I live in a society with a shallow social gradient in literacy. But a shallower gradient means that children whose parents had less education will fare better in some societies than others. You may well go home, happy, because your disadvantage has less chance of being passed on to your children, than if you lived somewhere else.

Figure 9.1 compared countries. There are similar findings from within Canada and the US. The disadvantage, in terms of literacy, of having parents with low education varies depending on which province or state your child is in. Northern American states tend to have higher average literacy scores with shallower gradients. Southern states, Texas particularly, have a steeper gradient with low literacy scores for children of parents with little education. California seems to be in between the north and the south. Doug Willms's next question is why: what is it about communities that modulates the effect of parents' position?

His answer is social capital. How this plays out is less clear. There appear to be at least three possible ways. First, children come to school with different degrees of readiness to learn. These different capacities will to some extent be related to what goes on inside the family home, but that in turn will be influenced by pressures on parents. Second, the wider social environment outside the school may be playing a role in how children fare in school: social disruption and hanging-out in gangs will affect children's school performance. Third, social capital may play out in the way parents relate to the school – Willms shows that schools that have more parental participation in governance and as volunteers have higher achievement scores. This last is particularly relevant for understanding the link with socioeconomic position. Schools which take in students from higher-than-average socioeconomic backgrounds have more parental participation. For a given level of parental background a child will do better in a school with more parental involvement than in one with less.

It is important to re-emphasise the point that the correlation of children's literacy with the education of their parents does not, by itself, mean that the important influence is in fact parents' education. Parents' education is a marker for socioeconomic position. It is a guide to income and living standards, jobs and leisure, attitudes and behaviours. All may be important. Parental education may also be a guide to genetic endowment. But even if you were inclined to believe that the social gradient in literacy could be explained principally by a social gradient in genetically determined abilities, the fact that the social gradient in literacy varies across countries most easily fits with the effects of the social environment on capabilities to benefit from schooling. These capabilities to benefit from schooling may have a genetic component, an environmental component and the effects of an interaction between them.

All very well that social capital matters, and parents' education matters, but what about the school itself? If schools did not matter, middle-class parents could save themselves a good deal of bother. At the extreme, the answer to whether schools matter is obvious. If there were no schools, children would learn a lot less. Or to be more precise, those who had knowledgeable parents with the skills, interest and time to teach their children would learn; the rest would suffer rather badly.

Given that everyone in advanced countries goes to school, for good or ill, it is easy enough to ask the question: would my child be better off if she went to school A or school B? But it is a bit trickier to answer it. The children who go to school A are different from those who go to school B in all the ways we have just been examining. We need a multi-level framework of thinking and data analysis to ask how much value is added by the school *per se* after taking into account the characteristics of the children who come there.

Willms's reports of research from Canada suggest that the school effect can be substantial. In British Columbia, for example, researchers looked at children's cognitive ability at the end of grade 3 and then observed how it grew over the next five years. Children in the three best-performing schools had a faster growth in cognitive ability than children in the four worst. The difference was equivalent to being a full school year ahead.[6] The quality of the teaching is only one contributor; the attitudes, expectations and behaviour of fellow pupils are crucial. Hence the argument about segregation in schools on the basis of ability. It is a fair bet that putting able students in one place helps their performance. The problem is that putting all the less able students in one place almost certainly hinders theirs.

If schools do make a difference, can they be social levellers? Not as much as we might like. If some children went to school and some did not, getting more children into school would improve their educa-

tion. But with everyone in school, might more spending on education, distributed equitably, reduce social inequalities in performance
on measures of educational 'output' such as literacy? Regrettably not.[7]
There is reason to believe that for a given amount of extra educational
input, across the board to children of all social backgrounds, social
inequalities in the outcome may increase. A moment's reflection
reveals this not to be quite as surprising as first it seems. Suppose you
have a new way of teaching history and teach it to everyone right
across the school system, who will benefit most? Those most ready to
take advantage of a new way of learning: the middle-class kids. Spend
a bit more on education and spread it equally, and you may well
increase inequalities in educational performance.

   We could try social levelling by not spending the money equitably,
or at least, defining 'equitable' as favouring those worst off. This could
be done by reducing the resources available to the better-off children.
But there are not too many middle-class parents, myself included,
who could muster much enthusiasm for that. There will, similarly,
always be a tension between the parents of more able children who
want their children to be stimulated by having other motivated
children around them, and those who see such selectivity in education
increasing the disadvantage of those not selected and fostering social
divisions. Spending even more money to bring the standard of
teaching and facilities of the worst schools up to the standard of
the best has to be part of the answer.

   But a big part of the answer will come from asking how children
can be helped to be in a better position to benefit from what schools
have to offer. We need, then, to return to the strong association of
children's educational performance with their parents' socioeconomic
position as measured by their education, and examine the role of the
family and wider social influences.

The family and social gradients in children's performance and behavioural problems

I once nearly spoilt an alpine walking holiday because my holiday
reading was about the murderous infants who inhabit Melanie Klein's
world of good and bad breasts and what the wicked breast-feeders

want to do to their parents, never mind what their parents might do to them. The parody of Freud suggests that the child either wants to kill you or copulate with you, depending on your sex relative to the child's. It has been a rough ride being a parent in the twentieth century. As the received wisdom of what determines who we are swings wildly between nature and nurture, between genes and environment, so the role of the parent has swung between innocent bystanders as the genetic destiny of their children unfolds, to all-important shapers of that destiny, and back again. It would be surprising if the pendulum came to rest, but I imagine that eventually it will allow for the shaping influence of parents and the wider social environment while acknowledging the crucial role genes play.

Every parent who has more than one child has marvelled over how different each appears to be from the other. Is it because the parents raised the children differently, because the second one had an older sibling, because the family circumstances changed, or is it something about the children, their genes, what happened to them *in utero*, or in infancy? Behavioural genetics use studies of twins and of adoption to sort out the role of genes, families and the wider social environment on children's personality and intelligence. These studies conclude that individual differences in personality and intelligence are about half due to the genes children inherit from their parents. As discussed in Chapter 2, the case has been made that these behavioural genetic studies understate the importance of environment because they do not sufficiently take into account the correlation between the two. Individuals with an aptitude for a particular skill, for example, will be likely to find themselves in an environment that fosters that skill. The behavioural genetic studies further break down the environmental component into family and wider social environment and conclude that the greater part of the variation comes from the wider environment.

What about families? Identical twins reared in the same family are no more similar than identical twins reared apart. Hence families don't matter for the development of personality or intelligence. However, the behavioural genetic studies that make the case that parents do not matter ask about the sources of *individual* differences within a given environment.[8] They are not set up to ask, for example, about why the higher social position of parents is linked to higher IQ of children. Here the role of parents may be quite different.

In fact, studies of differences between social groups show that families have big effects on children's abilities. In a sample of children from different centres in the USA, Jeanne Brooks-Gunn and colleagues at Columbia University characterised families according to the ratio between income and needs.[9] There was a remarkably graded relation. Marching progressively up the income scale, the higher the income relative to needs, the higher the IQ scores of children.

The evidence summarised by Brooks-Gunn suggests that this relation between family income and children's cognitive abilities can be attributed both to the family and to the community and neighbourhood. The family effects operate through nutrition and health behaviour, provision of learning experiences, parental interactions with children, parental and emotional and physical health, household stability, choice of schools and child care, use of health-care services. The community and neighbourhood operate through the effects of the peer group, exposure to violence and safety, toxins, neighbourhood spirit and connectedness, school characteristics, access to amenities.

How can it be that twin and adoptive studies show little effect of families and that studies of the social gradient – the differences between social groups – show big effects of family? There are two related answers. The first has to do with who gets into the behavioural genetic studies and the second to do with the important general rule that the explanation of differences between groups that differ markedly in their environmental characteristics may be different from the explanation of differences among individuals within relatively homogeneous groups. Steven Pinker explains these clearly when referring to the behavioural genetic studies:

Differences among homes don't matter within the samples of homes netted by these studies, which tend to be more middle-class than the population as a whole. But differences between those samples and other kinds of home could matter. The studies exclude cases of criminal neglect, physical and sexual abuse, and abandonment in a bleak orphanage, so they do not show that extreme cases fail to leave

scars. Nor can they say anything about the differences between cultures
– about what makes a child a middle-class American as opposed to a
Yanomamo warrior . . . or even a member of an urban street gang.[10]

It is likely then that adoption studies miss this phenomenon of the
social gradient in intelligence, because parents who adopt are, in
general, of higher social class than the average family in the population. There is, therefore, less environmental variation among these
families than there would be in the general population. The conclusion that families don't matter rests on studying individual differences
in a relatively standardised environment. The more standardised the
environment between families, the less will families appear to matter
in behavioural genetic studies.[11] If families into which children are
adopted are higher social class than the families of the biological
parents, and families mattered, you would expect that the adopted
children would have higher IQ and fewer behavioural problems than
their biological siblings, who were not adopted, and biological
parents. They do. On average, adoption appears to be associated
with about a twelve-point rise in IQ ($\frac{3}{4}$ of a standard deviation). In
adoption studies in Sweden and Denmark, adoptive children have
about half the lifetime prevalence of arrest by the police of their
biological fathers.[12]

Almost every social phenomenon that I have examined in this book
shows a social gradient – not bad effects for deprived children and
reasonable results for everyone else. I would expect it to be the same
for the effects of families on children. Pinker says that parents do
matter if the ones you have are pretty rotten or if you have not got
any. Apart from that, it is irrelevant if you have yours or somebody
else's. But why not a gradient? If parents do matter if they are absent or
totally hopeless, what about if they are a bit absent or a bit hopeless,
would you not expect them to matter a bit? I would. When we turn
our attention to differences among social groups – social variation –
that is what the data seem to indicate. Families do play a role.

Let me be clear about what is at issue. I do not question that genetic
inheritance is a big part of what parents pass to their children. The
question is whether they pass on anything else that is relevant to their
children's cognitive abilities and behaviour and hence to their sub-

sequent health as adults, as opposed to the environmental effect all coming from the wider society. The fact of the social gradient in IQ and behavioural problems according to parents' income does not by itself prove that families matter.

Here's the problem. Someone does a study that shows that maternal interactions, reading and use of language appear to be related to language skills of the child, and that such use of language is less the lower the income of the parents. Armed with the result of the behavioural genetic studies, you could argue: A family effect? Must be due to genes. This is, in my view, inappropriate precisely because the behavioural genetic designs do not study the social variation. They study relatively well-off families who volunteer to be in their studies. Yes, it may be that the fact that children of professional violinists are themselves more likely to be gifted on the violin has nothing to do with being made to practise from the age of three and all to do with genes. But it tells us little of why most professional violinists do not come from urban street gangs.

We seem, therefore, to have two sorts of conclusions. First, among middle-class families, variations in parental styles may matter less for children's cognitive ability and behaviour than either the parents' genes or the wider social environment. Second, when we turn our attention to the differences among social groups, parents may play a much bigger role in explaining these differences. The evidence suggests that the socioeconomic environment affects parents who, in turn, affect their children.

What is it with families?

In Hampstead in North London there are probably more psycho-analysts per square metre than in any other part of the planet except, I am told, a part of Buenos Aires. On a good day, I can cycle to work past Freud's house, doff my helmet to the memory of the master, then later walk the dog past the houses of the late John Bowlby and his son who lives next door. You know Freud, and he makes, shall we say, a subconscious contribution to this book, but who was Bowlby? A psychoanalyst, he articulated attachment theory[13]. The path that led to attachment theory was his observation of what happened to children who had been deprived of their mothers. Bowlby pointed to the crucial nature of the attachment between parent, usually mother, and child.

I read his book, *Child Care and the Growth of Love*, as a medical student and it had a big impact on me. It also now gives us a chance to bring these two heroes, Freud and Bowlby, together. In the book, Bowlby quotes a description by Freud's daughter Anna, who ran a nursery in Hampstead, of a well-developed easy child of two years of age who was placed in a residential nursery during the Second World War. When the mother gave up visiting, the child regressed severely.

> He became listless, often sat in a corner sucking and dreaming, at other times he was very aggressive. He almost completely stopped talking. He was dirty and wet continually, so that we had to put nappies on him. He sat in front of his plate eating very little without pleasure, and started smearing his food over the table. At this time the nurse who had been looking after him fell ill, and Bobby did not make friends with anyone else . . . He hardly ever said a word, had entirely lost his bladder and bowel control, sucked a great deal.[14]

Bowlby's thesis was that such maternal separation did not only have short-term effects on the infant but had long-term effects on the ability of the child to form secure relationships. Security of attachment as a child, in Bowlby's view, led to resilience in the face of stressful life events in later life. Crucially for our present concern, an infant with secure patterns of attachment becomes an adult with secure attachment.[15] This, in turn, is likely to lead to resistance to stress-induced illness.

If you want to see the grossest effects of maternal deprivation, visit your local prison. A large proportion of the inmates, you will find, were children in care and have low levels of literacy, not to mention a history of psychiatric illness. Richard Tremblay in Montreal traces a typical 'career' of a boy – it is usually a boy – from aggressive child, to disruptive in school, to juvenile delinquency, to fully fledged adult violent crime. This aggressive behaviour shows a clear socioeconomic gradient: the lower the status of the parents the greater the frequency of aggressive behaviour in their children. Interestingly, although girls as expected have less aggressive behaviour than boys, they too show a social gradient in the frequency of aggression.

This is not to argue that all poor people have children who are aggressive. In the first place, the phenomenon is not confined to people in poverty, it is graded – the greater the level of deprivation the more frequent the aggressive behaviour. Second, not all children follow this 'career'. The majority of children born to parents of low social position do not end up in crime. Even remembering the figure that I reported earlier – that 30 per cent of young black men in Washington DC will be arrested for drug-dealing between the ages of eighteen and twenty-four – the majority are not involved in violent crime. Tremblay traces the causes back to the general social environment and to a clear influence of the family.[16] He adopts the perspective of the behavioural geneticists, in trying to disaggregate the effect of the family from the effects of the wider social environment. He does this by looking at clustering within families of physically aggressive behaviour and other behaviour problems.

Tremblay is not blind to the obvious: that children inherit genes from their parents as well as a deprived environment. He draws an analogy with horticulture.

The differences among flowers that are growing in fertile ground will be mainly due to genotype differences, whereas differences among flowers growing in less fertile ground will be due to the quality of the added care (e.g. water, fertilizer) given to these flowers.

Rather than ask is it the wider environment or the family that is important, Tremblay and colleagues look at the interaction of these. They ask to what extent siblings within a family resemble each other with respect to aggressive behaviour and whether this degree of resemblance varies with the socioeconomic level of the parents. The results are interesting: the higher the socioeconomic position, the less the family appears to matter to the prevalence of aggressive behaviour. These are the flowers growing in fertile ground. The lower the socioeconomic position, the more important the family effect, for good or bad, on aggression.

Let's put some numbers on Tremblay's study. For families with high socioeconomic level, the family effect explained only 3 per cent of the variance in physical aggression scores of children. For families with the lowest socioeconomic position, the effect of the family on aggression explained 53 per cent of the variance. If all around you is going to hell, the family really matters.

Supermums in the forest of life

What about genes in all this? Perhaps the family matters because families pass on a cluster of genes that predispose to aggressive behaviour. An elegant series of studies by Steve Suomi shows the importance of gene–environment interactions for disturbed behaviour in their offspring.[17] The standard joke among scientists in the world of hypertension research is that the reason for studying humans is the better to understand hypertension in the laboratory-bred rat. Steve Suomi's studies in Old World rhesus monkeys (Macaca mulatta) draw heavily on Bowlby's attachment theory in humans to understand monkeys, but in turn, the rhesus studies illustrate the importance of early experience on long-term effects in adult life.

Rhesus monkey society has it all: hierarchies, strong females, courting males, devoted mothers and attached children, adolescent males roaming around in gangs in between leaving the parental troop and taking up with a new one. Human society might indeed help us understand monkeys.

Rhesus infants cling close to mum in the first weeks of life. To the observer, this bond of attachment represents a secure base from which the monkey can launch out into exploration of the immediate physical and social environment. There appear to be three distinct phases of this early development. First is attachment to mother. Next comes a stage of curiosity and exploration. This includes interactions with other young monkeys – their peers. During this time their play starts to mimic adult social activities, including dominance/aggressive interactions and reproductive behaviours. Sound familiar? Mother is important here. As the little monkey gets the courage to interact with others, if he gets frightened or tired, mother is around for a quick return to base, to her protective care. During stage two, the monkey has not developed sufficient ability to recognise when a situation might be threatening. Mother is there to save the day. The third stage is when the monkey develops his own anxiety around strangers. There is a maturation of social fears. Increasingly, then, they can stray from maternal care and look after themselves. Crucial for our story is that when the young monkey does not have a secure attachment to mother, its subsequent exploratory behaviour is compromised.

This is the normal developmental situation. It turns out that in the wild there are two variations on this. In both of these variants behavioural disturbances develop and there may be increased risk of death. One subgroup of the population, about 15 to 20 per cent, are high reactors. Take a stimulus that a normal monkey would explore with interest, other youngsters playing for example. The high reactors have profound behavioural disturbance and overactive physiological stress responses: high activity of the hypothalamic pituitary adrenal system and of the sympathetic nervous system. Because of this over-reaction to stimuli, the young high-reactive monkeys tend to avoid exploration and become shy and reserved. When mother is temporarily absent, a normal monkey reacts with agitation until he gets used to it and then adapts by expanding his interactions with others in the peer group. For the high reactors, separation from mother is a stress too far. They look like the young children in Anna Freud's nursery: lethargy and social withdrawal, eating and sleeping difficulties; they curl up into the foetal position and stay there for hours. In short, they are depressed. This state is accompanied by greater and longer physiological stress responses. Heritability is important for high reactivity – there appears to be a genetic predisposition.

The other variant subgroup makes up about 5 to 10 per cent of the population. These are impulsive monkeys who get carried away. Rough-and-tumble play can turn into downright aggression. They make impulsive leaps from treetops and commonly get injured in the process. It is hard to resist the temptation to see the living-dangerously aggressive behaviour of subgroups of young human males.

There are two experiments that show the potential importance of environment on these behavioural disturbances. If you take a youngster away from its mother and raise it with other youngsters, it will develop both the over-reactions of the high reactors and the aggressive behaviours of the impulsive monkeys. These peer-reared monkeys have normal motor development but are shy in interactions and slip down the social hierarchy. Suomi's interpretation is that this can be attributed to the missing attachment-relationship with the mother. In other words, maternal deprivation can mimic the effects of genetic predisposition. There is more. When females who were peer-reared become mothers themselves, they are more likely to neglect or abuse their offspring. Thus this environmentally induced behavioural disturbance can be passed to the next generation, just as a genetically induced one can be.

The second experiment involves a more positive intervention. Rather than take normal monkeys and make them behaviourally disturbed by maternal deprivation, this experiment seeks to go the other way. It takes monkeys presumed to be genetically predisposed to be high reactors to see if a good environment can avert genetic destiny. Some mothers are supermums. These are especially nurturant. One can picture them taking the rhesus equivalent of Suzuki lessons on the violin just to support their infants, while doing the school run, making brilliant birthday parties and being there for a cuddle and a kiss when knees get grazed, all the while being a successful investment banker. These supermums are recruited for a cross-fostering experiment.

First, though, there are the controls. Take normal monkeys and cross-foster them with a mother other than their own. Whether the mother is all right or a supermum appears to make little difference. The infants develop normally. This is consistent with the human behavioural geneticists' conclusions that individual parents who rear 'normally' do not have a big effect on children's personality. Now, take the genetically predisposed high reactors, the ones who would with their own mothers become shy, withdrawn, and slip down the social hierarchy, and cross-foster them with supermums. They do not just do well, they do super well. They have a secure relationship with the foster mother and they are behaviourally precocious. They cope well with temporary maternal separation. When they grow up, they become leaders of monkeys, especially adept at recruiting allies, and rise to the top of dominance hierarchies. When they become mothers, they adopt the style of their foster mothers and become especially nurturant.

It is, as I have noted, tempting to see the whole thing as a human society in microcosm. Behavioural disturbances can be induced either by the social environment or by genetic predisposition. Even when genetically induced, an especially supportive maternal environment can overcome this accident of birthright.

We are not monkeys

We are not rhesus macaques. Nevertheless, these rhesus studies suggest a biologically and socially plausible account of gene–environment interactions that show how early experiences may lead to behavioural disturbances that last a lifetime.[18] We cannot do such neat cross-fostering experiments with supermums in humans. There is ample evidence to suggest that the insights supplied by these rhesus studies do have wide applicability to the human situation. Genes matter and so does the environment. In asking the question about how much of early experience can be attributed to parents, and how much to the wider environment, there are two points to note. First, the earlier the experience the more likely is it that parents are involved. They form the social environment of the young child. Second, parents are affected by the social environment. Although they may be the proximal influence on the child, the social environment may be influencing the child through them.

As the rhesus studies make clear, effects on the young may last a lifetime. What we do to our children may change their risk of developing adult disease. There are at least three ways this can happen. The first is a latency model. What happens during a critical period has an enduring effect on disease risk in subsequent life. Second, there may be accumulation of advantage and disadvantage throughout life.[19] Third, where you start out affects where you end up – a pathway model. It is where you end up that matters for health. Early life experiences may be vital, not because they affect health directly, but because they change the child's chance of ending up in a favourable social situation in later life.

Let us look at each of these models. David Barker, working in the Medical Research Council unit in Southampton in England, has focused on life *in utero*. His idea is that what happens to the foetus during pregnancy can programme the body's metabolism to react in certain ways for the rest of the person's life. One way of determining what might have been happening to the foetus in the environment of the mother's body is to look at birth weight or thinness at birth. In a series of studies, Barker has shown that an infant with low birth weight, or who is thin at birth, and has low growth during the first year, fifty years later becomes an adult with high risk of high blood pressure, diabetes and cardiovascular disease.[20]

These findings were pretty startling. Something about the environment provided by the mother in pregnancy changed for the rest of their offspring's life their risk of developing diabetes or having a heart attack. When David Barker first produced his findings, there was a degree of polarisation in the scientific community. The 'early lifers' thought the effects of the social environment in adulthood had been overstated. Those concerned with the adult environment thought the opposite.

I was once invited to take part in a gladiatorial contest against David Barker. An unlikely gladiator, I am even less credible as a Christian or a lion. The venue for this proposed blood sport was the elegant rooms of Trinity College Cambridge. The only problem with this fight to the death is that I was not aware it was about to take place. I had been invited to a meeting 'to discuss David Barker's work'. Any preparation needed? No. Just turn up. The day before the meeting, the programme arrived: 10.00am D. Barker. 10.30am M. Marmot. We were supposed to fight over whether early life or adult circumstances were important for the development of risk of adult disease.

To my relief, David Barker decided to disappoint the blood lust of the crowd. A few hours before the meeting he sent me the unpublished manuscript of a paper of his reporting a long-term study from Finland.[21] It showed that both early life and adult social position were important. A boy with low birth weight became a man with an increased risk of heart disease. That risk showed up most clearly if in adulthood he was of low social position. Imagine a gladiatorial contest in which the supposed adversaries shake hands and agree that the position that the other holds is entirely reasonable. The closest David and I came to a spat was a friendly disagreement over whether the way to say this was that adult social class mattered most for heart disease risk if you had been a low birth weight infant; or low birth weight only really mattered if you were low social class in adulthood. Fundamentally, we were agreed that his data showed that both were important. A disadvantage from early life, combined with a disadvantage from later life, increased risk of heart disease.

Other data support this view. Mike Wadsworth has been conducting a long-term study of a sample of people born in one week in 1946 in Britain. He looked at the chance of having high blood pressure at forty-three years of age. The greatest risk was among people who were disadvantaged in childhood and became overweight in adult life.[22]

The Barker thesis is that programming occurs *in utero* and in the first year of life. It may not be limited to the metabolic pathways that he has studied so elegantly. Michael Meaney has no doubt about the importance of the family, or that what he shows in his rats has applicability to other animals, including humans. Meaney's work shows that environmental demand on a mother rat – stress – changes the quality of her maternal care. A rat pup exposed to inadequate maternal care develops an overactive stress response that stays with it for the rest of its life. In the jargon, there is an increase in the expression of the genes that determine activity of the hypothalamic-pituitary-adrenal axis. A high level of maternal licking and grooming reduces expression of these genes and leads to lower stress responses to stimuli in adulthood and higher quality of maternal care when the pup herself grows up and becomes a mother.[23]

Meaney thus shows that there is intergenerational transmission of inadequate mothering. Even if you were the sort that went around blaming bad mothers for their low-quality child care, it would be difficult to blame the first mother. Her low-quality mothering was induced by environmental stresses upon her. As with Suomi's studies, Meaney uses cross-fostering to show that this intergenerational transmission is not genetic. Offspring inherit the behaviour from the nursing mother, not from the biological mother.

Of direct relevance for our enquiry as to how the social gradient in adults affects their children is the extension of the Meaney work to humans. Schoolchildren in Canada were studied. At age six to ten, children of families with low social position had more biological evidence of being affected by stress than children of families with higher social position. The measure in question was salivary cortisol early in the morning.[24] High school seemed to have some levelling effect as no differences were then seen in cortisol level.

Families, or their lack, are important in programming in humans. The plight of Romanian orphans aroused the horror and sympathy of observers. When the Ceauşescu government fell at the end of the 1980s, the orphanages opened to show young children like those in Anna Freud's nursery. Many were later adopted in the West. Michael Rutter's studies show profound behavioural disturbances in these children that last as the children grow and develop. The degree of behavioural disturbance is crucially dependent on the age of adoption. The younger the children were when adopted, the more their development resembles children brought up in a secure family environment; the later the age of adoption, the greater the behavioural disturbance.[25]

In gross examples of child neglect or abuse such as these, it has been demonstrated that there are changes to the brain: what has been termed the neurobiology of child abuse.[26] If the developing brain is permanently changed by maltreatment, it provides a ready explanation for why early exposure may have long-lasting effects.

As we move to consider the second model – accumulation of advantage and disadvantage throughout life – please note that arguing for the importance of care, particularly maternal care, does not negate the importance of the wider environment. As with Meaney's rats so with human societies, maternal care is shaped by the influences on the mother, whether through the quality of care she herself received as an infant or through the pressures on her as an adult. It is not straightforward attributing effects to mother or to the fact that parents' socioeconomic level has a determining effect on the environment to which the child will be exposed.

To illustrate, here is one example from our own research. In a national study in England, we found that at ages four to fourteen, children of single mothers had more behavioural problems than children living with intact families made up of their two biological parents.[27] It may seem that this finding panders to the prejudices of those who are ready to blame single mothers for their plight, but what the data reveal is that there are single mothers and then there are single mothers. The children of single mothers who were not in poverty were no more likely to have behavioural problems than other children. It was the children of single mothers in poverty who were at risk. Poverty of these mothers was, in turn, strongly related to their lack of education. It is too simplistic to dismiss the results as the fault of feckless women. If women have the education and skills to live out of poverty, their single motherhood does not appear to be affecting their children on these measures of behavioural problems.

Disturbingly, children of 'reconstituted families', i.e. where one of the parents was not their biological parent, were at increased risk of behavioural problems regardless of the degree of poverty or otherwise of the family. This is part of a body of evidence that suggests that divorce takes its toll on children. Longitudinal studies that trace children though their experience of divorce and into adult life provide the best evidence. Best is to look at a birth cohort study that traces children from birth to adult life. There are five of these studies in Britain.

In the 1946 birth cohort, directed by Mike Wadsworth, women whose parents were divorced at some time had higher risk of depression, when they were restudied at age forty-three, than women whose parents remained together.[28] Why was the effect seen in women and not men? The investigators were not clear, but some studies show the effect in men as well. If you ask is it the marital disharmony that leads to divorce that harms children or the splitting up of the parents, the answer is almost certainly, yes. Both are important. The argument that it is not only divorce *per se* is supported by the fact that women whose parents divorced when the women were older than eighteen were at high risk of depression. This suggests it might have been what led up to the divorce not only the divorce itself. ('Why divorce, now?' asked the judge of the ninety-five-year-old couple. 'We had to wait till the children died, your Honour.')

Shelley Taylor brings together evidence from a range of studies, her own and others, that what she terms 'risky families' have a profound effect on children's emotional and physical health.[29] Families, of course, are not all there is to it. Not only is the social environment important because it has an impact on family life, but as the child grows, increasingly the environment outside the home assumes more importance.

Chris Power has been analysing data from the 1958 birth cohort for long enough, well into her second decade of work, to reach some fascinating conclusions. She and Clyde Hertzman looked at health at age thirty-three and asked about the importance of early life factors and those acting on adults. The results come from a huge regression model. You put in all the relevant variables that might be related to health at age thirty-three and see which appear to predict ill-health when the effect of the others is taken into account. By themselves, these associations do not prove causation but they are certainly consistent with the evidence that we have been reviewing. Health at age thirty-three is affected by a combination of effects from early life, cumulative life-course effects, and current circumstances, material and psychosocial.[30]

The third model of how what we do to our children affects their chance of disease as they become adults is the pathway model. In a way, much of the book has been about this. The argument here is that the circumstances impinging on adults are causally important in generating the social gradient in health. But people are not randomly allocated in adult life to high or low status, to jobs with high opportunity for control, to greater or lesser opportunities for social participation. Their chances of being in a favourable or unfavourable situation in adulthood will have much to do with what happened to them earlier in life: the security of attachment, pre-school environment, schooling, the neighbourhoods in which they grew up, opportunities for higher education, quite apart from genetic endowment. Even if the latency model were not operating, nor the accumulation of advantage and disadvantage, early life experiences could still influence adult disease risk by influencing where people ended up. The central point is that there is evidence for all three of these models and their interactions. The socioeconomic environment that affects us as adults has a profound effect on our children.

10. THE MORAL IMPERATIVE
AND THE BOTTOM LINE

To criticise inequality and to desire equality is not, as is sometimes suggested, to cherish the romantic illusion that men are equal in character and intelligence. It is to hold that, while their natural endowments differ profoundly, it is the mark of a civilised society to aim at eliminating such inequalities as have their source not in individual differences but in (social) organisation.

R. H. Tawney[1]

How do you get the press coverage of a scientific report about health moved from page seven of the newspaper to the front page? Get a government representative to ban the press conference. The story then becomes about how a government could have become so exercised about a scientific report. What facts about the health of the population are so scary to a government that they would rather keep them under wraps? Unethical experiments? Leakage of nuclear waste? Civilian casualties? It was worse than that.

The report was *The Health Divide* written by Margaret Whitehead, now professor of public health at the University of Liverpool.[2] Her 1987 report[3] summarised evidence on health inequalities from the 1980s.[4] As my research, showing health inequalities to be increasing in Britain (as they have been in the USA), was quoted in the report, I was asked to be on the panel at the press launch. On the very morning of the press conference, with panel and journalists assembled, we heard the news that the government-appointed chairman of the Health Education Council (HEC) (which had commissioned the report) had directed that the launch could not take place on HEC premises, and that the Director General, David Player, was forbidden to appear. A gaggle of scientists and journalists trooped off to some suitably down-at-heel location; the press conference went ahead; and the fuss moved the news from page seven to page one of the next day's newspapers. The type of headline was: Government attempts cover-up of report that shows widening health gap!

One lesson of this encounter was: thank goodness for a free press. A second, and it is the one that leads me into this final chapter, is that the science of understanding health inequalities is always going to be of great public concern because it goes to the heart of the way we live as individuals and of how we organise our affairs as societies. If a democratically elected government should care so much about this issue as to be wary of its being exposed to public view, we should pay attention. In this chapter I suggest that we should care about health inequalities because of the claims of social justice and of having a fairer society. We need, therefore, to consider what 'fairer' means. I will then go on to show that there is much we can do that would improve the quality of our lives as individuals and reduce the social gradient in health.

A restatement of the main idea: health and human flourishing

This book is about us: you and me. The conclusions from studying the links between health and status – the status syndrome – and populations as diverse as civil servants and ghetto residents, Swedish PhDs and young men in Chicago, Japanese and Keralans, Russians and Hungarians, is that the circumstances in which we live and work are crucial to health. How we organise our lives, or have them structured by society, affects our own health and that of the people around us.

All societies have rankings because individuals are unequal in a variety of ways; but not all societies have the same gradient in health. What matters is the degree to which inequalities in rankings lead to inequalities in capabilities – being able to lead the lives they most want to lead.[5] Central to these capabilities are autonomy and social participation. As I have shown, the lower in the hierarchy you are, the less likely it is that you will have full control over your life and opportunities for full social participation. Autonomy and social participation are so important for health that their lack leads to deterioration in health. Thus the gradient in health has led us to consider fundamental needs for living full and flourishing lives.

In this book I have spent little time on other determinants of health such as environmental influences and patterns of personal behaviour. It is not that I deem them to be unimportant. Rather, I subscribe to the argument put forward by Len Doyal and Ian Gough, an ethicist and social policy academic respectively, who argue that health and autonomy are basic human needs, which cut across all societies.[6] Autonomy includes opportunities for social participation and to fill social roles. This view of basic human needs is close to Aristotelian philosophy, as described by Martha Nussbaum.[7] The evidence I have reviewed shows clearly that these needs are linked: control over one's life and opportunities for meaningful social engagement are necessary for health. It is also likely that the relationship goes the other way: without good health it is harder to achieve autonomy and full social engagement.

Whatever affects risk of health and disease will, therefore, be important in addition to autonomy and social engagement in meeting basic needs. In poor communities risks to health will be basic sanitation, shelter and nutrition; in richer communities, the quality of the environment, and personal behaviours such as diet, smoking, alcohol consumption and patterns of activity. We need to keep two ideas in mind. First, some determinants of health exert their influence regardless of social position. Improvement in environment and health behaviours will benefit the health of everybody whether high status, low, or in between. They are important for everyone's health. Second, this set of determinants does not explain the health gradient. They were the obvious places to look first in seeking to understand why health follows a social gradient. The reason that autonomy and social engagement came to the fore is because the health gradient could not be attributed, in the main, to differences in diet, smoking or other aspects of 'lifestyle'.

The social gradient was not only a way of coming to understand the importance of autonomy and social engagement; but it demonstrated that these factors are distributed unequally in society. They are not randomly distributed among individuals. There are social forces at work that lead to social groups lower in the hierarchy having worse health than higher groups. Where these systematic differences be-tween social groups differ in magnitude it is likely that we can take actions to meliorate their effects. Before focusing on what we can do, let us consider first why we should do it.

Why care?

In the early 1990s, the British government was, for the first time, developing a health policy for the nation: not a policy about health care, i.e. how to organise and deliver medical and surgical services, but about setting goals for the nation's health and setting out means to achieve those goals.[8] I had been asked to write the background paper on prevention of coronary heart disease. I summarised the strong and consistent evidence on the importance of quitting smoking, improving diet, increasing physical activity, and lowering obesity, blood pressure and plasma cholesterol levels. The question I asked myself was whether I should put into my paper the dramatic facts about health inequalities. After all, we still had a Conservative government whose representatives had tried to suppress a scholarly report on health inequalities, as I showed at the beginning of this chapter. Like most academics, I was troubled by having two hands. On the one hand, were I to put something in my paper about the importance of social inequalities in cardiovascular disease, and the paper was rejected as a result, what would happen to the recommendations on smoking and diet? Emphasising inequalities might lead to my paper being ignored with consequent damage to the other recommendations. On the other hand, if I exercised self-censorship and refrained from all mention of social inequalities, it would seem that the year was 1984 not 1991, in fact: the Party had won. I metaphorically sucked my pencil.

In the end, I decided this was not a time for half-measures. We need to address social inequalities in cardiovascular disease, I said, for three reasons: efficiency, tactics and morality. The argument for efficiency relates to the achievement of targets. The government planned to set a target for reduction of heart disease in the whole population. But if only half the population benefited from action to reduce heart disease, that half would have to get a huge reduction to make up for the lack of benefit in the less fortunate half. Therefore, even if you did not care who got disease and who did not – its social distribution – you would want the benefit to be more evenly spread. I assumed that it is more efficient to have all social groups achieve a 30 per cent reduction than one group achieve 60 per cent and another none. I wonder now if the efficiency argument was correct. If you simply wanted bang for your buck and did not care who benefited, the most efficient strategy might be to concentrate on those who were already healthiest and improve them even more. Forget about the unhealthy ones and consign them to the scrap heap; they would not appreciate advice to eat more fruit and vegetables or join another gym. By this stage of the book, you will appreciate that I find little appeal in an efficiency argument that ignores fairness. I had two further arguments for considering inequalities.

The argument for tactics proceeded from a knowledge of what had been happening with smoking. In the 1950s, smoking was equally common in all social classes.[9] Subsequently, the 'middle classes' responded to the 'smoking kills' message more readily than those lower in the social scale. We therefore had the situation of a social gradient in smoking: higher smoking rates lower in the social scale. A policy maker, therefore, had a choice about actions to reduce smoking levels. It was likely that health education messages might increase social inequalities in smoking and other health behaviours, if they were heeded more by the health-conscious, educated groups in society. A policy of taxing tobacco might be more likely to affect consumption of lower-income people.[10] One should, at the very least, take the social distribution of heart disease into account when formulating strategies to deal with its prevention.

The moral argument was that social inequalities in disease are wrong. We should not tolerate a society where inequalities that are remediable are left unchecked. Bold and rather unsubtle, I know. I now have a slightly more nuanced account of when inequalities are unfair and therefore should be the subject of social action.

Back in 1991, I felt better having written it down. But it had little effect. Conservative politicians at the time were not going to make this a centrepiece of their health strategy. The health strategy document was published as *The Health of the Nation*.[11] I don't think the word 'inequalities' appeared anywhere in the document. It was transmuted into the blander 'variations'. In an obscure appendix, there was a reference to the complex nature of ethnic, geographical and social variations; as these were little understood, there was no action that could be taken to reduce them. So much for my agonising. As it turned out, it took a change in government for reduction of health inequalities to become an aim of policy. I shall come to that shortly.

It was put to me at the time, by a senior government official (one of the civil servants in our study, as it happened) that we should not worry about the distribution of health as long as everyone was improving. Focus not on inequalities, therefore, but on moving everyone up. But is that right?

Consider this oft-quoted example of health inequality: the *Titanic* disaster. Drowning rates varied with the class of passenger: highest in the third class, lower in the second class, lowest in the first.[12] There are at least two reasons why we should care: personal and moral. The personal is that 'there but for the grace of God, go I'. Most of us, although we don't travel through life in steerage, don't travel first class either. It could have been me going down with the *Titanic*. If we generalise from the *Titanic* to the health problems that plague us, the personal concern is that most of us are not in the top social group. The status syndrome therefore applies to us: we are suffering from a higher risk of worse health than those who travel through life in luxury class.

The moral reason for caring about the gradient, in the case of the *Titanic*, hits us in the face. Are we going to say, if we are second class, that we simply do not care if some third-class passengers drown, as long as we survive? And, if first class, that it is of no interest if people below us go under – it is their fault if they are silly enough to choose to travel third class? Of course not, at least not in public. If we think it is wrong that people lower in the hierarchy have a higher rate of death by drowning, why do we behave as if we don't care that people lower than us in the social hierarchy have a higher rate of death from heart disease, stroke, lung cancer, chronic lung disease, accidents and violence including suicide? Our inaction suggests that we seem not to care that life is more likely to be blighted by illness and prematurely shortened if people are lower in the hierarchy. I care and, put like this, I suspect that you care too.

A response might be that you care about all sorts of problems, but you want to know if anything can be done to put it right and at what cost. If providing enough lifeboats for everyone on the *Titanic* added immeasurably to the cost, given the rarity of colliding with icebergs, you might decide not to do it. The same money might be better spent providing better education for poor children rather than more life-boats for sea travellers.

Figure 10.1 A theoretical model showing that the social gradient in mortality could bcome steeper when overall mortality rates are falling.

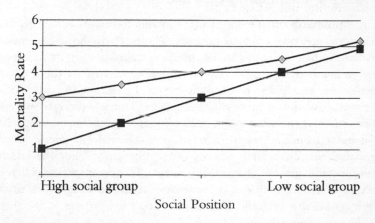

Note: The two graphs show mortality according to social position. In the bottom line, every social group has lower mortality than in the top graph, but the gradient is steeper. The absolute and relative differences between high and low social groups are bigger in the second graph than in the first.

A different response from the senior official I quoted earlier might be, if there were better navigation no one would have drowned; the issue of the gradient in drowning would not therefore have arisen. Hence his argument: improve health for everyone. I agree, with a caveat. Had the *Titanic* reached the other side of the Atlantic, average lifespan for all classes of passenger would have improved – a very welcome benefit – but the third-class passengers would have died earlier on average than the first-class from other causes: tu-berculosis and the like. Given that the gradient in health has, in the last thirty years, become steeper in the US, Britain, and some other developed countries, we need to consider explicitly the distribution of health.

In my view, we should care about inequalities in health where they are the result of unfairness that could be put right. Whether we have the will to put them right will depend on whether we have the means and what we have to give up to put them right. It will also depend on our philosophy of how we wish to organise our affairs.

Reducing inequalities of what?

I drew the two graphs in Figure 10.1 during a conversation with the Princeton economist Angus Deaton. The top one shows the social gradient in health for five social groups: increasing mortality rates as one goes down the social scale. As I have drawn it, there is an absolute mortality difference of just over 2 per cent (5.1 minus 3) between lowest and highest social group. The relative rate of low versus high is $5.1 \div 3 = 1.7$. Let us say that a social change occurred that moved our society from the top to the bottom graph. Here mortality for all social groups is lower, but the higher the social position, the greater the improvement. Hence inequalities have increased: absolute difference between lowest and highest is now 4 per cent (5 minus 1) and the lowest group has 5 times the mortality of the top group $(5 \div 1)$.

Angus Deaton asked me which of the two graphs I would prefer: the bottom one where everyone is better off, or the top one where inequalities are narrower. I demurred. He was in no doubt that all economists would choose the bottom graph because everyone is better off. In fact, a highly prevalent notion of fairness comes from Harvard philosopher John Rawls' theory of justice as fairness.[13] In the Rawls system, if the worst off improve then things have become fairer. This implies that the bottom graph is fairer than the top one. This makes me uncomfortable. How could a situation with dramatically increased inequality be deemed to have become fairer! Angus Deaton suspected that I went for the one with less inequality where everyone suffered more. The implication of such a choice is that those in high social positions should be deprived of benefit in order for there to be less inequality. No, I am not comfortable with greater fairness and bigger inequalities going together. But I am also not comfortable with the idea that everyone in society should be deprived of benefit in order for there to be less inequality.

I rejected both alternatives. I justify this rejection for the reasons set out in Chapters 1 and 2 of this book. There is no reason why the health of today's lowest social group should not, tomorrow, be as good as the health of today's highest social group. It is my view that we should reject both alternatives and aim for a society where health for everyone has improved *and* inequality is less.

In drawing Figure 10.1 with mortality as the 'outcome' I have glossed over a crucial distinction, that between equality of opportunity and equality of condition. Health is a condition. As a doctor, with a public health focus, I am concerned with health of populations. Hence I am concerned with equality of condition. I have argued throughout this book, however, that health functions as a kind of social accountant. If health suffers it tells us that human needs are not being met. Health may be a condition, but inequalities in health are telling us about more general social inequalities in the crucial influences on health.

An alternative approach for those who wish to see progress in reducing inequality is to argue for equality of opportunity. The argument here is that equality of condition or outcome can never be guaranteed because, as Tawney wrote, individuals have different natural endowments. The role of a just society is to guarantee equality of opportunity. The Rawls argument would be to guarantee a fair distribution of primary goods, not to guarantee equality of outcome.

We can use education to illustrate the tension between an approach to fairness and social justice that emphasises equality of opportunity and one that has regard to equality of outcomes. Education is highly relevant to the discussion for all the reasons that we have seen: the link between low education and worse health. Suppose we had new resources to put into education and we decided to spend it according to a principle of fairness: equal amounts for every child regardless of socioeconomic or ethnic background. This is a fine egalitarian programme according to a principle of equality of opportunity. The result would be increasing inequality of outcome: educational performance.[14] Why? Suppose the new money were spent on new computer training for every child. The middle-class children would benefit more. As we saw in Chapter 9, the more advantaged the background the more are children able to take advantage of what schools have to offer – they benefit more.

An egalitarian approach to the distribution of educational opportunity had therefore led to increased inequality in the outcome. I do not want to argue that middle-class children should be deprived of the best education, in order to equalise things out. Not at all. I do claim, however, that we have to have regard to the outcome, in this case educational performance. An analysis that looks at conditions therefore reveals whether or not a policy that focuses on equality of opportunity is achieving a reduction in inequalities. In the case of education, such an analysis leads to recommending investment in preschool education and support for low-income families, not to making schools worse in middle-class areas.

This tension between equality of opportunity and equality of condition has been well characterised by the Nobel prize-winning economist Robert Fogel.[15] He describes four 'great awakenings' in American society to the idea of equality. (The first, in the eighteenth century, emphasised 'new birth' at revival meetings with an emergence of an ethic of benevolence and challenge to church authority.) In particular, the second great awakening, which began in the early nineteenth century, argued strongly for egalitarianism of opportunity, e.g. female franchise, prohibition, and universal primary education. It was appropriate to a predominantly rural society with small businesses, that was relatively homogeneous ethnically and in terms of religion. When society changed dramatically, with urbanisation, immigration and the rise of industrialisation, equality of opportunity was no longer sufficient to achieve egalitarian advances.

The third great awakening began at the end of the nineteenth century and argued for equality of economic and social conditions. Fogel characterises it as modern egalitarianism. It raised equality of condition over equality of opportunity. Modern egalitarianism saw the state as a primary instrument of promoting equality of material conditions, and it had remarkable success in reducing differences in health. Better nutrition for all reduced social and ethnic differences in height. I have expressed profound unease over the size of the differences in life expectancy between black and white that we see in the US today. Nevertheless, the gap was much bigger at the beginning of the twentieth century than at the end of it.

If the third great awakening, modern egalitarianism, dealt with a fairer distribution of material goods, the need now, says Fogel, is for a postmodern egalitarian agenda: the major challenge for egalitarian progress is in spiritual resources. I have been out of California too long to be comfortable with the word 'spiritual', but my research on psychosocial factors fits well with the Fogel formulation. I speak of the need for autonomy and social engagement. Fogel speaks of achieving self-realisation. They are very close. Just as, in the past, access to material resources was the aim of egalitarian progress, so in the future egalitarianism of self-realisation will be the watchword.

Where does that leave me on the spectrum of equality of condition, achieved through social action and equality of opportunity? Somewhere in the middle, endorsing Amartya Sen's concept of capabilities. It is important to guarantee equality of opportunity, but that is not enough. Equality of opportunity may be more apparent than real. The opportunity to go to Harvard or Oxbridge is simply not equally available, not only because there are inequalities of natural endowment, but because there are inequalities in the possibility to develop natural talents to their fullest. We need to pay attention not only to what is available to people but what they can do with what is available, their capabilities. A more just distribution of capabilities – control and social engagement – will lead to a more equal distribution of health. The aim should be to focus on the conditions for good health. These will be material, yes, but more they will have to do with self-realisation: control over life in the sense of being able to lead the life we most want to lead.

What is to be done?

This is not utopian dreaming. It can be achieved, but it will require action of individuals and society. A society, or its leaders, cannot push a recalcitrant population where it does not want to go, without great human misery. If individuals do not want to take action to increase their sense of autonomy and social engagement, the institutions and activities of society can do little to take them in that direction. Equally, individuals cannot achieve this solely for themselves. The circumstances in which we live and work determine, to a large extent, how we as individuals function. There are things you and I can do in our everyday lives, but there is much that we want the organs of society to develop and improve.

One important role for individuals is in changing the political agenda. My view of our political leaders is that they do not see their role as providing leadership in changing social views. At best, they capture a mood of the population, or sections of it to which they are in thrall, and translate it into political reality. Much has been made of the fact that Margaret Thatcher and Ronald Reagan captured a mood of individualism in sections of their populations and turned it into a political credo. We need now to develop a mood that emphasises autonomy and full social engagement, not just for the privileged, but for everyone regardless of status. Conservative or anarchist political philosophers often champion individual rights as against those of an interfering state. I am not using autonomy in that sense of the individual against the state. Social action is fundamental to ensure that people lower in the social hierarchy, as well as higher, enjoy autonomy and social engagement in their jobs, their communities and their schools.

Does this all sound a bit starry-eyed? It need not. We need to use the scientific findings as set out here in three ways: to act ourselves, to change the social and political agenda and to push social institutions to move. Recent experience in Britain makes me optimistic that we can push governments to move in this direction.

I described at the beginning of this chapter how a Conservative British government was unwilling even to recognise the problem of social inequalities in health, let alone take action. Such a situation is familiar to American colleagues. But this situation changed in Britain. I was one among a small number of scientists who had been doing research on health inequalities for two decades before the election of the New Labour government of Tony Blair in 1997. Our research was 'pure' in the sense that no one appeared particularly concerned with the policy implications. Then, suddenly, yesterday's pure research became today's applied research because the new government declared two headline health targets: to improve health for everyone, and to reduce the gap in health between those worst off and the average.

The government set up an Independent Inquiry into Inequalities in Health under the chairmanship of a former Chief Medical Officer, Sir Donald Acheson.[16] I was a member of the small scientific advisory group that reviewed the evidence and prepared the report. Parenthetically, as a young researcher, I used to think that if ever I got to the stage where I thought government committees, or even independent committees, were important, heaven help me. The business of research was to publish a paper. If the question, 'now what?', arose at the end of a piece of research, the answer was to do more research and publish another paper. Yet here am I about to tell you why I think the Acheson Report is so important. I now think that the purpose of research is to find things out, certainly, but in my area at least, it is to use that new knowledge to change things for the better – to improve the lives of all of us, and to reduce health inequalities. That was the mission the government set for the Acheson Inquiry. I told my younger self to see sense and stop giving me such a hard time. The possibility to have research findings feed directly into policy was not to be missed.

Place yourself on such a group. The first question to confront is that most people see the inequalities problem as one of bad health among the poor. The challenge is to take on the entire health gradient. Given the research findings from Whitehall and elsewhere, it seems entirely reasonable to attack the health gradient.

A second question for you to consider is what you are going to recommend about living standards for the worst off. Are you going to bite the bullet and recommend redistribution of income? In the US, the government has been pursuing a policy of income redistribution, but not in the direction the Acheson group had in mind. I note that those who chorus most vigorously against fiscal policies that aim at redistribution from rich to poor, are curiously silent at tax changes that redistribute to the benefit of the rich. On Acheson we did indeed endorse redistribution such that the living standards of the worst off were brought closer to the average.

The discussion in this book in Chapters 3 and 4 was informed by precisely this question of living standards. I had been writing that relative position in the hierarchy was important for health. It was put to me that it was illogical for me then to endorse a recommendation that supported an absolute improvement in income and living conditions. It was at that point that reading Amartya Sen, whom I quoted in Chapter 3, gave me the answer: a relative difference in income can translate into an absolute difference in capabilities. If having a low income means lack of control and participation, then one step along the way of redressing that problem is to improve relative living conditions.

A third point for you to consider as a member of the Acheson group is where to direct your recommendations. Every area of public life potentially has an impact on the lives people are able to lead and hence on health and health inequalities. Therefore although your topic is health inequalities, your recommendations need to span the whole of government, not just the health department.

The Acheson group made thirty-nine recommendations. These are listed in the Appendix. Only three of the thirty-nine related to health care. The others covered the tax and benefit system; education; employment; housing and environment; mobility, transport and pollution; nutrition. We also oriented our recommendations to stages of the life course: mothers, children and families; young people and adults of working age; and older people. We examined the potential impact of our recommendations on ethnic and gender differences in health. It is not stretching the concept I have laid out to describe our recommendations as fitting in to the three categories that I have been using: health, autonomy and full social engagement.

Government committees have their function and help, slowly, to move things along. I want, though, to come back to things we can all do that would make a difference. Our actions will be helped if we can push local and central governments along. There are four areas worth highlighting because they are important and show how the research covered in this book can lead to actions for improvement: children, workplaces, communities, and support for older people.

Children

It is little short of heartbreaking that children's voyage through the educational system should be blighted from the moment they enter the school. But that is the implication of the research covered in Chapter 9. Children from disadvantaged backgrounds do worse in school. The social circumstances of adults affect their children, such that inequalities can be 'transmitted' socially and psychologically, rather than biologically. A prime way of giving children a good start in life is to help their parents. There has been a move to get women with young children back to work and off welfare. Whether this is a good policy depends on the quality of the work, and the alternatives available for child care. If a single mother comes off welfare to go into a low-paid, uncertain job with low control and imbalance between efforts and rewards, she is unlikely to benefit. Nor is her child, unless good-quality, affordable child care is available.

We need therefore first, to provide appropriate financial, social and emotional support for parents; second, to provide high-quality programmes for pre-school children, third to identify and address the physical and psychological needs of children who are looked after by others. The aim should be to prepare the child for school. Without such preparation money spent on education is unlikely to have an effect in reducing inequalities in educational performance. There is much to do improve the standard of education for all.

Employment

The workplace also offers the opportunity either to make life harder for people with bad effects on health or to make life richer and more meaningful with consequent health improvement. What you and I want for ourselves we should want for everyone in society: work that is characterised by a degree of control over the way we manage the job, and the inevitable psychological demands. We also want appropriate rewards for the efforts we expend – be those rewards money, self-esteem or status in the eyes of the world. (See Chapter 5.) We also want not to feel insecure about losing the job. The old style of management of managing by fear should be long gone. It is bad for employees and, therefore, probably bad for business.

Does this sound utopian? I shall tell you in a moment what happened as a result of our research recommendations on the work-place.

Communities

It is easy to know what we want in the way of a healthy community; less easy to know how to get it. There is no question that environmental planning and design are crucial, but so are you and I. We want to create safe, secure environments in which people of all generations can flourish. There is a movement across the world that the World Health Organization has sponsored: Healthy Cities. Selected cities have been trying to improve urban environments, including housing quality, access to goods and services, promotion of social networks and economic regeneration.

There is a catch in attempts to improve urban environments. When the middle classes move into a hitherto run-down area, they use their financial and other resources to 'improve' the area. While such gentrification may make the area habitable for them, if the former, more deprived residents end up moving out, their lot may not have been improved at all. No one quite knows how to improve social capital in an area (see Chapter 7). Presumably we want to feel that we are connected with our neighbours without that leading to exclusion of those outside the circle.

Older people

Much of the Acheson group's concern was with the maintenance of independence and quality of life. A few weeks after we published the Inquiry Report in 1998, I was at a health policy meeting where a distinguished elder statesman of the health policy fraternity stopped me in the street and harangued me. How, he wanted to know, could I possibly justify putting my name to this string of unsubstantiated recommendations. He illustrated the sheer fatuousness of what we had done by asking rhetorically how it could possibly do anything for anyone's health to subsidise public transport for older people – he actually said, old buffers like him.

When I could eventually get a word in, I offered the opinion that subsidised public transport for older people was one of our better evidence-based recommendations. The evidence shows clearly (see Chapter 6) that lack of social contacts kills older people, and is not so good for younger ones either. The evidence also shows that reducing the fare increases usage of public transport. This was, therefore, a policy that had high likelihood of increasing quality and length of lives of older people. He invited me to lunch.

What happened next?

I have described the fate of a previous report on health inequalities. The government of the day tried to bury it.[17] This, of course, led to huge merriment on the part of the press, much public discussion, anger among activists and little action. When we produced the Acheson Report, the government issued a report saying they welcomed it. My heart sank; killed with blandness. Welcoming the report seemed like a clever way of doing nothing at all, while talking correctly. In the event they did more, much more. We reviewed the policies that were set in motion in the wake of Acheson, that may have impact on health inequalities, and they are substantial.[18] The degree to which these policies do what they set out to do, in reversing the trend of wider health inequalities, remains a matter of intense interest.

I do want to pick out three areas where action has been taken, whether or not as a result of our report is difficult to say. They may have already been on the government agenda. Either way, they are consistent with what a recommendation to reduce health inequalities would wish to see.

Income inequalities have been increasing in many countries including Britain and the US. The reasons for this are not altogether clear. Hence there is not much governments can do on inequalities in gross income. Governments do, however, mitigate the effects of inequalities in gross income by taxation and distributing benefits. Quietly in the UK, the Chancellor of the Exchequer (Minister of

Finance elsewhere) has been redistributing income. The Institute of
Fiscal Studies has calculated the effects of the Chancellor's annual
budgets on income and the results are shown in Figure 10.2.[19] The
higher the starting income in 1997, the less benefit someone had from
changes to fiscal policy. This is redistribution of income, and it is
graded; it is not only the poor who benefit, but the lower the initial
income the greater the benefit. This was recommendation 3 of the
Acheson Report, although we cannot claim credit for the Chancellor's actions.

**Figure 10.2 The effects on disposable incomes of changes to tax and benefits
between 1997 and 2002, by income decile group**

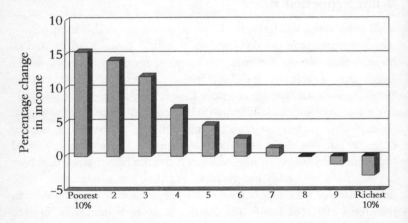

Note: The chart shows how changes in personal taxes and benefits and in
expenditure taxes have affected disposable incomes on average in tenths of the
population ranked according to disposable (measured before taking account of
reforms announced between 1997 and 2002). Proportional gains in income due to
these fiscal reforms have tended to be larger for those with the lower incomes.

Source: Bond and Wakefield (2003)

A second area of note relates to early child development. Head Start
in the USA has had a mixed press – the idea that by investing in pre-
school education one can give disadvantaged children a better chance
when they get into the school system. The UK government has put
significant resources into a new programme called Sure Start, aimed at

children up to three years old, from relatively deprived backgrounds. As I write, it is being implemented and, eventually, will be evaluated.

The 'music to my ears' development centres on work. Stress at work is now an area of major national concern. That's not the good news. The welcome development is that a government-sponsored organisation, the Health and Safety Executive, is taking it seriously. As spelled out in Chapter 5, most people view work stress as having to do with pressure, deadlines, too much to do. The new view that high demands are bad for health when in the presence of low control, and imbalance between efforts and rewards increases risk of mental and physical illness, has now taken hold. The Health and Safety Executive has a strong record of concern with physical and chemical hazards at work. They have now included the psychosocial work environment within their purview. Based on our research, they are working with organisations to try to change work climate so that employees have more control, more controllable demands and better support in the workplace.

We have made the case that there should be no trade-off between a healthy workplace and a wealthy one. It is likely that paying attention to the working conditions that lead to better health will lead to more productivity. Everyone stands to benefit. It is a virtuous circle.

Making it real

This is, of course, not a recipe book. There are no prescriptions telling you what to do when you get up in the morning – the social-determinants equivalent of the low-carbohydrate diet or the one-minute manager. I am not going to tell you how to treat your neighbour with the respect she deserves, how to raise your children to be self-aware people with a passion for social justice that goes along with their efforts at self-realisation, how to treat your employees as individuals who, given a sense of autonomy and engagement, will have better health and be more productive. Would it help if you fostered a neighbourhood spirit or joined a club as a mark of your social engagement? Yes, probably, but it is not for me to prescribe how that should be done. Would it be beneficial if you started a movement that agitated to give people more control in the workplace, and to enhance their sense of engagement? Almost certainly, but what that means in practice needs to be tailored to the specific situation.

It is not only my reluctance to prescribe that leads me to refrain from giving 'how-to' instructions. This has been a book about science, but science with clear implications for what should happen next. My purpose has been to alert you to the existence of basic human needs – health, autonomy and social engagement – that are intimately related. How these are met will differ among cultures and societies; hence a recipe is inappropriate.

Each of us has several roles, whether as parent, partner, child, employer, employee, resident, citizen, opinion former, opinion consumer, older person, group member. What we do in these roles has an important influence on our own opportunities for self-realisation, in Fogel's phrase, or autonomy and social participation, in mine. What we do also has effects on others' autonomy and opportunities for social engagement. These are not just pleasant things to have, but they are so fundamental that health suffers if these needs are thwarted. The fact that we systematically thwart them for people lower in the hierarchy means that status syndrome is a stain on a civilised society. In order to do something about that, we need to have regard not only to what we can do to make life better for ourselves and those around us, but how we move the organs of society in the direction of improving opportunities for control and engagement for all. My hope is that we all become agents for change: changing ourselves, changing the debate about the kind of society we want, and taking steps to improve it.

There will always be inequalities in society but the magnitude of their effects on health is within our control. Why not make things better? It is in all our interests.

APPENDIX:
Recommendations from the Independent Inquiry into Inequalities in Health

Chair
  Donald Acheson
Scientific Advisory Group
  David Barker
  Jacky Chambers
  Hilary Graham
  Michael Marmot
  Margaret Whitehead
Secretary
  Ray Earwicker
  Catherine Law

General recommendations

1. We recommend that as part of health impact assessment, all policies likely to have a direct or indirect effect on health should be evaluated in terms of their impact on health inequalities, and should be formulated in such a way that by favouring the less well off they will, wherever possible, reduce such inequalities.

  1.1 We recommend establishing mechanisms to monitor inequalities in health and to evaluate the effectiveness of measures taken to reduce them.

  1.2 We recommend a review of data needs to improve the capacity to monitor inequalities in health and their determinants at a national and local level.

  2. We recommend a high priority is given to policies aimed at improving health and reducing health inequalities in women of childbearing age, expectant mothers and young children.

Poverty, income, tax and benefits

3. We recommend policies which will further reduce income inequalities, and improve the living standards of households in receipt of social security benefits. Specifically:

3.1 We recommend further reductions in poverty in women of childbearing age, expectant mothers, young children and older people should be made by increasing benefits in cash or in kind to them.

3.2 We recommend uprating of benefits and pensions according to principles which protect and, where possible, improve the standard of living of those who depend on them and which narrow the gap between their standard of living and average living standards.

3.3 We recommend measures to increase the uptake of benefits in entitled groups.
We recommend further steps to increase employment opportunities (recommendation 8.1).

Education

4. We recommend the provision of additional resources for schools serving children from less well off groups to enhance their educational achievement. The Revenue Support Grant formula and other funding mechanisms should be more strongly weighted to reflect need and socioeconomic disadvantage.

5. We recommend the further development of high-quality pre-school education so that it meets, in particular, the needs of disadvantaged families. We also recommend that the benefits of pre-school education to disadvantaged families are evaluated and, if necessary, additional resources are made available to support further development.

6. We recommend the further development of 'health-promoting schools', initially focused on, but not limited to, disadvantaged communities.

7. We recommend further measures to improve the nutrition provided at school, including: the promotion of school food policies; the development of budgeting and cooking skills; the preservation of free school meals entitlement; the provision of free school fruit; and the restriction of less healthy food.

Employment

8. We recommend policies which improve the opportunities for work and which ameliorate the health consequences of unemployment. Specifically:

8.1 We recommend further steps to increase employment opportunities.

8.2 We recommend further investment in high-quality training for young and long-term unemployed people.

We recommend policies which will further reduce income inequalities, and improve the living standards of households in receipt of social security benefits (recommendation 3).

We recommend an integrated policy for the provision of affordable, high-quality day care and pre-school education with extra resources for disadvantaged communities (recommendation 21.1).

9. We recommend policies to improve the quality of jobs, and reduce psychosocial work hazards. Specifically:

9.1 We recommend employers, unions and relevant agencies take further measures to improve health through good management practices which lead to an increased level of control, variety and appropriate use of skills in the workforce.

9.2 We recommend assessing the impact of employment policies on health and inequalities in health (see also recommendation 1).

Housing and environment

10. We recommend policies which improve the availability of social housing for the less well off within a framework of environmental improvement, planning and design which takes into account social networks, and access to goods and services.

11. We recommend policies which improve housing provision and access to health care for both officially and unofficially homeless people.

12. We recommend policies which aim to improve the quality of housing. Specifically:

12.1 We recommend policies to improve insulation and heating systems in new and existing buildings in order to reduce further the prevalence of fuel poverty.

12.2 We recommend amending housing and licensing conditions and housing regulations on space and amenity to reduce accidents in the home, including measures to promote the installation of smoke detectors in existing homes.

13. We recommend the development of policies to reduce the fear of crime and violence, and to create a safe environment for people to live in.

We recommend policies which will further reduce income inequalities, and improve the living standards of households in receipt of social security benefits (recommendation 3).

Mobility, transport and pollution

14. We recommend the further development of a high-quality public transport system which is integrated with other forms of transport and is affordable to the user.

15. We recommend further measures to encourage walking and cycling as forms of transport and to ensure the safe separation of pedestrians and cyclists from motor vehicles.

16. We recommend further steps to reduce the usage of motor cars to cut the mortality and morbidity associated with motor vehicle emissions.

17. We recommend further measures to reduce traffic speed, by environmental design and modification of roads, lower speed limits in built-up areas, and stricter enforcement of speed limits.

18. We recommend concessionary fares should be available to pensioners and disadvantaged groups throughout the country, and that local schemes should emulate high-quality schemes, such as those of London and the West Midlands.

Nutrition and the Common Agricultural Policy

19. We recommend a comprehensive review of the Common Agricultural Policy (CAP)'s impact on health and inequalities in health.

19.1 We recommend strengthening the CAP Surplus Food Scheme to improve the nutritional position of the less well off.

20. We recommend policies which will increase the availability and accessibility of foodstuffs to supply an adequate and affordable diet. Specifically:

20.1 We recommend the further development of policies which will ensure adequate retail provision of food to those who are disadvantaged.

We recommend policies which will further reduce income inequalities, and improve the living standards of households in receipt of social security benefits (recommendation 3).

We recommend the further development of a high-quality public transport system which is integrated with other forms of transport and is affordable to the user (recommendation 14).

20.2 We recommend policies which reduce the sodium content of processed foods, particularly bread and cereals, and which do not incur additional cost to the consumer.

Mothers, children and families

21. We recommend policies which reduce poverty in families with children by promoting the material support of parents; by removing barriers to work for parents who wish to combine work with parenting; and by enabling those who wish to devote full-time to parenting to do so. Specifically:

21.1 We recommend an integrated policy for the provision of affordable, high-quality day care and pre-school education with extra resources for disadvantaged communities (see also recommendation 5).

We recommend further reductions in poverty in women of childbearing age, expectant mothers, young children and older people should be made by increasing benefits in cash or in kind to them (recommendation 3.1).

We recommend measures to increase the uptake of benefits in entitled groups (recommendation 3.3).

22. We recommend policies which improve the health and nutrition of women of childbearing age and their children with priority given to the elimination of food poverty and the prevention and reduction of obesity. Specifically:

We recommend further reductions in poverty in women of childbearing age, expectant mothers, young children and older people should be made by increasing benefits in cash or in kind to them (recommendation 3.1).

We recommend further measures to improve the nutrition provided at school, including: the promotion of school food policies; the development of budgeting and cooking skills; the preservation of free school meals entitlement; the provision of free school fruit; and the restriction of less healthy food (recommendation 7).

We recommend a comprehensive review of the Common Agricultural Policy (CAP)'s impact on health and inequalities in health (recommendation 19).

We recommend policies which will increase the availability and accessibility of foodstuffs to supply an adequate and affordable diet (recommendation 20).

22.1 We recommend policies which increase the prevalence of breast-feeding.

22.2 We recommend the fluoridation of the water supply.

22.3 We recommend the further development of programmes to help women to give up smoking before or during pregnancy, and which are focused on the less well off.

23. We recommend policies that promote the social and emotional support for parents and children. Specifically:

23.1 We recommend the further development of the role and capacity of health visitors to provide social and emotional support to expectant parents, and parents with young children.

23.2 We recommend local authorities identify and address the physical and psychological health needs of looked-after children.

Young people and adults of working age

We recommend policies which improve the opportunities for work and which ameliorate the health consequences of unemployment (recommendation 8).

We recommend policies to improve the quality of jobs, and reduce psychosocial work hazards (recommendation 9).

24. We recommend measures to prevent suicide among young people, especially among young men and seriously mentally-ill people.

25. We recommend policies which promote sexual health in young people and reduce unwanted teenage pregnancy, including access to appropriate contraceptive services.

26. We recommend policies which promote the adoption of healthier lifestyles, particularly in respect of factors which show a strong social gradient in prevalence or consequences. Specifically:

26.1 We recommend policies which promote moderate intensity exercise including: further provision of cycling and walking routes to school, and other environmental modifications aimed at the safe separation of pedestrians and cyclists from motor vehicles; and safer opportunities for leisure.

26.2 We recommend policies to reduce tobacco smoking including: restricting smoking in public places; abolishing tobacco advertising and promotion; and community, mass media and educational initiatives.

26.3 We recommend increases in the real price of tobacco to discourage young people from becoming habitual smokers and to encourage adult smokers to quit. These increases should be introduced in tandem with policies to improve the living standards of low-income households and polices to help smokers in these households become and remain ex-smokers.

26.4 We recommend making nicotine replacement therapy available on prescription.

26.5 We recommend policies which reduce alcohol-related ill-health, accidents and violence, including measures which at least maintain the real cost of alcohol.

Older people

27. We recommend policies which will promote the material well being of older people. Specifically:

We recommend policies which will further reduce income inequalities, and improve the living standards of households in receipt of social security benefits (recommendation 3).

We recommend uprating of benefits and pensions according to principles which protect and, where possible, improve the standard of living of those who depend on them and which narrow the gap between their standard of living and average living standards (recommendation 3.2).

We recommend measures to increase the uptake of benefits among entitled groups (recommendation 3.3).

28. We recommend the quality of homes in which older people live be improved. Specifically:

We recommend policies to improve insulation and heating systems in new and existing buildings in order to reduce further the prevalence of fuel poverty (recommendation 12.1).

We recommend amending housing and licensing conditions and housing regulations on space and amenity to reduce accidents in the home, including measures to promote the installation of smoke detectors in existing homes (recommendation 12.2).

29. We recommend policies which will promote the maintenance of mobility, independence, and social contacts. Specifically:

We recommend the development of policies to reduce the fear of crime and violence, and to create a safe environment for people to live in (recommendation 13).

We recommend the further development of a high-quality public transport system which is integrated with other forms of transport and is affordable to the user (recommendation 14).

We recommend concessionary fares should be available to pensioners and disadvantaged groups throughout the country, and that local schemes should emulate high-quality schemes, such as those of London and the West Midlands (recommendation 18).

30. We recommend the further development of health and social services for older people, so that these services are accessible and distributed according to need. *We recommend a review of data needs to improve the capacity to monitor inequalities in health and their determinants at a national and local level (recommendation 1.2).*

Ethnicity

31. We recommend that the needs of minority ethnic groups are specifically considered in the development and implementation of policies aimed at reducing socioeconomic inequalities. Specifically:

We recommend policies which will further reduce income inequalities, and improve the living standards of households in receipt of social security benefits (recommendation 3).

We recommend policies which improve the opportunities for work and which ameliorate the health consequences of unemployment (recommendation 8).

We recommend policies which improve the availability of social housing for the less well off within a framework of environmental improvement, planning and design which takes into account social networks, and access to goods and services (recommendation 10).

We recommend policies which aim to improve the quality of housing (recommendation 12).

We recommend the development of policies to reduce the fear of crime and violence, and to create a safe environment for people to live in (recommendation 13).

We recommend the further development of a high-quality public transport system which is integrated with other forms of transport and is affordable to the user (recommendation 14).

We recommend further measures to encourage walking and cycling as forms of transport and to ensure the safe separation of pedestrians and cyclists from motor vehicles (recommendation 15).

We recommend further steps to reduce the usage of motor cars to cut the mortality and morbidity associated with motor vehicle emissions (recommendation 16).

We recommend further measures to reduce traffic speed, by environmental design and modification of roads, lower speed limits in built-up areas, and stricter enforcement of speed limits (recommendation 17).

We recommend concessionary fares should be available to pensioners and disadvantaged groups throughout the country, and that local schemes should emulate high-quality schemes, such as those of London and the West Midlands (recommendation 18).

32. We recommend the further development of services which are sensitive to the needs of minority ethnic people and which promote greater awareness of their health risks.

33. We recommend the needs of minority ethnic groups are specifically considered in needs assessment, resource allocation, health-care planning and provision. Specifically:

We recommend a review of data needs to improve the capacity to monitor inequalities in health and their determinants at a national and local level (recommendation 1.2).

Gender

34. We recommend policies which reduce the excess mortality from accidents and suicide in young men (see also recommendation 24). Specifically:

We recommend policies which improve the opportunities for work and which ameliorate the health consequences of unemployment (recommendation 8).

We recommend policies which improve housing provision and access to health care for both officially and unofficially homeless people (recommendation 11).

We recommend further measures to encourage walking and cycling as forms of transport and to ensure the safe separation of pedestrians and cyclists from motor vehicles (recommendation 15).

We recommend further steps to reduce the usage of motor cars to cut the mortality and morbidity associated with motor vehicle emissions (recommendation 16).

We recommend further measures to reduce traffic speed, by environmental design and modification of roads, lower speed limits in built-up areas, and stricter enforcement of speed limits (recommendation 17).

We recommend measures to prevent suicide among young people, especially among young men and seriously mentally-ill people (recommendation 24).

We recommend policies which reduce alcohol-related ill-health, accidents and violence, including measures which at least maintain the real cost of alcohol (recommendation 26.5).

35. We recommend policies which reduce psychosocial ill health in young women in disadvantaged circumstances, particularly those caring for young children. Specifically:

We recommend further reductions in poverty in women of childbearing age, expectant mothers, young children and older people should be made by increasing benefits in cash or in kind to them (recommendation 3.1).

We recommend uprating of benefits and pensions according to principles which protect and, where possible, improve the standard of living of those who depend on them, and which narrow the gap between their standard of living and average living standards (recommendation 3.2).

We recommend measures to increase the uptake of benefits among entitled groups (recommendation 3.3).

We recommend policies which improve the availability of social housing for the less well off within a framework of environmental improvement, planning and design which takes into account social networks, and access to goods and services (recommendation 10).

We recommend the further development of a high-quality public transport system which is integrated with other forms of transport and is affordable to the user (recommendation 14).

We recommend policies which will increase the availability and accessibility of foodstuffs to supply an adequate and affordable diet (recommendation 20).

We recommend policies which reduce poverty in families with children by promoting the material support of parents; by removing barriers to work for parents who wish to combine work with parenting, and by enabling those who wish to devote full-time to parenting to do so (recommendation 21).

We recommend an integrated policy for the provision of affordable, high-quality day care and pre-school education with extra resources for disadvantaged communities (recommendation 21.1).

We recommend policies which improve the health and nutrition of women of childbearing age and their children with priority given to the elimination of food poverty and the prevention and reduction of obesity (recommendation 22).

We recommend policies which promote the social and emotional support for parents and children (recommendation 23).

We recommend the further development of the role and capacity of health visitors to provide social and emotional support to expectant parents, and parents with young children (recommendation 23.1).

We recommend policies which promote sexual health in young people and reduce unwanted teenage pregnancy, including access to appropriate contraceptive services (recommendation 25).

36. We recommend policies which reduce disability and ameliorate its consequences in older women, particularly those living alone. Specifically: *We recommend further reductions in poverty in women of childbearing age, expectant mothers, young children and older people should be made by increasing benefits in cash or in kind to them (recommendation 3.1).*

We recommend uprating of benefits and pensions according to principles which protect and, where possible, improve the standard of living of those who depend on them, and which narrow the gap between their standard of living and average living standards (recommendation 3.2).

We recommend measures to increase the uptake of benefits among entitled groups (recommendation 3.3).

We recommend the development of policies to reduce the fear of crime and violence, and to create a safe environment for people to live in (recommendation 13).

We recommend the further development of a high-quality public transport system which is integrated with other forms of transport and is affordable to the user (recommendation 14).

We recommend concessionary fares should be available to pensioners and disadvantaged groups throughout the country, and that local schemes should emulate high-quality schemes, such as those of London and the West Midlands (recommendation 18).

We recommend the quality of homes in which older people live be improved (recommendation 28).

We recommend the further development of health and social sevices for older people, so that these services are accessible and distributed according to need (recommendation 30).

The National Health Service

37. We recommend that providing equitable access to effective care in relation to need should be a governing principle of all policies in the NHS. Priority should be given to the achievement of equity in the planning, implementation and delivery of services at every level of the NHS. Specifically:

37.1 We recommend extending the focus of clinical governance to give equal prominence to equity of access to effective health care.

37.2 We recommend extending the remit of the National Institute for Clinical Excellence to include equity of access to effective health care.

37.3 We recommend developing the National Service Frameworks to address inequities in access to effective primary care.

37.4 We recommend that performance management in relation to the national performance management framework is focused on achieving more equitable access, provision and targeting of effective services in relation to need in both primary and hospital sectors.

37.5 We recommend that the Department of Health and NHS Executive set out their responsibilities for furthering the principle of equity of access to effective health and social care, and that health authorities, working with Primary Care Groups and providers on local clinical governance, agree priorities and objectives for reducing inequities in access to effective care. These should form part of the Health Improvement Programme.

38. We recommend giving priority to the achievement of a more equitable allocation of NHS resources. This will require adjustments to the ways in which resources are allocated and the speed with which resource allocation targets are met. Specifically:

38.1 We recommend reviewing the 'pace of change' policy to enable health authorities that are furthest from their capitation targets to move more quickly to their actual target.

38.2 We recommend extending the principle of needs-based weighting to non-cash limited General Medical Services (GMS) resources. The size and effectiveness of deprivation payments in meeting the needs and improving the health outcomes amongst the most disadvantaged populations, including ethnic minorities, should be assessed.

38.3 We recommend reviewing the size and effectiveness of the Hospital and Community Health Service (HCHS) formula and deprivation payments in influencing the health-care outcomes of the most disadvantaged populations, and to consider alternative methods of focusing resources for health promotion and public health care to reduce health inequalities.

38.4 We recommend establishing a review of the relationship of private practice to the NHS with particular reference to access to effective treatments, resource allocation and availability of staff.

39. We recommend Directors of Public Health, working on behalf of health and local authorities, produce an equity profile for the population they serve, and undertake a triennial audit of progress towards achieving objectives to reduce inequalities in health.

39.1 We recommend there should be a duty of partnership between the NHS Executive and regional government to ensure that effective local partnerships are established between health, local authorities and other agencies and that joint programmes to address health inequalities are in place and monitored.

We recommend that as part of health impact assessment, all policies likely to have a direct or indirect effect on health should be evaluated in terms of their impact on health inequalities, and should be formulated in such a way that by favouring the less well off they will, wherever possible, reduce such inequalities (recommendation 1).

NOTES

Introduction

1 Murray, Michaud, McKenna and Marks (1998).
2 Marmot, Rose, Shipley and Hamilton (1978); Marmot, Shipley and Rose (1984); Marmot and Shipley (1996).
3 Farmer (1999).
4 Sen (1999).
5 Sen (1999).
6 Farmer (1999).
7 Farmer (2003).

Chapter 1 Some Are More Equal than Others

1 Maugham (1949).
2 I am not the only one moved by *La Bohème*. A friend who is a professional musician said that she played in the orchestra in a five-week season of *La Bohème* and cried every night when Mimi died!
3 McDonough, Duncan, Williams and House (1997).
4 Redelmeier and Singh (2001).
5 Osler (1910).
6 Friedman and Rosenman (1974).
7 Marmot, Adelstein, Robinson and Rose (1978).
8 Farmer (1999).
9 Stevenson (1928).
10 Drever and Whitehead (1997).
11 US Department of Health and Human Services (1998).
12 For a brilliant introduction to this way of thinking and its application to a number of contemporary issues, see Gladwell (2000).
13 Collis and Greenwood (1921) in Davey Smith, Dorling and Shaw (2001).
14 Quoted in Farmer (1999).
15 McKeown (1976).
16 Szreter (1988).
17 Farmer (1999).
18 See Booth in Davey Smith, Dorling and Shaw (2001).
19 Rose (1992).
20 Daly and Wilson (1988).
21 Cronin (1991).

Chapter 2 Men and Women Behaving Badly?

1 Shakespeare, *Julius Caesar*, Act I, Scene II.
2 The original for this is Shakespeare's *Twelfth Night*: 'Be not afraid of greatness: some are born great, some achieve greatness and some have greatness thrust upon them' (Act II, Scene V).
3 In the best British tradition, the first Whitehall study was arranged over lunch at a London gentlemen's club by Donald Reid, one of my predecessors as Professor of Epidemiology at the University of London. He sought to study a population of employees of a large organisation because it made it easier to find them and organise the medical examinations.
4 Marmot and Shipley (1996).
5 The first Whitehall study was started in 1967. Over 18,000 men, initially aged forty to sixty-nine, underwent a medical screening examination in London. They were then followed using the national death registry. The data shown come from the twenty-five-year follow-up.
6 Acheson (1998).
7 OPCS (1978).
8 It has recently changed to a new system, the Office for National Statistics Socio-economic Classification, that groups occupations according to measures that are closer to differences in span of control in the workplace, i.e. more like Whitehall employment grades.
9 Marmot, Bosma, Hemingway, Brunner and Stansfeld (1997).
10 Britton, Shipley, Marmot and Hemingway (under review, unpublished).
11 Moser, Pugh and Goldblatt (1988).
12 Sacker, Firth, Fitzpatrick, Lynch and Bartley (2000).
13 Klein (2000).
14 Klein (2000).
15 Van Rossum, Shipley, Van de Mheen, Grobbee and Marmot (2000).
16 Acheson (1998), p. 84.
17 Graham (1993).
18 See Satel (2000) for a critique of what she sees as politically correct medicine.
19 Marmot, Shipley and Rose (1984); Marmot, Shipley, Brunner and Hemingway (2001).
20 Plomin (1990).
21 Fogel (2000).
22 Komlos and Baur (2004).
23 Jencks (1972).
24 Marmot, Shipley, Brunner and Hemingway (2001).
25 Singh-Manoux (2003)
26 Plomin (1990).
27 Dickens and Flynn (2001). *http://www.apa.org/journals/rev/rev1082346.htm*
28 Jencks (1972).
29 Jencks (1972).
30 Marmot, Shipley, Brunner and Hemingway (2001).
31 Gould (2000), p. 258.
32 Gould (2000).
33 Morris (1974).
34 Adda and Marmot (unpublished); Smith (1999).

35 Bartley and Plewis (1997).
36 Blane, Harding and Rosato (1999).
37 Wadsworth (1986).

Chapter 3 Poverty Enriched

1   Cited in Sen (1999).
2   J. K. Galbraith, 'Economics and the Quality of Life', reproduced in Galbraith (2001).
3   Infant mortality was 247/1,000 live births. Rowntree (1901) in Davey Smith, Dorling and Shaw (2001).
4   Infant mortality of Social Class V was 8/1,000 live births.
5   Orwell (1937).
6   US Department of Health and Human Services (2002).
7   Infant mortality among the servant-keeping class of York in 1900 was 94/1,000 live births. Rowntree (1901).
8   World Bank (2001).
9   Anand and Ravallion (1993).
10 United Nations Development Programme (2003).
11 The income figures are gross domestic product per head, adjusted for purchasing power, i.e. it takes into account the fact that US$1 will buy different amounts in different countries and adjusts for this.
12 Williams (1999).
13 US Department of Health and Human Services (2001).
14 Geronimus, Bound, Waidmann, Hillemeier and Burns (1996).
15 Rose (1981).
16 Sen (1992).
17 Sen (1999).
18 Gordon and Townsend (2000).
19 World Bank (2003); World Bank Gender and Development Group (2003).
20 United Nations Development Programme (2003). The figures make interesting reading. Among the twenty most developed countries, the prevalence of poverty, by this definition, ranges from 3.9 per cent in Luxembourg, to 5.4 per cent in Finland, 6.6 per cent in Sweden, 7.5 per cent in Germany, 8.0 per cent in France, 12.5 per cent in the United Kingdom, 12.8 per cent in Canada, 14.3 per cent in Australia, and, the prize, 17.0 per cent in the USA.
21 Sen (1992).
22 Lynch, Davey Smith, Kaplan and House (2000).
23 Marmot and Wilkinson (2001).
24 Erikson (2001).
25 Martikainen, Adda, Ferrie, Davey Smith and Marmot (2003).
26 Kawachi and Kennedy (2002).
27 There is an approximately constant relative difference in mortality throughout the income scale. This is seen in Figure 1.1 in Chapter 1 from the US Panel Study of Income Dynamics (p. 17). The relative measure means that as you move from the top income to the $30–50,000 range, mortality is multiplied about 1.6 times. As you move down two further categories, to the $15–20,000 range it is multiplied by about 1.9 again to give three times higher mortality than the highest income group. But this approximately constant relative increase must correspond to an increasing mortality

disadvantage if measured on an absolute scale. To illustrate, suppose that the annual mortality rates in the three income categories just described were 10/1,000, 16/1,000 and 30/1,000. The increase in mortality in going from the richest to the $30–50,000 range is 6 per year. The further increase in going down to the $15–20,000 is 14 – more than twice as great.

28 Wilkinson (1996).
29 Wilkinson (2000).
30 Wilkinson (1996).
31 Deaton (2003).
32 Ross, Wolfson, Dunn, Berthelot, Kaplan and Lynch (2000), Wolfson, Kaplan, Lynch, Ross, Backlund, Gravette, and Wilkinson (1999).
33 Kawachi, Kennedy and Wilkinson (1999).
34 Deaton (2003).

Chapter 4 Relatively Speaking

1 Galbraith (1998)
2 Layard (2003).
3 Diener and Oishi (2000).
4 Marmot, Ryff, Bumpass, Shipley and Marks (1997).
5 Diener and Oishi (2000).
6 Cited in Frank (1999).
7 Galbraith (1999).
8 Kitayama and Marcus (2000).
9 Pinker (1998).
10 Shakespeare, *Merchant of Venice*, Act III, Scene I.
11 Cronin (1991).
12 Miller (2000).
13 Shively (2000).
14 Buss (1999).
15 Erdal and Whiten (1996).
16 Wright (2001).
17 Ridley (1996).
18 Quoted in deWaal (1996).
19 Wright (2001).
20 Miller (2000).
21 Frank (1999).
22 Frank (1999).
23 Alesina (2004).
24 Edmonds and Eidinow (2001).
25 Dash (1998).
26 Majors cited in Dash (1998), p. 198.
27 Newman (1999).
28 Daly, Wilson and Vasdev (2001).
29 Daly and Wilson (1988).
30 Daly, Wilson and Vasdev (2001).
31 MacCoun and Reuter (2001), p. 113.
32 Wilson and Daly (1997).

Chapter 5 Who's in Charge?

1 Sen (1999).
2 Witte, Bots, Hoes and Grobbee (2000).
3 Home (1941).
4 Meisel, Dayan, Pauzner, Chetboun, Arbel, David, and Kutz (1991).
5 Trichopoulos, Katsouyanni, Zavitsanos, Tzonou and Dalla-Vorgia (1983).
6 Sapolsky (1999) in Kahneman (1999).
7 Sapolsky (1998), Sapolsky (2001).
8 Sapolsky (1999) in Kahneman (1999).
9 LeDoux (1998).
10 Steptoe and Marmot (2001).
11 Sapolsky, Romero and Munck (2000).
12 Shively (2000).
13 Kaplan, Manuck, Adams, Weingand and Clarkson (1987).
14 Brunner, Marmot, Nanchahal, Shipley, Stansfeld, Juneja and Alberti (1997).
15 Bjorntorp and Rosmond (2000).
16 Marmot, Siegrist, Theorell and Feeney (1999).
17 Karasek and Theorell (1990).
18 Siegrist and Marmot (2004).
19 Wolfe (1987).
20 Kuper, Marmot, Hemingway, Nicholson, Brunner and Stansfeld (1997).
21 Bosma, Marmot, Hemingway, Nicholson, Brunner and Stansfeld (1997).
22 Kuper, Marmot and Hemingway (2002).
23 Stansfeld, Fuhrer, Shipley and Marmot (1999).
24 Bosma, Marmot, Hemingway, Nicholson, Brunner and Stansfeld (1997).
25 Marmot, Bosma, Hemingway, Brunner and Stansfeld (1997).
26 Marmot, Bosma, Hemingway, Brunner and Stansfeld (1997).
27 Stansfeld, Fuhrer, Shipley and Marmot (1999).
28 Stansfeld, Head, Fuhrer, Wardle and Cattell (2003).
29 Womack, Jones and Roos (1990).
30 Griffin, Fuhrer, Stansfeld and Marmot (2002).
31 Chandola, Kuper, Singh-Manoux, Bartley and Marmot (2004).
32 Jahoda (1979).
33 Bartley (1992).
34 Moser, Fox and Jones (1984).
35 Bartley, Ferrie and Montgomery (1999).
36 Ferrie, Shipley, Stansfeld and Marmot (2002).
37 Karasek and Theorell (1990).
38 Ridley (1997).
39 Dawkins (1989).
40 Siegrist (1996).
41 Bosma, Peter, Siegrist and Marmot (1998).

Chapter 6 Home Alone

1 Conrad (1904), 1960 edn, pp. 395–6.
2 Taylor, Klein, Lewis, Gruenewald, Gurung and Updegraff (2000).
3 Taylor (2002).

4 Taylor (2002), p. 28
5 Shively (2000).
6 de Tocqueville (1835 and 1840; 2000).
7 Putnam (2000), p. 146.
8 Dunbar (1998).
9 Cassel (1976).
10 Tolstoy (1869), 1968 edn, pp. 942–4.
11 Weinberg (1998).
12 Farmer (1999), p. 186.
13 Farmer (1999), pp. 201–2.
14 McKeown (1976).
15 Borges (1970).
16 Selye (1956).
17 Cassel (1976).
18 Syme and Berkman (1976).
19 Marmot, Shipley and Rose (1984).
20 Van Rossum, Shipley, Van de Mheen, Grobbee and Marmot (2000).
21 Davey Smith, Leon, Shipley and Rose (1991).
22 Stansfeld and Fuhrer (2001).
23 Bosma, Marmot, Hemingway, Nicholson, Brunner and, Stansfeld (1997).
24 Stansfeld, Hood, Fuhrer, Wardle and Cattell (2003).
25 Marmot, Bosma, Hemingway, Brunner and Stansfeld (1997).
26 Stansfeld, Fuhrer, Shipley and Marmot (1999).
27 Cited in Charlton and Murphy (1997).
28 Durkheim (1951).
29 Hu and Goldman (1990).
30 Goldman (1993).
31 Jonson, Backlund, Sorlie and Loveless (2000).
32 Van Poppel and Joung (2001).
33 Kravdal (2001).
34 Fuhrer, Stansfeld, Chemali and Shipley (1999).
35 Fuhrer and Stansfeld (2002).
36 Bartley, Sacker, Firth and Fitzpatrick (1999).
37 Cohen, Doyle, Skoner, Rabin and Gwaltney (1997).
38 Berkman and Glass (2000).
39 Berkman and Syme (1979).
40 Putnam (2000).
41 Joint Health Surveys Unit (1999).

Chapter 7 Trusting Together

1 Forster (1921), p. 42.
2 Williams, Haney, Lee, Kong, Blumenthal and Whalen (1980).
3 Williams R. cited in Marmot (2000).
4 Ironically, Philadelphia has a Greek origin, meaning 'brotherly love'.
5 Putnam (2000).
6 Lynch, Due, Muntaner and Davey Smith (2000).
7 Lynch, Davey Smith, Kaplan and House (2000).
8 Marmot and Wilkinson (2001).

9 Durkheim (1951).
10 Durkheim (1951).
11 Ridley (2003), p. 206.
12 Pinker (2002).
13 Sen (1999).
14 Reid (2000), p. 68.
15 World Health Organization (2000b).
16 Marmot and Davey Smith (1989).
17 Sekikawa, Satoh, Hayakawa, Ueshima and Kuller (2001).
18 Sekikawa, Satoh, Hayakawa, Ueshima and Kuller (2001).
19 Ueshima, Tatara and Asakura (1987).
20 Okayama, Ueshima, Marmot, Elliott, Yamakawa and Kita (1995).
21 Marmot and Davey Smith (1989)
22 The Economist 10 Aug. 2002.
23 Reid (2000), p. 23.
24 Putnam (2000).
25 Dore (2002).
26 Dore, Lazonick and O'Sullivan (1999).
27 The Economist 17 Aug. 2002.
28 World Bank (2001).
29 Gordon (1967).
30 Hosokawa (1969).
31 Kagan, Harris, Winkelstein, Johnson, Kato, Syme, Rhoads, Gay, Nichaman, Hamilton and Tillotson (1974)
32 Marmot, Syme, Kagan, Kato, Cohen and Belsky (1975).
33 Matsumoto (1970).
34 Marmot and Syme (1976).
35 Sen (1999).
36 Measham, Rao, Jamison, Wang and Singh (1999).
37 Kerala figures from Murthi, Guio, and Drèze (1995).
38 Caldwell (1986).
39 Thankappan (2001).
40 Sen (1999), pp. 45–8.
41 Sen (1999), p. 46.
42 Cattell and Herring (2002).
43 Sixsmith and Boneham (2002).
44 Sixsmith and Boneham (2002).
45 Diez Roux, Merkin, Arnett, Chambless, Massing, Nieto, Sorlie, Szklo, Tyroler and Watson (2001).
46 Geronimus, Bound, Waidmann, Hillemeier and Burns (1996).
47 Macintyre, Ellaway and Cummins (2002).
48 Newman (1999).
49 Kawachi, Kennedy, Lochner and Prothrow-Smith (1997).
50 Putnam (2000), p. 360.

Chapter 8 The Missing Men of Russia

1 Bellow (1988).
2 Cornia and Paniccia (2000b).

3 World Health Organisation (2000). Strictly, the figures quoted are for a present fifteen-year-old, not for a fifteen-year-old forty years ago.
4 Sen (1999).
5 Marmot and Bobak (2000)
6 Bobak, Hertzman, Skodova and Marmot (1998).
7 UNICEF (2003).
8 Marmot and Bobak (2000).
9 Bobak (1996).
10 Marmot and Bobak (2000).
11 Fox, Goldblatt and Jones (1990).
12 Giddens (1991).
13 Hiscock, Kearns, Macintyre and Ellaway (2001).
14 Giddens (1991).
15 Hiscock, Kearns, Macintyre and Ellaway (2001).
16 Bobak, Hertzman, Skodova and Marmot (1998).
17 Bobak, Pikhart, Hertzman, Rose and Marmot (1998).
18 Bobak, Pikhart, Rose, Hertzman and Marmot (2000).
19 Mikhail Gorbachev, 'The way ahead – more democracy and openness'. *Guardian*, Mon. 2 Feb. 1987, cited in Wilkinson (1996).
20 Rose (1995).
21 Bobak, Hertzman, Skodova and Marmot (1998).
22 Cornia and Paniccia (2000a).
23 Cornia and Paniccia (2000b), p. 31.
24 Pikhart, Bobak, Siegrist, Pajak, Rywik, Kyshegyi, Grostautas, Skodova and Marmot (2001).
25 Bobak, Skodova and Marmot (2000).
26 Malyutina, Bobak, Kurilovitch, Gafarov, Simonova, Nikitin and Marmot (2002).
27 Tunstall-Pedoe, Vanuzzo, Hobbs, Mahonen, Cepaitis, Kuulasmaa and Keil (2000).
28 Blazek and Dzurova (2000).

Chapter 9 The Travails of the Fathers . . . and Mothers

1 Attributed to George Bernard Shaw.
2 Juster (1964).
3 Blane, Morris and White (1996).
4 Willms (1999a).
5 Willms (1999).
6 Willms (1999).
7 Mortimore and Whitty (1997).
8 Pinker (2002).
9 Brooks-Gunn, Duncan and Britto (1999).
10 Pinker (2002).
11 Stoolmiller (1999).
12 Cited in Stoolmiller (1999).
13 Bowlby (1988).
14 Bowlby (1965).
15 Fonagy (2000).
16 Tremblay in Keating and Hertzman (1999).
17 Suomi (1997).

18 Maugham and McCarthy (1997).
19 Power and Hertzman (1997).
20 Barker (1998).
21 Barker, Forsen, Uutela, Osmond and Eriksson (2001).
22 Hardy, Wadsworth, Langenberg and Kuh (in press).
23 Champagne and Meaney (2001).
24 Lupien, Kings Meaney and McEwen (2001).
25 Rutter, Kreppner, O'Connor on behalf of the English and Romanian Adoptees
    (ERA) study team (2001).
26 Teicher (2002).
27 McMunn, Nazroo, Marmot, Boreham, Goodman (2001).
28 Rodgers (1994).
29 Taylor (2002).
30 Hertzman, Power, Matthews and Manor (2001).

Chapter 10 The Moral Imperative and the Bottom Line

1 Tawney (1931) 1964 edition.
2 Whitehead, Townsend and Davidsen (1992).
3 It was commissioned by Dr David Player, head of the Health Education Council, a
   quasi-non-governmental organisation, the work of which was overseen by a council
   chaired by a government appointee.
4 It followed the Black Report, the product of a committee set up by the British Labour
   government in 1978 to report on why health inequalities had been increasing despite
   the establishment of the NHS, thirty years previously. It was chaired by a prestigious
   physician, Sir Douglas Black. By the time the committee reported, the government
   had changed and the Conservative government of Margaret Thatcher rejected the
   report. There was then a vigorous newspaper coverage of the report's rejection.
5 Sen (1992); Sen (1999).
6 Doyal and Gough (1991).
7 See for example Nussbaum (1992).
8 HMSO (1992).
9 Marmot, Adelstein, Robinson and Rose (1978).
10 I have subsequently had deep concern about the regressive nature of tobacco taxation.
   Because smoking is a behaviour that is more common in lower-income groups, they
   pay a bigger tax.
11 HMSO (1992).
12 Hall (1986).
13 Rawls 1971. Justice as fairness.
14 Mortimore and Whitty (1997).
15 Fogel (2000).
16 Acheson (1998).
17 See footnote 4 for what happened next to a previous report – the Black Report.
18 Exworthy, Stuart, Blane and Marmot (2003).
19 Bond and Wakefield (2003).

BIBLIOGRAPHY

Acheson, D. *Inequalities in Health: Report of an Independent Inquiry.* 1998. London: HMSO.

Adda, J. and M. Marmot. (unpublished). *Income and Health over the Life Cycle: A Dynamic Approach to Evaluate the Importance of Selection and Social Causation.*

Alesina, A. R. Di Tella, R. MacCulloch. (forthcoming). 'Inequality and Happiness: Are the Europeans and Americans Different?' *Journal of Public Economics.*

Anand, S. and M. Ravallion. 1993. 'Human Development in Poor Countries: On the Role of Private Incomes and Public Services', in *Journal of Economic Perspectives* 7:133–50.

Barker, D. J. P. 1998. *Mothers, Babies and Health in Later Life.* Edinburgh: Churchill Livingstone.

Barker, D. J. P., T. Forsen, A. Uutela, C. Osmond and J. G. Eriksson. 2001. 'Size at Birth and Resilience to Effects of Poor Living Conditions in Adult Life: Longitudinal Study', in *British Medical Journal* 323:1273–6.

Bartley M. *Authorities and Partisans.* 1992. Edinburgh: Edinburgh University Press.

Bartley, M., J. E. Ferrie and S. Montgomery. 1999. 'Living in a High Unemployment Economy: Understanding the Consequences', in *Social Determinants of Health*, ed. M. Marmot and R. Wilkinson. Oxford: Oxford University Press.

Bartley, M. and I. Plewis. 1997. 'Does Health-selective Mobility Account for Socioeconomic Differences in Health? Evidence from England and Wales, 1971 to 1991', in *Journal of Health and Social Behaviour* 38:376–86.

Bartley, M., A. Sacker, D. Firth and R. Fitzpatrick. 1999. 'Social Position, Social Roles and Women's Health in England: Changing Relationships 1984–1993', in *Social Science and Medicine* 48:99–115.

Bellow, S. 1988. *More Die of Heartbreak.* London: Penguin.

Berkman, L. F. and T. Glass. 2000. 'Social Integration, Social Networks, Social Support, and Health', in *Social Epidemiology*, ed. L. F. Berkman and I. Kawachi. Oxford: Oxford University Press.

Berkman, L. F. and S. L. Syme. 1979. 'Social Networks, Host Resistance and Mortality: A Nine-year Follow-up of Alameda County Residents', in *American Journal of Epidemiology* 109:186–204.

Bjorntorp, P. and R. Rosmond. 2000. 'Obesity and Cortisol', in *Nutrition* 16:924–36.

Blane, D., S. Harding and H. Rosato. 1999. 'Does Social Mobility Affect the Size of the Socioeconomic Mortality Differential?', in *Journal of the Royal Statistical Society*, Series A: *Statistics in Society* 162 [Part 1], 59–70.

Blane, D., J. N. Morris and I. R. White. 1996. 'Education, Social Circumstances and Mortality', in *Health and Social Organisation: Towards a Health Policy for the 21st Century*, ed. D. Blane, E. Brunner and R. Wilkinson. London: Routledge.

Blazek, J. and D. Dzurova. 2000. 'The Decline of Mortality in the Czech Republic during the Transition: A Counterfactual Case Study', in *The Mortality Crisis in Transitional Economies*, ed. G. A. Cornia and R. Paniccia. WIDER Studies in Development Economies. Oxford: Oxford University Press.

Bobak, M. 1996. 'Determinants of the Epidemic of Coronary Heart Disease in the Czech Republic'. PhD Thesis, London School of Hygiene and Tropical Medicine, London.

Bobak, M., C. Hertzman, Z. Skodova and M. Marmot. 1998. 'Association between Psychosocial Factors at Work and Non-fatal Myocardial Infarction in a Population Based Case-control Study in Czech men', in *Epidemiology* 9:43–7.

Bobak, M., H. Pikhart, C. Hertzman, R. Rose and M. Marmot. 1998. 'Socioeconomic Factors, Perceived Control and Self-reported Health in Russia. A Cross-sectional Survey', in *Social Science and Medicine* 47:269–79.

Bobak, M., H. Pikhart, R. Rose, C. Hertzman and M. Marmot. 2000. 'Socioeconomic Factors, Material Inequalities, and Perceived Control in Self-rated Health: Cross-sectional Data from Seven Post-communist Countries', in *Social Science and Medicine* 51:1343–50.

Bobak, M., Z. Skodova and M. Marmot. 2000. 'Effect of Beer Drinking on Risk of Myocardial Infarction: Population Based Case-control Study', in *British Medical Journal* 320:1378–9.

Bond, S. and M. Wakefield. 2003. Distributional effects of fiscal reforms since 1997. In *The IFS Green Budget: January 2003*, Commentary No. 92, edited by Chote, R., C. Emmerson, and H. Simpson (London: Institute for Fiscal Studies).

Booth, C. 1902–3. 'On the City: Physical Pattern and Social Structure.' *In Poverty, Inequality and Health in Britain, 1800–2000: A Reader*, 2001, ed. G. Davey Smith, D. Dorling, and M. Shaw, Bristol: The Policy Press.

Borges, J. L. 1970. 'The Library of Babel', in *Labyrinths: Selected Stories and Other Writings*. London: Penguin.

Bosma, H., M. G. Marmot, H. Hemingway, A. Nicholson, E. J. Brunner and S. Stansfeld. 1997. 'Low Job Control and Risk of Coronary Heart Disease in the Whitehall II (Prospective Cohort) Study'; in *British Medical Journal* 314:558–65.

Bosma, H., R. Peter, J. Siegrist and M. G. Marmot. 1998. 'Two Alternative Job Stress Models and the Risk of Coronary Heart Disease', in *American Journal of Public Health* 88:68–74.

Bowlby, J. 1965. *Child Care and the Growth of Love*. London: Penguin.

Bowlby, J. A. 1988. *A Secure Base: Clinical Applications of Attachment Theory*. London: Routledge.

Britton, A., M. S. Shipley, M. Marmot and H. Hemingway (unpublished). 'Does Low Social Position and South Asian Ethnicity Influence Access to Cardiac Investigation and Treatment'. The Whitehall II Prospective Cohort Study.

Brooks-Gunn, J., G. J. Duncan and P. Rebello Britto. 1999. 'Are Socioeconomic Gradients for Children Similar to Those for Adults?: Achievement and Health of Children in the United States', in *Developmental Health and the Wealth of Nations*, ed. D. P. Keating and C. Hertzman. New York: The Guilford Press.

Brunner, E. J., M. G. Marmot, K. Nanchahal, M. J. Shipley, S. A. Stansfeld, M. Juneja and K. G. M. M. Alberti. 1997. 'Social Inequality in Coronary Risk: Central Obesity and the Metabolic Syndrome. Evidence from the WII Study', in *Diabetologia* 40:1341–9.

Buss, D. M. 1999. *Evolutionary Psychology: The New Science of the Mind*. Boston: Pearson Allyn & Bacon.

Caldwell, J. C. 1986. 'Routes to Low Mortality in Poor Countries', in *Population and Development Review* 2:171–220.

Cassel, J. 1976. 'The Contribution of the Social Environment to Host Resistance', in *American Journal of Epidemiology* 104:107–23.

Cattell, V. and R. Herring. 2002. 'Social Capital, Generations and Health in East

London', in *Social Capital for Health*, ed. C. Swann and A. Morgan. London: Health Development Agency.

Champagne, F. and M. J. Meaney. 2001. 'Like Mother, Like Daughter: Evidence for Non-genomic Transmission of Parental Behaviour and Stress Responsivity', in *Progress in Brain Research* 133:287–302.

Chandola, T., H. Kuper, A. Singh-Manoux, M. Bartley and M. Marmot. (2004). 'The Effect of Control at Home on CHD Events in the Whitehall II Study: Gender Differences in Psychosocial Domestic Pathways to Social Inequalities in CHD', in *Social Science and Medicine* 58, 1501–09.

Charlton, J. and M. Murphy, 1997. *The Health of Adult Britain 1841–1994*, vol 1. London: Office for National Statistics.

Cohen, S., W. J. Doyle, D. P. Skoner, B. S. Rabin and J. M. Gwaltney. 1997. 'Social Ties and Susceptibility to the Common Cold', in *Journal of the American Medical Association* 277:1940–44.

Collis, E. L. and M. Greenwood. 1921. 'The Health of the Industrial Worker 1921', in *Poverty, Inequality and Health in Britain, 1800–2000: A Reader*, ed. G. Davey Smith, D. Dorling, and M. Shaw, 2001. Bristol: The Policy Press.

Conrad, J. 1904. *Nostromo*. 1960 edn. New York: The New American Library.

Cornia, G. A. and R. Paniccia. eds. 2000a. *The Mortality Crisis in Transitional Economies*. Oxford: Oxford University Press.

Cornia, G. A. and R. Paniccia. 2000b. 'The Transition Mortality Crisis: Evidence, Interpretation and Policy Responses', in *The Mortality Crisis in Transitional Economies*, ed. G. Cornia and R. Paniccia. Oxford: Oxford University Press.

Cronin, H. 1991. *The Ant and the Peacock*. Cambridge: Cambridge University Press.

Daly, M. and M. Wilson. 1988. *Homicide*. Hawthorne, NY: Aldine de Gruyter.

Daly, M., M. Wilson, and S. Vasdev. 2001. 'Income Inequality and Homicide Rates in Canada and the United States', in *Canadian Journal of Criminology* 43:219–36.

Dash, L. 1998. *Rosa Lee*. London: Profile Books.

Davey Smith, G., D. Dorling and M. Shaw. 2001. *Poverty, Inequality and Health in Britain, 1800–2000: A Reader*. Bristol: The Policy Press.

Davey Smith, G., C. Hart, D. Blane, C. Gillis and V. Hawthorne. 1997. 'Lifetime Socioeconomic Position and Mortality: Prospective Observational Study', in *British Medical Journal* 314:547–52.

Davey Smith, G., D. Leon, M. J. Shipley and G. Rose. 1991. 'Socioeconomic Differentials in Cancer among Men', in *International Journal of Epidemiology* 20:339–45.

Dawkins, R. 1989. *The Selfish Gene*. Oxford: Oxford University Press.

de Tocqueville, A. 1835/1840. *Democracy in America*. 2000 edn. Indianapolis: Hacket.

de Waal, F. 1996. *Good Natured*. Cambridge, MA: Harvard University Press.

Deaton, A. 2003. 'Health, Inequality, and Economic Development', in *Journal of Economic Literature* 41:113–58.

Department of the Environment, Transport and the Regions. 2000. *Road Accidents Great Britain 1999: The Casualty Report*. London: The Stationery Office.

Dickens, W. T. and J. R. Flynn. 2001. 'Heritability Estimates Versus Large Environmental Effects: The IQ Paradox Resolved', in *Psychological Review* 108:346–69.

Diener, E. and S. Oishi. 2000. 'Money and Happiness: Income and Subjective Well-being across Nations', in *Culture and Subjective Well-being*, ed. Diener, E. and E. M. Suh. Cambridge; MA: MIT Press.

Diez Roux, A. V., S. S. Merkin, D. Arnett, L. Chambless, M. Massing, F. J. Nieto, P. Sorlie, M. Szklo, H. A. Tyroler and R. L. Watson. 2001. 'Neighborhood of Residence and Incidence of Coronary Heart Disease', in *New England Journal of Medicine* 345(2):99–106.

Dore, R. 2002. 'Will Global Capitalism be Anglo-Saxon Capitalism?', in *Asian Business and Management* 1:9–18.

Dore, R., W. Lazonick and M. O'Sullivan. 1999. 'Varieties of Capitalism in the Twentieth Century', in *Oxford Review of Economic Policy* 15:102–20.

Doyal, L. and I. Gough. 1991. *A Theory of Human Need*. London: Macmillan.

Drever, F. and M. Whitehead. 1997. *Health Inequalities: Decennial Supplement*. Series DS No. 15, 1–257. London: The Stationery Office, Office for National Statistics.

Dunbar, R. I. M. 1998. *Grooming, Gossip and the Evolution of Language*. Boston: Harvard University Press.

Durkheim, E. 1951. *Suicide: A Study in Sociology*. New York: Free Press.

Edmonds, D. and J. Eidinow. 2001. *Wittgenstein's Poker: The Story of a Ten Minute Argument between Two Great Philosophers*. London: Faber and Faber.

Erdal, D. and A. Whiten. 1996. 'Egalitarianism and Machiavellian Intelligence in Human Evolution', in *Modelling the Early Human Mind*, ed. P. Mellars and K. Gibson. Cambridge: McDonald Cambridge.

Erikson, R. 2001. 'Why Do Graduates Live Longer?', in *Cradle to Grave: Life-course Change in Modern Sweden*, ed. J. O. Jonsson and C. Mills. Durham: Sociology Press.

Exworthy, M., M. Stuart, D. Blane and M. Marmot. 2003. *Tackling Health Inequalities since the Acheson Inquiry*. Bristol: The Policy Press.

Farmer, P. 1999. *Infections and Inequalities*. Berkeley: University of California Press.

Farmer, P. 2003. *Pathologies of Power: Health, Human Rights, and the New War on the Poor*. Berkeley: University of California Press.

Ferrie, J. E., M. Shipley, S. Stansfeld and M. G. Marmot. 2002. 'Effects of Chronic Job Insecurity and Change in Job Security on Self-reported Health, Minor Psychiatric Morbidity, Physiological Measures and Health Related Behaviours in British Civil Servants: The Whitehall II Study', in *Journal of Epidemiology and Community Health* 56:450–4.

Fogel, R. W. 2000. *The Fourth Great Awakening and the Future of Egalitarianism*. Chicago: University of Chicago Press.

Fonagy, P. 2000. 'Early Influences on Development and Social Inequalities', in *The Society and Population Health Reader – A State and Community Perspective*, ed. A. Tarlov and R. St Peter. New York: The New Press.

Forster, E. M. 1910 (1921 edn.). *Howards End*. New York: Vintage.

Fox, J., P. Goldblatt and D. Jones. 1990. 'Social Class Mortality Differentials: Artifact, Selection or Life Circumstances?', in *Longitudinal Study – Mortality and Social Organisation*, ed. P. Goldblatt. London: HMSO.

Frank, R. 1999. *Luxury Fever*. New York: Free Press.

Friedman, M. and R. H. Rosenman. 1974. *Type A Behavior and Your Heart*. London: Wildwood House.

Fuhrer, R., M. J. Shipley, J. F. Chastang, A. Schmaus, I. Niedhammer, S. A. Stansfeld, M. Goldberg and M. G. Marmot. 2002. 'Socioeconomic Position, Health and Possible Explanations: A Tale of Two Cohorts', in *American Journal of Public Health* 92(8):1290–94.

Fuhrer, R. and S. A. Stansfeld. 2002. 'How Gender Affects Patterns of Social Relations and Their Impact on Health: A Comparison of One or Multiple Sources of Support from "Close Persons",' in *Social Science and Medicine* 54:811–25.

Fuhrer, R., S. A. Stansfeld, J. Chemali and M. J. Shipley. 1999. 'Gender, Social Relations and Mental Health: Prospective Findings from an Occupational Cohort (Whitehall II Study)', in *Social Science and Medicine* 48:77–87.

Galbraith, J. K. 1998. *The Affluent Society*. (40th anniversary edn) New York: Houghton Mifflin.

Galbraith, J. K. 1999. *Name-dropping*. New York: Houghton Mifflin.

Galbraith, J. K. 2001. *The Essential Galbraith*. New York: Houghton Mifflin.

Galton, F. 1883. *Inquiries into Human Faculty and Its Development*. London: Macmillan.

Geronimus, A. T., J. Bound, T. A. Waidmann, M. M. Hillemeier and P. B. Burns. 1996. 'Excess Mortality among Blacks and Whites in the United States', in *New England Journal of Medicine* 335:1552–58.

Giddens, A. 1991. *Modernity and Self Identity: Self and Society in the Late Modern Age*. Cambridge: Polity Press.

Gladwell, M. 2000. *The Tipping Point*. Boston: Little Brown and Co.

Goldman, N. 1993. 'Marriage Selection and Mortality Patterns: Inferences and Fallacies', in *Demography* 30:189–208.

Gordon, D. and P. Townsend. 2000. *Breadline Europe: The Measurement of Poverty*. Bristol: The Policy Press.

Gordon, T. 1967. 'Further Mortality Experience among Japanese Americans', in *Public Health Report* 82:973–84.

Gould, S. J. 1981. *The Mismeasure of Man*. New York: W. W. Norton.

Gould, S. J. 2000. *The Lying Stones of Marrakech: Penultimate Reflections in Natural History*. London: Jonathan Cape.

Graham, H. 1993. *Hardship and Health in Women's Lives*. London: Harvester Wheatsheaf.

Griffin, J., R. Fuhrer, A. Stansfeld and M. Marmot. 2002. 'The Importance of Low Control at Work and Home on Depression and Anxiety: Do These Effects vary by Gender and Social Class? In *Social Science and Medicine* 54:783–98.

Hall, W. 1986. 'Social Class and Survival on the S. S. *Titanic*'. *Social Science and Medicine*. 22:687–90.

Hardy, R. J., M. E. J. Wadsworth, C. Langenberg and D. J. Kuh. (in press). 'Birth Weight, Childhood Growth and Blood Pressure at 43 Years in a British Birth Cohort', in *International Journal of Epidemiology*.

Hertzman, C., C. Power, S. Matthews and O. Manor. 2001. 'Using an Interactive Framework of Society and Lifecourse to Explain Self-rated Health in Early Adulthood', in *Social Science and Medicine* 53:1575–85.

Hiscock, R., A. Kearns, S. Macintyre and A. Ellaway. 2001. 'Ontological Security and Psycho-social Benefits from the Home: Qualitative Evidence on Issue of Tenure', in *Housing Theory and Society* 18:50–66.

HMSO. 1992. *The Health of the Nation*. London: HMSO.

Home, E. 1941. 'A Short Account of the Author's Life by his Brother-in-law, Everard Home', in *Cardiac Classics*, ed. F. A. Willius and T. E. Keys. St Louis, MO: C.V. Mosby.

Hosokawa, B. 1969. *Nisei: The Quiet Americans*. New York: William Morrow.

Hu, Y. and N. Goldman. 1990. 'Mortality Differentials by Marital Status: An International Comparison', in *Demography* 27:233–250.

Jahoda, M. 1979. 'The Impact of Unemployment in the 1930s and the 1970s', in *Bulletin of the British Psychological Society* 32:309–14.

Jencks, C. 1972. *Inequality*. New York: Harper Colophon.

Joint Health Surveys Unit. 1999. *Health Survey for England 1999*. London: The Stationery Office.

Jonson, N. J., E. Backlund, P. D. Sorlie and C. A. Loveless. 2000. 'Marital Status and Mortality: The National Longitudinal Mortality Study', in *Annals of Epidemiology* 10:224–38.

Juster, N. 1964. *The Phantom Tollbooth*. New York: Random House.

Kagan, A., B. R. Harris, W. Winkelstein, K. G. Johnson, H. Kato, S. L. Syme, G. G. Rhoads, M. L. Gay, M. Z. Nichaman, H. B. Hamilton and J. Tillotson, 1974. 'Epidemiologic Studies of Coronary Heart Disease and Stroke in Japanese Men Living in Japan, Hawaii and California: Demographic, Physical, Dietary and Biochemical Characteristics', in *Journal of Chronic Diseases* 27:345–64.

Kahneman, D., E. Diener and N. Schwarz, ed. 1999. *Well-being: The Foundations of Hedonic Psychology*. New York: Russell Sage Foundation.

Kaplan, J. R,, S. B. Manuck, M. R. Adams, K. W. Weingand and T. B. Clarkson. 1987. 'Inhibition of Coronary Atherosclerosis by Propranolol in Behaviorally Predisposed Monkeys Fed an Atherogenic Diet', in *Circulation* 76: 1364–72.

Karasek, R. and T. Theorell. 1990. *Healthy Work: Stress, Productivity, and the Reconstruction of Working Life*. New York: Basic Books.

Kawachi, I. and B. P. Kennedy. 2002. *The Health of Nations: Why Inequality Is Harmful to Your Health*. New York: The New Press.

Kawachi, I., B. P. Kennedy, K. Lochner and D. Prothrow-Smith. 1997. 'Social Capital, Income Inequality, and Mortality', in *American Journal of Public Health* 87:1491–98.

Kawachi, I., B. P. Kennedy and R. G. Wilkinson. 1999. *The Society and Population Health Reader: Income Inequality and Health*. New York: The New Press.

Keating, D. and C. Hertzman. 1999. (eds) *Developmental Health: The Wealth of Nations in the Information Age*. New York: Guilford Press.

Kitayama, S. and H. R. Markus. 2000. 'The Pursuit of Happiness and the Realization of Sympathy: Cultural Patterns of Self, Social Relations, and Well-being', in *Culture and Subjective Well Being*, ed. E. Diener and E. M. Suh. Cambridge, MA. MIT Press.

Klein, R. 2000. 'Health Inequalities: Bringing the Hidden Assumptions into the Open', in *Health Economics* 9:569–70.

Komlos, J. and M. Baur. 2004. 'From the Tallest to (One of) the Fattest: The Enigmatic Fate of the American Population in the 20th Century', in *Economics and Human Biology* 2(1). (in press).

Kravdal, O. 2001. 'The Impact of Marital Status on Cancer Survival', in *Social Science and Medicine* 52:357–68.

Kuper, H., M. Marmot and H. Hemingway. 2002. 'Psychosocial Factors in the Aetiology and Prognosis of Coronary Disease: A Systematic Review', in *Seminars in Vascular Medicine* 2(3):267–314.

Layard, R. 2003. 'Happiness: Has Social Science a Clue?' (Lionel Robbins Memorial Lectures.) Centre for Economic Performance, London School of Economics.

LeDoux, J. 1998. *The Emotional Brain*. London: Phoenix.

Lupien, S. J., S. King, M. J. Meaney and B. S. McEwen. 2001. 'Can Poverty Get under Your Skin? Basal Cortisol Levels and Cognitive Function in Children from Low and High Socioeconomic Status', in *Developmental Psychopathology* 13:653–76.

Lynch, J., P. Due, C. Muntaner, A. and G. Davey Smith. 2000. 'Social Capital – Is It Good Investment Strategy for Public Health?', in *Journal of Epidemiology and Community Health* 54:404–8.

Lynch, J. W., G. Davey Smith, G. A. Kaplan and J. S. House. 2000. 'Income Inequality and Mortality: Importance to Health of Individual Income, Psychosocial Environment, or Material Conditions', in *British Medical Journal* 320:1200–04.

MacCoun, R. J. and P. Reuter. 2001. *Drug War Heresies: Learning from Other Vices, Times, and Places*. Cambridge: Cambridge University Press.

McDonough, P., G. J. Duncan, D. Williams and J. S. House. 1997. 'Income Dynamics and Adult Mortality in the United States, 1972 through 1989', in *American Journal of Public Health* 87:1476–83.

Macintyre, S., A. Ellaway and S. Cummins. 2002. 'Place Effects on Health: How Can We Conceptualise, Operationalise and Measure Them?', in *Social Science and Medicine* 55:125–39.

McKeown, T. 1976. *The Role of Medicine: Dream, Mirage or Nemesis?* London: Nuffield Provincial Hospitals Trust.

McMunn A., J. Y. Nazroo, M. G. Marmot, R. Boreham and R. Goodman. 2001. 'Children's emotional and behavioural well-being and the family environment: findings from the Health Survey for England, in *Social Science and Medicine* 53: 423–440.

Malyutina, S., M. Bobak, S. Kurilovitch, V. Gafarov, G. Simonova, Y. Nikitin and M. Marmot. 2002. 'Relation between Heavy and Binge Drinking and All-cause and Cardiovascular Mortality in Novosibirsk, Russia: A Prospective Cohort Study', in *Lancet* 360:1448–54.

Marmot, M. 2000. 'Inequalities in Health Causes and Policy Implications', in *The Society and Population Health Reader: A State and Community Perspective*, ed. A. R. Tarlov and R. F. St Peter. New York: The New Press.

Marmot, M. and M. Bobak. 2000. 'International Comparators and Poverty and Health in Europe', in *British Medical Journal* 321:1124–28.

Marmot, M., M. Shipley, E. Brunner and H. Hemingway. 2001. 'Relative Contribution of Early Life and Adult Socioeconomic Factors to Adult Morbidity in the WII Study', in *Journal of Epidemiology and Community Health* 55(5):301–7.

Marmot, M., J. Siegrist, T. Theorell and A. Feeney. 1999. 'Health and the Psychosocial Environment at Work', in *Social Determinants of Health*, ed. M. Marmot and R. G. Wilkinson. Oxford: Oxford University Press.

Marmot, M. and R. G. Wilkinson. 2001. 'Psychosocial and Material Pathways in the Relation between Income and Health: A Response to Lynch et al., in *British Medical Journal* 322:1233–36.

Marmot, M. G., A. M. Adelstein, N. Robinson and G. Rose. 1978. 'The Changing Social Class Distribution of Heart Disease', in *British Medical Journal* 2:1109–12.

Marmot, M. G., H. Bosma, H. Hemingway, E. Brunner and S. Stansfeld. 1997. 'Contribution of Job Control and Other Risk Factors to Social Variations in Coronary Heart Disease', in *Lancet* 350:235–40.

Marmot, M. G. and E. J. Brunner. 1991. 'Alcohol and Cardiovascular Disease: The Status of the U-shaped Curve', in *British Medical Journal* 303:565–8.

Marmot, M. G. and G. Davey Smith. 1989. 'Why Are the Japanese Living Longer?', in *British Medical Journal* 299:1547–51.

Marmot, M. G., G. Rose, M. Shipley and P. J. S. Hamilton. 1978. 'Employment Grade and Coronary Heart Disease in British Civil Servants', in *Journal of Epidemiology and Community Health* 32:244–9.

Marmot, M. G., C. Ryff, L. Bumpass, M. J. Shipley and N. F. Marks. 1997. 'Social Inequalities in Health: Next Questions and Converging Evidence', in *Social Science and Medicine* 44:901–10.

Marmot, M. G. and M. J. Shipley. 1996. 'Do Socioeconomic Differences in Mortality Persist after Retirement? 25.Year Follow up of Civil Servants from the First Whitehall Study', in *British Medical Journal* 313:1177–80.

Marmot, M. G., M. J. Shipley and G. Rose. 1984. 'Inequalities in Death – Specific Explanations of a General Pattern', in *Lancet* 323:1003–6.

Marmot, M. G. and S. L. Syme. 1976. 'Acculturation and Coronary Heart Disease in Japanese Americans', in *American Journal of Epidemiology* 104:225–47.

Marmot, M. G., S. L. Syme, A. Kagan, H. Kato, J. B. Cohen and J. Belsky. 1975. 'Epidemiologic Studies of Coronary Heart Disease and Stroke in Japanese Men Living in Japan, Hawaii and California: Prevalence of Coronary and Hypertensive Heart Disease and Associated Risk Factors', in *American Journal of Epidemiology* 102:514–25.

Martikainen, P., J. Adda, J. E. Ferrie, G. Davey Smith and M. Marmot. 2003. 'Effects of Income and Wealth on GHQ Depression and Poor Self-rated Health in White Collar Women and Men in the Whitehall II Study', in *Journal of Epidemiology and Community Health* 57:718–23.

Matsumoto, Y. S. 1970. 'Social Stress and Coronary Heart Disease', in *Milbank Memorial Fund Quarterly* 48:9–36.

Maugham, B. and G. McCarthy. 1997. Childhood adversities and psychosocial disorders. In *British Medical Bulletin. Foetal and early childhood environment: long-term health implications. Vol 53. No. 1.*, edited by Marmot, M. and M. E. J. Wadsworth (London: Royal Society of Medicine Press Limited).

Maugham, W. Somerset. 1949. *A Writers' Notebook*. London: William Heineman.

Measham, A. R., K. D. Rao, D. T. Jamison, J. Wang and A. Singh. 1999. 'Reducing Infant Mortality and Fertility, 1975–1990: Performance at All-India and State Levels', in *Economic and Political Weekly*, 34, no. 22:1359–1367.

Meisel, S. R., I. Kutz, K. I. Dayan, H. Pauzner, I. Chetboun, Y. Arbel and D. David. 1991. 'Effect of Iraqi Missile War on Incidence of Acute Myocardial Infarction and Sudden Death in Israeli Civilians. *Lancet* 338:660–1.

Miller, G. F. 2000. *The Mating Mind. How Sexual Choice Shaped the Evolution of Human Nature*. New York: Doubleday.

Morris, J. N. 1974. *Uses of Epidemiology*. 3rd edn. London: Churchill Livingstone.

Mortimore, P. and G. Whitty. 1997. *Can School Improvement Overcome the Effects of Disadvantage?* London: Institute of Education.

Moser, K. A., A. J. Fox and D. R. Jones. 1984. 'Unemployment and Mortality in the OPCS Longitudinal Study', in *Lancet* 2:1324–29.

Moser, K. A., H. S. Pugh, and P. O. Goldblatt. 1988. 'Inequalities in women's health: looking at mortality differentials using an alternative approach'. *British Medical Journal* 296:1221–1224.

Murray, C. J. L., C. M. Michaud, M. T. McKenna and J. S. Marks. 1998. U.S. *Patterns of Mortality by County and Race*: 1965–94. Cambridge, MA: Harvard Center for Population and Development Studies.

Murthi, M, A. C. Guio, and J. Drèze, 1995. 'Mortality, Fertility and Gender Bias in India: A District Level Analysis'. *DEP* No. 61, London: London School of Economics.

Newman, K. S. 1999. *No Shame in My Game*. New York: Alfred A. Knopf and Russell Sage.

Nussbaum, M. C. 1992. 'Human Functioning and Social Justice', in *Political Theory* 20:202–46.

Office for National Statistics. 1997. *The Health of Adult Britain 1841–1994*, ed. J. Charlton and M. Murphy. Vol. 1. London: The Stationery Office.

Okayama, A., H. Ueshima, M. G. Marmot, P. Elliott, M. Yamakawa and Y. Kita. 1995. 'Different Trends in Serum Cholesterol Levels among Rural and Urban Populations Aged 40–59 in Japan from 1960 to 1990', in *Journal of Clinical Epidemiology* 48:329–37.

OPCS. 1978. *Occupational Mortality 1970–1972, Decennial Supplement*. London: HMSO.

Orwell, G. 1937. *The Road to Wigan Pier*. London: Secker.

Osler, W. 1910. 'The Lumleian Lectures on Angina Pectoris', in *Lancet* i:839–44.

Pikhart, H., M. Bobak, J. Siegrist, A. Pajak, S. Rywik, J. Kyshegyi, A. Gostautas, Z. Skodova and M. Marmot. 2001. 'Psychosocial Work Characteristics and Self-Rated Health in Four Post-communist Countries', *Journal of Epidemiology and Community Health* 55: 624–30.

Pinker, S. 1998. *How the Mind Works*. London: Allen Lane.

Pinker, S. 2002. *The Blank Slate*. London: Allen Lane.

Plomin, R. 1990. *Nature and Nurture, An Introduction to Human Behavioural Genetics*. Pacific Grove, CA: Brooks–Cole.

Power, C. and C. Hertzman. 1997. 'Social and Biological Pathways Linking Early Life and Adult Disease', in *British Medical Bulletin. Fetal and Early Childhood Environment: Long-term Health Implications*. Vol. 53. No. 1., ed. M. Marmot and M. E. J. Wadsworth. London: Royal Society of Medicine Press Limited.

Putnam, R. 2000. *Bowling Alone: The Collapse and Revival of American Community*. New York: Simon and Schuster.

Rawls, J. 1971. *A Theory of Justice*. Cambridge, MA: Harvard University Press.

Redelmeier, D. A. and S. M. Singh. 2001. 'Survival in Academy Award-winning Actors and Actresses', in *Annals of Internal Medicine* 134(10):955–62.

Reid, T. R. 2000. *Confucius Lives Next Door*. New York: Vintage.

Ridley, M. 1996. *Origins of Virtue: Human Instincts and the Evolution of Cooperation*. London: Penguin Books.

Ridley, M. 1999. *Genome: The Autobiography of a Species in 23 Chapters*. London: Fourth Estate.

Ridley, M. 2003. *Nature via Nurture*. London: Fourth Estate.

Rodgers, B. 1994. 'Pathways between Parental Divorce and Adult Depression', in *Journal of Child Psychology and Psychiatry* 35:1289–1308.

Rose, G. 1981. 'Strategy of Prevention: Lessons from Cardiovascular Disease', in *British Medical Journal* 282:1847–51.

Rose, G. 1992. *The Strategy of Preventive Medicine*. Oxford: Oxford University Press.

Rose, R. 1995. 'Russia as an Hour-glass Society: A Constitution without Citizens', in *East European Constitutional Review* 4:34–42.

Ross, N. A., M. C. Wolfson, J. R. Dunn, J. M. Berthelot, G. Kaplan and J. W. Lynch. 2000. 'Relation between Income Inequality and Mortality in Canada and in the United States: Cross Sectional Assessment Using Census Data and Vital Statistics', in British Medical Journal 320:898–902.

Rowntree, B. S. 1901. 'Poverty: A Study of Town Life,' in *Poverty, Inequality and Health in Britain, 1800–2000: A Reader*, 2001 ed. G. Davey Smith, D. Dorling and M. Shaw. Bristol: The Policy Press.

Rutter, M. L., J. M. Kreppner and T. G. O'Connor on behalf of the English and Romanian Adoptees (ERA) study team. 2001. 'Specificity and Heterogeneity in Children's Responses to Profound Institutional Privation'. *British Journal of Psychiatry* 179:97–103.

Sapolsky, R. 1999. 'The Physiology and Pathophysiology of Unhappiness', in *Well-being: The Foundations of Hedonic Psychology*, ed. D. Kahneman, E. Diener and N. Schwarz. New York: Russell Sage Foundation.

Sapolsky, R. M. 1998. *Why Zebras Don't Get Ulcers: An Updated Guide to Stress, Stress-related Diseases, and Coping*. New York: W. H. Freeman.

Sapolsky, R. M. 2001. *A Primate's Memoir*. London: Jonathan Cape.

Sapolsky, R. M., M. Romero and A. U. Munck. 2000. 'How Do Glucocorticoids Influence Stress Responses? Integrating Permissive, Suppressive, Stimulatory and Preparative Actions?', in *Endocrine Reviews* 21:55–89.

Sacker, A., D. Firth, R. Fitzpatrick, K. Lynch and M. Bartley, 2000. 'Comparing health inequality in men and women: prospective study of mortality, 1986–96. *British Medical Journal* 320: 1303–1307.

Satel, S. 2000. *PC, M.D.: How Political Correctness Is Corrupting Medicine*. New York: Basic Books.

Sekikawa, A., T. Satoh, T. Hayakawa, H. Ueshima and L. H. Kuller. 2001. 'Coronary Heart Disease Mortality among Men Aged 35–44 Years by Prefecture in Japan in 1995–1999 Compared with That among White Men Aged 35–44 by State in the United States in 1995–1998: Vital Statistics Data in a Recent Birth Cohort,' in *Japanese Circulation Journal* 65:887–92.

Selye, H. 1956. *The Stress of Life*. New York: McGraw-Hill.

Sen, A. 1992. *Inequality Reexamined*. Oxford: Oxford University Press.

Sen, A. 1999. *Development As Freedom*. New York: Alfred A. Knopf, Inc.

Shively, C. A. 2000. 'Social Status, Stress and Health in Female Monkeys', in *The Society and Population Health Reader – A State and Community Perspective*, ed. A. R. Tarlov and R. F. St Peter. New York: The New Press.

Siegrist, J. 1996. 'Adverse Health Effects of High-effort/Low-reward Conditions,' in *Journal of Occupational Health Psychology* 1:27–41.

Siegrist, J. and M. Marmot. (2004). 'Health Inequalities and the Psychosocial Environment – Two Scientific Challenges'. *Social Science and Medicine* 58:1463–73.

Singh-Manoux, A., M. Richards and M. Marmot. 2003. 'Leisure Activities and Cognitive Function in Middle Age: Evidence from the Whitehall II Study'. *Journal of Epidemiology and Community Health*. 57:907–913.

Sixsmith, J. and M. Boneham. 2002. 'Men and Masculinities', in *Social Capital for Health*, ed. C. Swann and A. Morgan. London: Health Development Agency.

Smith, J. P. 1999. 'Healthy Bodies and Thick Wallets: The Dual Relationship between Health and Socioeconomic Status', in *Journal of Economic Perspectives* 13(2):145–66.

Stansfeld, S. A. and R. Fuhrer. 2001. 'Depression and Coronary Heart Disease', in *Stress and the Heart: Psychosocial Pathways to Heart Disease*, ed. S. A. Stansfeld and M. G. Marmot. London: BMJ Books.

Stansfeld, S. A., R. Fuhrer, M. J. Shipley and M. G. Marmot. 1999. 'Work Characteristics Predict Psychiatric Disorder: Prospective Results from the Whitehall II Study', in *Occupational and Environmental Medicine* 15:302–7.

Stansfeld, S. A., J. Head, R. Fuhrer, J. Wardle and V. Cattell. 2003. 'Social Inequalities in Depressive Symptoms and Physical Functioning in the Whitehall II Study: Exploring a Common Cause Explanation', in *Journal of Epidemiology and Community Health* 57:361–7.

Steptoe, A. and M. Marmot. 2001. 'The Role of Psychobiological Pathways in Socio-economic Inequalities in Cardiovascular Disease Risk', in *European Heart Journal*. 23:13–25.

Stevenson, T. H. C. 1928. 'The Vital Statistics of Wealth and Poverty, in *Journal of the Royal Statistical Society*', in *British Medical Journal* i:354.

Stoolmiller, M. 1999. 'Implications of the Restricted Range of Family Environments for Estimates of Heritability and Nonshared Environment in Behaviour-genetic Adoption Studies', in *Psychological Bulletin* 125:392–409.

Suomi, S. J. 1997. 'Early Determinants of Behaviour: Evidence from Primate Studies', in *British Medical Bulletin. Fetal and Early Childhood Environment: Long-term Health Implications*, ed. M. Marmot and M. E. J. Wadsworth. London: Royal Society of Medicine Press Limited.

Syme, S. L. and L. F. Berkman. 1976. 'Social Class, Susceptibility, and Sickness', in *American Journal of Epidemiology* 104:1–8.

Szreter, S. 1988. 'The Importance of Social Intervention in Britain's Mortality Decline c.1850–1914: A Re-interpretation of the Role of Public Health', in *Social History of Medicine* 1:1–37.

Tawney, R. H. 1931. *Equality*. 1964 edn. London: Unwin.

Taylor, S. E. 2002. *The Tending Instinct*. New York: Henry Holt and Company.

Taylor, S. E., L. C. Klein, B. P. Lewis, T. L. Gruenewald, R. A. R. Gurung and J. A. Updegraff. 2000. 'Biobehavioural Responses to Stress in Females: Tend-and-befriend, Not Fight-or-flight', in *Psychological Review* 107:411–29.

Teicher, M. H. 2002. 'Scars That Won't Heal: The Neurobiology of Child Abuse', in *Scientific American*, March Issue 68–75.

Thankappan, K. R. 2001. 'Some Health Implications of Globalization in Kerala, India', in *Bulletin of the World Health Organization* 79:892–3.

Tolstoy, L. 1869 (1968). *War and Peace*. New American Library 1968 edn. New York: New American Library.

Tremblay, R. E. 1999. 'When Children's Social Development Fails'. in *Developmental Health and the Wealth of Nations. Social, Biological and Educational Dynamics*, ed. Keating, D. and C. Hertzman. New York: Guilford Press.

Trichopoulos, D., K. Katsouyanni, X. Zavitsanos, A. Tzonou and P. Dalla-Vorgia. 1983. 'Psychological Stress and Fatal Heart Attack: The Athens (1981) Earthquake Natural Experiment', in *Lancet* 321, no. 8322:441–4.

Tunstall-Pedoe, H., D. Vanuzzo, M. S. Hobbs, M. Mahonen, Z. Cepaitis, K. Kuulasmaa and U. Keil. 2000. 'Estimation of Contribution of Changes in Coronary Care to Improving Survival, Event Rates, and Coronary Heart Disease Mortality across the WHO MONICA Project Populations', in *Lancet* 355:688–700.

Ueshima, H., K. Tatara, and S. Asakura. 1987. 'Declining Mortality from Ischaemic Heart Disease and Changes in Coronary Risk Factors in Japan, 1956–1980', in *American Journal of Epidemiology* 125:62–72.

UNICEF. 2003. *Social Monitor 2003*. Florence: UNICEF Innocenti Research Centre.

United Nations Development Programme. 2003. *Human Development Report*. New York: Oxford University Press.

US Department of Health and Human Services. Health, United States, 1998. Socio-economic Status and Health Chartbook.

US Department of Health and Human Services. Health, United States, 2001.

US Department of Health and Human Services. Health, United States, 2002.

van Poppel, F. and I. Joung. 2001. 'Long Term Trends in Marital Status Mortality Differences in the Netherlands, 1850–1970', in *Journal of Biosocial Science* 33:279–303.

van Rossum, C. T. M., M. J. Shipley, H. Van de Mheen, D. E. Grobbee and M. G. Marmot. 2000. 'Employment Grade Differences in Cause-specific Mortality. A 25 Year Follow Up of Civil Servants from the First Whitehall Study', in *Journal of Epidemiology and Community Health* 54:178–84.

Wadsworth, M. E. J. 1986. 'Serious Illness in Childhood and Its Association with Later-life Achievement', in *Class and Health*, ed. R. G. Wilkinson. London: Tavistock Publications Ltd.

Weinberg, R. A. 1998. *One Renegade Cell*. London: Weidenfeld and Nicolson.

Whitehead, M., P. Townsend and N. Davidsen. 1992. *Inequalities in Health: The Black Report/The Health Divide*. London: Penguin.

Wilkinson, R. 1986. *Class and Health*. London: Tavistock.

Wilkinson, R. G. 1996. *Unhealthy Societies: The Afflictions of Inequality*. London: Routledge.

Wilkinson, R. G. 1999. 'The Culture of Inequality', in *Income Inequality and Health. The*

Society and Population Health Reader. Volume 1, ed. I. Kawachi, B Kennedy and R. G. Wilkinson. New York: The New Press.

Wilkinson, R. G. 2000. *Mind the Gap. Hierarchies, Health and Human Evolution*. London: Weidenfeld and Nicolson.

Williams, D. R. 1999. 'Race, Socioeconomic Status and Health. The Added Effects of Racism and Discrimination', in *Socioeconomic status and health in industrial nations. Social and biological pathways. Annals of the New York Academy of Sciences, Vol. 896*, ed. N. E. Adler, M. Marmot, B. S. McEwen, and J. Stewart. New York: New York Academy of Sciences.

Williams, R., T. Haney, K. Lee, Y. Kong, J. Blumenthal and R. Whalen. 1980. 'Type A Behavior, Hostility and Coronary Heart Disease', in *Psychosomatic Medicine* 42:539–49.

Willms, J. D. 1999a. *Inequalities in Literacy Skills among Youth in Canada and the United States. (International Adult Literacy Survey No 6)*. Ottawa: Human Resources Development Canada and National Literacy Secretariat.

Willms, J. D. 1999. 'Quality and Inequality in Children's Literacy: The Effects of Families, Schools and Communities', in *Developmental Health and the Wealth of Nations: Social, Biological, and Educational Dynamics*, ed. D. Keating and C. Hertzman. New York: Guilford Press.

Wilson, M. and M. Daly. 1997. 'Life Expectancy, Economic Inequality, Homicide and Reproductive Timing in Chicago Neighbourhoods', in *British Medical Journal* 314:1271–74.

Witte, D. R., M. L. Bots, A. W. Hoes and D. E. Grobbee. 2000. 'Cardiovascular Mortality in Dutch Men during 1996 European Football Championship: Longitudinal Population Study', in *British Medical Journal* 321:1552–4.

Wolfe, T. 1987. *Bonfire of the Vanities*. New York: Farrar, Straus and Giroux.

Wolfson, M., G. Kaplan, J. Lynch, N. Ross, E. Backlund, H. Gravelle, and R. G. Wilkinson. 1999. 'Relation between Income Inequality and Mortality: Empirical Demonstration', in *British Medical Journal* 319:953–7.

Womack, J. P., D. T. Jones and D. Roos. 1990. *The Machine That Changed the World*. Don Mills: Collier Macmillan Canada, Inc.

World Bank. *World Development Report 2000/2001*. 2001. New York: Oxford University Press.

World Bank. *World Development Report 2003*. 2003. New York: The World Bank and Oxford University Press.

World Bank Gender and Development Group. 2003. *Gender Equality and the Millennium Development Goals*. New York, Gender and Development Group, The World Bank.

World Health Organization. 2000a. *Health for All*. Copenhagen: World Health Organization.

World Health Organization. 2000b. *World Health Report 2000*. Geneva: World Health Organization.

World Health Organization. 2001. World Health Report 2001. Geneva, World Health Organization.

Wright, R. 2001. *Non Zero – The Logic of Human Destiny*. New York: Vintage.

ACKNOWLEDGEMENTS

There are two myths about academic life that my experience comfortably contradicts. The first is that academic existence, up in the ivory tower, is measured out in cups of tea taken at leisurely pace in the common room. Somewhere perhaps, but not among the people with whom it has been my privilege to work. Extraordinary dedication and hard work by a large number of colleagues gave rise to the research on which this book is based.

The second, propounded by those who are eager to debunk the ivory tower myth, is that academic life is riddled with rivalry and jealousy, personal attack and vaunting ambition. Indeed, I allude to some of this behaviour in the book. But the people with whom I have worked have been generous in all the important ways. Ambitious, to be sure, but ambitious to do good work and make a contribution, not to walk over others to get ahead. I have not studied the question systematically but I am willing to hazard a guess that generosity is a concomitant of success in academic life. Certainly, the people who have been most generous with me of their ideas, time and effort have been wonderfully successful academics.

My first academic debt is to Dr Peter Harvey. He was consultant chest physician at Royal Prince Alfred Hospital in Sydney when I was a junior doctor. It was he who steered me into epidemiology. He came back from a meeting on the health of migrants organised by his friend (and subsequently my friend) Dr Ian Prior – a self-made epidemiologist – and said: 'I have just the thing for you: it's called epidemiology. Doctors, social scientist, statisticians, all work together to understand why health patterns differ depending on the type of society. There are two fantastic men, Len Syme at Berkeley and John Cassel at Chapel Hill. You should go and study with one of them.' I had heard of Berkeley and not Chapel Hill, so I went to Len Syme, and he changed my life.

Symes's general point was that just because I had studied medicine did not mean I had any special reason for understanding health in society. I needed to understand society as well as biomedicine. It was Syme who invited me to work on the study of Japanese migrants, reported in Chapter 7. It was only after I had moved to London and started working on the Whitehall studies that I realised that the idea that the gradient was important, and not just poverty had, of course, come from Len Syme. All the best ideas come from someone else.

It was Syme who introduced me to the ideas of Durkheim. Interestingly, Geoffrey Rose who I went to work with at the London School of Hygiene and

Tropical Medicine was, in his own way, a Durkheimian. Rose was a wonderful model of sticking close to the data, in the best spirit of British empirical enquiry, while making imaginative syntheses. He reached the conclusion that the causes of population rates of disease might be different from the causes of individual differences in who gets sick. Geoffrey Rose and Professor Donald Reid (the man who offered me a job in London) had started the first Whitehall study and invited me to examine the differences in mortality among men in the different employment grades. The invitation was almost accidental. I have been obsessed with the social gradient ever since.

When I moved from the London School of Hygiene to University College London, two successive provosts, James Lighthill and Derek Roberts, were very supportive of the work I was trying to do. They saw it as not quite fitting the mould of a traditional medical school. It therefore needed support from the centre. I am very grateful to them for that support and investment.

Fraser Mustard, founding president of the Canadian Institute of Advanced Research (CIAR), more than anybody, taught me the lesson that generosity helps everybody and 'the cause' of improving population health. He was responsible for setting up the programme in population health of the CIAR and involving me in it at its earliest phase. I was beavering away in London doing the Whitehall studies, but it was Fraser, with Len Syme, who took the view that the implications of Whitehall were fundamental to how we think of health in society. Owing to Fraser, Whitehall had more public airing and discussion in policy circles in Canada than it did in the UK. Fraser called in to see the provost of UCL, Derek Roberts, and asked him if it would be all right if Fraser raised funds to support my work. Slightly surprised by this Canadian visitation, Derek agreed.

This led to the establishment at UCL of the International Centre for Health and Society. The colleagues who founded it with me, Richard Wilkinson, David Blane, Mel Bartley, Chris Power, Aubrey Sheiham, Mike Wadsworth, Eric Brunner, Stephen Stansfeld, Di Kuh, and latterly also, James Nazroo, Jane Ferrie, Archana Singh-Manoux, Annie Britton, Meena Kumari, and Tarani Chandola, formed a mutually supportive network of researchers who fostered each other's ideas and helped with research and publishing. Donald Acheson assumed the chair of the Centre and was a powerful advocate for our work as well as supportive of everything we were trying to do. This is one of a number of books for which the International Centre can take considerable credit.

In the interim between leaving the London School of Hygiene and Tropical Medicine and taking up my chair at UCL, I spent a three-month mini-sabbatical with Tores Theorell and colleagues at National Institute for Psychosocial factors and Health at the Karolinska Institute in Stockholm. When I was wondering how to take forward research on psychosocial factors and health, the intellectual shot in the arm that I received from Tores and colleagues was vital. They showed me how important the psychosocial work environment might be for health. As a result, I went home to London and started the Whitehall II study.

Tores, along with Johannes Siegrist, and I nourished each other's work with an association that has spanned more than two decades. Whatever your political views on European integration, the possibility of having wonderfully supportive colleagues in different European countries, with frequent exchange, is something that one country alone would not provide.

The opportunity to use research findings to influence policy in a direct way is to be cherished. In 1997, Donald Acheson, former Chief Medical Officer of the British Government was asked by the government to conduct an Independent Inquiry into Inequalities in Health. The Scientific Advisory Group was chaired by Sir Donald, and consisted of David Barker, Jacky Chambers, Hilary Graham, Margaret Whitehead and me. Catherine Law was the scientific secretary and Ray Earwicker the administrative secretary. I learnt an enormous amount about health inequalities from these colleagues and from the distinguished scientists we consulted.

I have been fortunate to be part of two interdisciplinary research networks supported by the MacArthur Foundation. The first, chaired by Bert Brim, was on successful midlife development. For several years, these friends gave me a post-graduate education in aspects of science I had not known existed: Paul Baltes, Bert Brim (Orville Gilbert Brim), Larry Bumpass, Paul Cleary, David Featherman, William Hazzard, Ronald Kessler, Margie Lachman, Hazel Rose Markus, Alice Rossi, Carol Ryff, Richard Shweder. The second is on socio-economic status and health, chaired by Nancy Adler. The task set for this group of scholars has been to decide what is important and pursue research on it. Can you imagine that! I enjoy my interactions with the group: Nancy Adler, Sheldon Cohen, Mark Cullen, Ana Diez-Roux, Ichiro Kawachi, Bruce McEwen, Karen Matthews, Katherine Newman, Chris Paxson, Joseph Schwartz, Teresa Seeman, Shelley Taylor, David Williams. In addition to providing support for the Whitehall studies, this was a wonderfully generative group of colleagues. My thanks to them and to the Foundation.

I had been urged for some time to make these research findings more generally available to a wider audience. My stimulus, finally, for putting this research into book form was an invitation from the University of California, Berkeley, to be a Hitchcock Professor in 2002. My task was to give two, non-specialist, public lectures to the university community. Given that I had about 18 months between invitation and lectures, it seemed a bit churlish simply to report whatever research results I happened to have to hand at the time. I had time to work out what I really thought about the subject reported in this book. Two lectures seemed a trifle evanescent for 18 months of thinking on top of 30 years of research. The first decision, therefore, was to write it down in book form. The second was that the lectures should come out of the book. The book should not be, simply, a record of the lectures. My thanks to the Hitchcock committee and the University of California, Berkeley.

I planned the book during a spell as a visiting professor in the Department of Health and Social Behavior at Harvard School of Public Health. My thanks to Dean Barry Bloom and to Lisa Berkman for this hospitality and for providing an environment where the most enjoyable and obvious thing to

ACKNOWLEDGEMENTS

do was to integrate thoughts and plan a book. Kathy Newman of the Kennedy School at Harvard introduced me to many interesting colleagues and helped educate me in the difference between writing scientific papers and a book like this.

Starting the book at Harvard set the pattern for how it would be written. It is, after all, a book that encompasses research on a number of countries and parts of the book were written while on the road in Japan, Siberia, Washington DC, Santa Monica, Miami, Sydney, Dusseldorf, Stockholm, the Rockefeller Foundation villa in Bellagio, Sicily, Harvard again, Prague, Krakow. Thanks to colleagues in all these places for their hospitality.

The book was revised during 2003 while enjoying a Visiting Fellowship at Trinity College Cambridge. My thanks to Amartya Sen, then the master, and the fellows of Trinity for affording me this opportunity. Having been educated and worked at big public universities in Sydney, Berkeley and London, I had never experienced the special charms of Oxbridge, both academic and of the wonderful setting. The contradiction of writing about social inequalities while enjoying the specialness of this environment was not lost on me. Good environments help people to function, even flourish. While on the subject of contradictions, none could be more apparent than going to Buckingham Palace to receive a knighthood from the Queen, the citation for which read: 'for services to epidemiology and understanding health inequalities'. For doing research highlighting the lot of those with low status, I get my relative position enhanced!

Many friends helped with the book itself. Kathy Newman helped with the plans. Len Syme, Angus Deaton and Harry Hemingway, heroically, read complete drafts and gave me incisive and constructive comments. Helena Cronin and Archana Singh-Manoux read selected chapters and commented extensively. I am enormously grateful to them for their time, generosity and insights.

My agent Rob McQuilkin gave inordinately of his time and insight at every stage. Heather Rodino and Robin Dennis at Henry Holt, and Bill Swainson and his colleagues at Bloomsbury, made this a much better book by their thorough attention, care and general supportiveness. I had been told that editorial attentiveness like this was a thing of the past. I am grateful that it is alive and well and represented by these talented professionals.

Most important in producing the research that is described in these pages have been my colleagues in the Department of Epidemiology and Public Health of University College London. All the scientists who worked on the Whitehall studies made important contributions. These are: Jerome Adda, Nicola Armstrong, Mel Bartley, Hans Bosma, Annie Britton, Eric Brunner, Christine Buxton, Douglas Carroll, Tarani Chandola, Paul Clarke, George Davey Smith, Elisa Diaz Martinez, Amanda Feeney, Jane Ferrie, Rebecca Fuhrer, Anne Golden, Anne Gosling, Jenny Head, Harry Hemingway, Melvyn Hillsdon, Maneesh Juneja, Meena Kumari, Hannah Kuper, Claudia Langenberg, Noel McCarthy, Pekka Martikainen, Gill Mein, Kim Morgan, Kiran Nanchahal, James Nazroo, Amanda Nicholson, Fiona North, Chandra Patel, Elizabeth Rael,

302 STATUS SYNDROME

Kirsten Rennie, Helen Rice, David Sheffield, Beverly Shipley, Martin Shipley, Archana Singh-Manoux, Janet Sorel, Mai Stafford, Stephen Stansfeld, Andrew Steptoe, Ian White, Christopher Whitty, Jing-Hua Zhao. Several visitors to the study made important contributions: Birgit Greiner, Joan Griffin, Jody Heyman, Mika Kivimaki, Yuko Morikawa, Annhild Mosdol, Michikazu Sekine, Burt Singer. Administrative and research support for Whitehall II has been provided by: Comfort Adeoba, Ellena Badrick, Margaret Beksinska, Floriana Bortolotti, Katrina Brown, Therese Butler, Rob Canner, Mo Chaudhury, Ndidi Duru, Angela Ezekiel, Alan Harding, Miriam Harris, Patricia Johnson, Michael Kimpton, Jean Persaud, Tania Salter, Amit Shukla, Stephanie Smith, Lynn Toon, Susan Yazdgerdi. I am grateful to all of them.

The research in Central and Eastern Europe has been carried out with the enthusiastic co-operation of Martin Bobak, Hynek Pikhart and Anne Peasey. We now have a research collaboration with Sofia Malyutina, Yuri Nikitin, Mikhail Voevoda in Novosibirsk; Andzrej Pajak and Roman Topor in Krakow; Ruzena Kubinova, Rudolf Poledne, Jaroslav Hubacek in the Czech Republic. They are an excellent group of colleagues. The Wellcome Trust and the MacArthur Foundation have supported this work and we have been pleased to collaborate with Clyde Hertzman, Andrea Cornia, Denny Vagero, Mike Murphy and Richard Rose.

None of this research could take place without funding. For the last several years I have been supported by the Medical Research Council as an MRC Research Professor and MRC have supported the Whitehall II study with a long-term programme of support. We have been fortunate in that the NIH of the American government has supported our studies of British government workers. I am grateful to successive committees at NHLBI and NIA for agreeing with our view that the Whitehall studies of the social gradient in health were highly relevant to the US situation. We were supported by grants: HL36310, AG13196, HS06516.

The British Heart Foundation has provided long-term support and successive grants from the Health and Safety Executive made much possible. Research support was also received from the Department of Health, as well as the John D. and Catherine T. MacArthur Foundation Research Networks on Successful Midlife Development and Socio-economic Status and Health. Specific studies were supported by the Economic and Social Research Council, Health Development Agency, Volvo Foundation, European Union, The New England Medical Centre, Division of Health Improvement; Institute for Work and Health, Toronto. The European Science Foundation supported a network of researchers on social variations in health expectancy, in which several of my colleagues and I were active participants.

We study the work/home interface. Administrative staff have made work seem more like a family, and my family have lived with the work of producing this book through every minute of it. The work family consists of the best possible university administrator, Paul Phibbs; my personal assistant, Elaine Reinertsen, and before her Julia Hum: they make working life a pleasure.

Patricia Crowley, Sandy Persaud, Floriana Bortolotti and Catherine Conroy make everything work smoothly and add the crucial element of care. For years I never did anything in research or writing without the help of Mandy Feeney. Her support, anticipation and wise counsel were irreplaceable until Ruth Bell, her successor, likewise became irreplaceable. I am grateful to all of these wonderful people for making it all work.

My family could, no doubt, tell you the content of every chapter of this book. André, Daniel and Deborah have been wonderfully responsive, tolerant, amused and irreverent. Alexi has been the long-term support without which none of this could have happened. The fact that she could do that while pursuing her own successful career, producing books of her own, and being the nurturing mother is no surprise to those who know her, but a continuing source of wonderment and appreciation to me. Thank you.

Michael Marmot, London, 23 December 2003

Extract from: the Acheson Report, Donald Acheson, *Inequalities in Health: Report of an independent inquiry*. 1998. HMSO: Crown copyright material is reproduced with the permission of the Controller of HMSO and the Queen's Printer for Scotland; *More Die of Heartbreak* by Saul Bellow reproduced with permission of the Wylie Agency (UK) Ltd, London on behalf of copyright © Saul Bellow 1988. Published by Secker & Warburg. Used by permission of The Random House Group Limited; *Child Care and the Growth of Love* by John Bowlby, Penguin edition 1965, edited by Margery Fry, page 30. (Pelican Books 1953, Second Edition 1965, Reprinted in Penguin Books 1990). Copyright © John Bowlby, 1953, 1965 and (part III) Mary Salter Ainsworth, 1965. Reproduced by permission of Penguin Books Ltd; Cornia, G. A. and R. Paniccia. 2000. 'The Transition Mortality Crisis: Evidence, Interpretation and Policy Responses', in *The Mortality Crisis in Transitional Economies*, edited by Cornia, G. A. and R. Paniccia (New York: Oxford University Press) reproduced by permission of Oxford University Press; the article 'Income inequality and homicide rates in Canada' by Martin Daly, Margo Wilson and Shawn Vasdev reproduced by permission of the *Canadian Journal of Criminology* 43 (2): 219–236. Copyright by the Canadian Criminal Justice Association; *Rosa Lee: A Mother and Her Family in Urban America*, by Leon Dash, published in the United States by Basic Books, 1996, Copyright © Leon Dash 1996, 1997, 1998, reprinted with permission of Perseus Books Group. UK, Profile Books, 1998, reproduced by permission; the article 'Will Global Capitalism be Anglo-Saxon Capitalism?' by Ronald Dore, in *Asian Business and Management* 1:9–18, 2002, reproduced by permission of Nature Publishing Group; Emile Durkheim, *Suicide: A Study in Sociology*, translated by John A. Spaulding and George Simpson. Edited by George Simpson: copyright © 1951 by the Free Press. Copyright © renewed 1979 by the Free Press, a Division of Simon and Schuster Adult Publishing Group. All rights reserved; Paul Farmer, *Infections and Inequalities*, University of California Press, 1999, reproduced by permission of University of California Press; *Howard's End* by E. M. Forster, Vintage Books, Alfred A. Knopf, Inc. and Random

Wealth of Nations: Social, Biological, and Educational Dynamics, edited by Keating, D. and C. Hertzman (New York: Guilford Press) used by permission of Guilford Publications, Inc.; Richard G. Wilkinson, *Unhealthy Societies: the Afflictions of Inequality*, Routledge, used by permission of Thomson Publishing Services.

Figure 1.1 used data from McDonough, P., G. J. Duncan, D. Williams, and J. S. House. 1997. 'Income dynamics and adult mortality in the United States, 1972 through 1989.' *American Journal of Public Health* 87:1476–1483, with permisison from the American Public Health Association; Figure 1.2 used data from Drever, F. and M. Whitehead, *Health Inequalities: Decennial Supplement*. Series DS No.15, 1–257. 1997. London: The Stationery Office, Office for National Statistics. Crown copyright material is reproduced with the permission of the Controller of HMSO and the Queen's Printer for Scotland; Table 1.1 used data from Department of the Environment, Transport and the Regions. 'Road accidents Great Britain 1999: the Casualty Report'. 2000. London, The Stationery Office. Crown copyright material is reproduced with the permission of the Controller of HMSO and the Queen's Printer for Scotland; Figure 2.1 data calculated from data in Marmot, M. G. and M. J. Shipley. 1996. 'Do socioeconomic differences in mortality persist after retirement? 25-year follow-up of civil servants from the first Whitehall study'. *British Medical Journal* 313:1177–1180. Modified from figure in Marmot, M. and Wilkinson, R. (eds). *Social Determinants of Health*. Oxford University Press, reprinted by permission of Oxford University Press; Figure 3.1 used data from Erikson, R. 2001. 'Why do graduates live longer?' In *Cradle to Grave: Life-course Change in Modern Sweden*, edited by Jonsson, J. O. and C. Mills (Durham: Sociology Press), used by permission of Sociology Press; Table 3.1 used data from *The Human Development Report* 2003 by United Nations Development Programme, copyright © 2003 by the United Nations Development Programme, used by permission of Oxford University Press, Inc.; Table 7.1 adapted from chart on p. 23 of *Confucius Lives Next Door* by T. R. Reid, copyright © 1999 by T. R. Reid, used by permission of Random House, Inc.; Table 7.2 used data from *World Bank, World Development Report 2000/2001*. Oxford University Press. 2001. New York, used by permission of Oxford University Press, Inc.; Table 7.3 used data from Measham, A. R., K. D. Rao, D. T. Jamison, J. Wang, and A. Singh. 1999. 'Reducing Infant Mortality and Fertility, 1975–1990: Performance at All-India and State Levels'. *Economic and Political Weekly* 34, no. 22:1359–1367, used by permission of the *Economic and Political Weekly*; Figure 9.1 was adapted from Figure A in the Statistics Canada publication *Inequalities in Literacy Skills Among Youth in Canada and the United States* by J. Douglas Willms, Catalogue no. 89-552-MPE, no 6, September 1999. Used with the permission of the Minister of Industry, as Minister responsible for Statistics Canada; Figure 10.2 from Bond, S. and M. Wakefield. 2003. 'Distributional effects of fiscal reforms since 1997.' In *The IFS Green Budget: January 2003*, Commentary No. 92, edited by Chote, R., C. Emmerson, and H. Simpson (London: Institute for Fiscal Studies), used by permission of the Institute for Fiscal Studies.

INDEX

INDEX

309

La Bohème (Puccini) 13, 16, 20
labour market 140, 180–1, 216
language 148–9
Latvia 214; Fig 8.2
Lebanon 68
Libya 68
life chances 123, 223–4, 225
life expectancy 2–3, 104, 200; in Central and
  Eastern Europe 199, 202, Fig 8.1; and education
  15; in Europe 200–2; Fig 8.1; and income
  inequality 80; in poor countries 6, 10–11, 65–6,
  187; in rich countries 66–8, 176, 189, Table 3.1;
  and self-esteem 22; and social class 26, Fig 1.2;
  and social integration 174
lifestyle 14, 43–5, 70, 177, 249; social differentials in
  45–7; of unmarried 162–3
literacy 225, 226–30, 231, 236; Fig 9.1
Lithuania 204, 207, 214, 217
love 13–14, 16
loyalty 178, 180, 181
lung cancer 28, 30, 44
lung disease, chronic 23, 27, 30, 64
Luxembourg 75, 279n

McKeown, Thomas 29–30, 152
Macmillan, Harold 91
Malawi 65
malnutrition 5, 52, 65
Malta 66; Table 3.1
marriage 112, 157–64, 172–3, 186, 216–17, Table
  7.3; as social support 157, 162–3, 210, 215
Marx, Karl 5
material conditions 64–6, 68, 69, 75–6, 79, 82, 137;
  in Central and Eastern Europe 211; equality of
  256–7; material deprivation 5, 18, 63, 64, 67, 70–
  1, 207–8, 214; material possessions 210–12; and
  social participation 76, 210–11; unmarried women
  163
Matsumoto, Scott 184
Meaney, Michael 243, 244
medical care 14, 176–7, 186, Table 7.3; in Central
  and Estern Europe 220; disparities in 8, 42; lack
  of access to 7, 18, 30; and money 62–3
Mencken, H. L. 86
mental illness 5, 6, 30, 59, 130–1, 138, 142, 156,
  162
metabolic syndrome 118, 121
migrants 182–5, 191
Miller, Geoffrey 92, 96, 97
money 11, 16, 22, 23, 61, 62–70, 73–4, 82, 140,
  261; and happiness 85–6; *see also* income
morality 96, 252
Morris, Jerry 226
mortality: causes of death 150–1, 208; and
  education 78, 205–6, Fig 3.1; and homicide rate
  104; and income 16–17, 77, 79, 81–2, 194–5,
  207, Fig 1.1; infant and child 1, 6, 64–6, 75,
  79–80, 185–7, 200, 204, 207–8, Table 7.3;
  male, premature 199, 200, 202–4, 209; and
  marriage 160, 161, 162, 210; and material
  possessions 211; and poverty 16, 64, 185; and
  social class 155, 254, Fig 10.1; and social
  relationships 165–6; in Soviet Union 9; and
  unemployment 135, 136–7, 161
Moynihan, Daniel Patrick 9
murder, *see* homicide

Napoleon Bonaparte 150
National Health Service 8, 175, 275–6
nature/nurture debate 48–9, 54, 84, 232, 239
necessaries 62, 73, 75–6, 77, 210–11
Netherlands 56, 106–7, 161, 200; Table 3.1
New York 188–9, 191
New Zealand 18, 66; Table 3.1
NiHonSan study 184
Norway 162; Table 3.1
Novosibirsk, Siberia 217–18, 219
Nussbaum, Martha 249
nutrition 18, 30, 51, 52–3, 64, 66, 152–3, 249, 270;
  see also diet

Oates, Captain Lawrence 19, 21
obesity 5, 44, 121, 199
occupation 15–16, 89, 124; hierarchy 26, 38–44, Fig
  2.1; occupational prestige 41, 50, 58; and social
  class 26, 41, 43; and status 124; stratification 41;
  see also work
older people 262–3, 272
ontological security 211–12
opportunity, equality of 72, 223–4, 255–6
Orwell, George: *The Road to Wigan Pier* 64, 70, 133
Oscar winners 21–3
Osler, Sir William 24, 25
overindulgence 6, 44
overweight 70, 121, 243

Pakistan 202
Panama 68
parents 232–5, 241, 261; educational levels 225–31;
  mothers 270; single 244–5, 261
participation, *see* social participation
personality 168, 169, 171
Phantom Tollbooth, The 222–3
Pinker, Steven 233, 234; *The Blank Slate* 174
Player, David 247, 285n
pleasure:pain ratio 112, 124
Poland 203, 206, 207, 210–12, 214, 217; Fig 8.2
polar explorers 19–20
politics 71–2, 172, 258; health policy 250–2, 263–4;
  income redistribution 263–4, Fig 10.2; social
  policy 18–19; and unemployment 133–6
Portugal Table 3.1
positional goods 97–8
poverty 4–5, 13, 18, 31, 51, 63, 167; Acheson
  Report 267–8; and behavioural problems 245;
  diseases of poor 5, 6, 25, 28–9, 36; and ill-health
  59, 63; and inequality 72; material deprivation 5,
  18, 64–6, 137, 188, 208; mortality rate 16, 64,
  185; poor communities 189–92, 249; poor
  countries 9–10, 63, 65–6, 185–8; relative 69–71,
  73–5; threshold 70; and social participation 70–1,
  73, 75–6, 82, 137–8; and unemployment 133,
  137
power 61, 62, 106–41
Power, Chris 246
predictability 114
prestige 23, 77, 212; occupational 41, 50, 58
privilege 21
protection 212
psychology 7, 20, 97, 113, 166; evolutionary 89–91,
  102, 173–4
psychosocial factors 123, 125, 128, 212, 219–20,
  257, 265
public health 32, 66, 72, 187, 250

A NOTE ON THE AUTHOR

Sir Michael Marmot is Professor of Epidemiology and Public Health and Director of the International Centre for Health and Society, University, College, London, and Adjunct Professor of Health and Social Behavior at the Harvard School of Public Health.